PHYSICAL AGENTS
FOR PHYSICAL THERAPISTS

PHYSICAL AGENTS
FOR PHYSICAL
THERAPISTS

By

JAMES E. GRIFFIN, Ph.D.
Professor of Physical Therapy
School of Health Related Professions
State University of New York at Buffalo

and

TERENCE C. KARSELIS, M.S.
Associate Professor of Medical Technology
School of Allied Health Professions
Medical College of Virginia
Virginia Commonwealth University
Richmond, Virginia

CHARLES C THOMAS · PUBLISHER
Springfield · Illinois · U.S.A.

Published and Distributed Throughout the World by

CHARLES C THOMAS • PUBLISHER

BANNERSTONE HOUSE

301-327 East Lawrence Avenue, Springfield, Illinois, U.S.A.

© *1978, by* CHARLES C THOMAS • PUBLISHER

ISBN 0-398-03706-X

Library of Congress Catalog Card Number: 77-22332

Printed in the United States of America

N-11

Library of Congress Cataloging in Publication Data

Griffin, James E
    Physical agents for physical therapists.

    Bibliography: p.
    Includes index.
    1. Physical therapy. 2. Medicine, Physical—Equipment and supplies.
Karselis, Terence, joint author. II. Title. [DNLM: 1. Physical therapy
—Methods. 2. Physical Therapy—Instrumentation WB460 G851p]
RM701.G75   615'.82   77-22332
ISBN 0-398-03706-X

PREFACE

THIS book deals with the clinical application of physical agents. It is intended as a text for the baccalaureate-level physical therapy student. It is assumed that the student has a reasonable background in undergraduate-level biology, chemistry, pathology, and physics and that the material contained herein will be supplemented by appropriate lectures and demonstrations.

The reason for writing the book is that nowhere in recent years has any physical therapist made an attempt to bring together and apply the advances in physiology and electronics which have evolved from clinical or laboratory research. These advances permit more logical use of cold, heat, nerve and muscle stimulating currents, diathermy, and ultraviolet and ultrasonic energy in helping the patient to be relieved of pain and to regain independence in activities of daily living.

A wealth of material has been reported in various journals within the last several decades. The literature cited in the book is in no way complete or exhaustive. It has been chosen as representative of developing new concepts of disease and treatment, or as confirming older concepts that have withstood the test of time.

Sections of the various chapters dealing with treatment technics do not spell out details that are more effectively learned within practice classes. Technics are given in detail when the described procedure can lead to improved patient care.

Chapters on electronic instrumentation design, hazards, and safety requirements reflect the major changes in federal regulations which are presently or soon to be in effect. Conceptual knowledge of modern apparatus design and of advances in physiological rationale for choice of physical agent to alleviate a problem should minimize the occasion for the physical therapist to become involved in malpractice suits because of use of defective equipment or because of misapplication of good equipment and/ or technics.

J.E.G.
T.C.K.

CONTENTS

PHYSICAL AGENTS
FOR PHYSICAL THERAPISTS

Chapter 1

PAIN

PERHAPS the simplest definition of pain is that "it is a hurt that we feel."[1] The standard medical dictionary definition of pain is that it is a more or less localized sensation of discomfort, distress, or agony, resulting from the stimulation of specialized nerve endings.[2]

If a physical therapist wishes to be useful in the relief of pain, he needs to know as much as possible about the biophysical effects of physical agents. If a patient is limited in his activities of daily living because of pain, or because he perceives his pain as a major factor during his waking hours, it is unlikely that he will make much progress in regaining control over range of motion, use of assistive devices, or gaining in strength until such time as the pain has been relieved, or at least reduced to a tolerable level.

Regular administration of the appropriate physical agent can be highly effective in relieving pain in properly selected patients. Physical agents may also be used in conjunction with medication and/or postsurgically. Frequently, the patient will derive greater benefit from therapeutic exercise if the exercise is preceeded by a carefully selected physical agent.

CAUSES OF PAIN

Causes of pain are myriad. Quite often there will be abnormal activity of muscle, peripheral circulation, and/or the nervous system, either as a cause or the result of the patient's perception of pain.

Spasm may be defined as an abnormal and continuing hyperactivity of any type of contractile tissue, such as skeletal, smooth, or cardiac muscle. Although far less common than spasm in either

3

skeletal or smooth muscle, the cardiac muscle spasm, which is a dominant feature in true angina pectoris, is one of the most severe forms of pain. If this abnormal cardiac muscle contraction can be relaxed, the accompanying pain will be diminished.

When pain is present, there is often concomitant local circulatory impairment. One known cause of such impairment is skeletal muscle spasm, which can significantly limit venous return. Such flow deficit can give rise to additional pain because the deficit leads to inadequate local removal of metabolic waste products.

Vasospasm is the abnormal continuing hyperactivity of smooth muscles in the walls of blood vessels. It is of particular importance in arterial vessels with a diameter of a few millimeters. The ratio of muscle to other tissues is especially high in arterial vessels of small diameter. Vasospasm can be triggered by peripheral or central irritation of sympathetic nerves, or by edema formation. In all cases, vasospasm leads to the reduction or cessation of arterial flow. Significant reduction gives rise to pain, and in extreme cases to irreversible damage, in the tissues supplied by the malfunctioning vessels. Organic occlusive peripheral vascular diseases can cause severe chronic impairment of circulation and give rise to steadily increasing pain over weeks and months.

Furthermore, diminished circulation, either arterial or venous, can give rise to skeletal or cardiac muscle spasm because of inadequate local nutrition or ineffective removal of waste products from the local area served by the malfunctioning vessels.

The nervous system can also play a major role in pain production. The sensory portions of the nervous system must be functioning and have functioning connections to the spinal cord and on up to higher (cortical) levels before the patient can be aware of noxious stimuli. The rare infant with a congenital lesion such that he cannot perceive pain seldom survives his infancy. He dies as a consequence of injury or disease of which no one is aware. Skeletal muscle hyperactivity, vasospasm, and nervous system malfunction can all occur without the patient feeling pain if pain pathways to the cortex are interrupted by trauma or disease. The abnormal activity without pain can be just as much or more of a handicap to activities of daily living. Abnormal muscular hyperactivity without pain is commonly seen in the chronic phase of the traumatic paraplegic or quadriplegic patient. In such patients, the primary lesion is usually in the spinal cord; more rarely, it occurs within the cranial vault. Usually, the peripheral nervous system remains largely intact, but because of edema, anatomical cord severance, or other lesion in the cord, pain pathways are interrupted. Because of neuroanatomical relationships within the spinal cord, pain and other sensation is more apt to be lost than is motor nerve control over skeletal muscle or sympathetic nerve control over smooth muscle in blood vessel walls.

CLASSIFICATION OF PAIN

The clinical physician usually classifies pain into three major categories. One type is often called a fast-onset, pricking type of pain. A second category is frequently described as of slow onset, leading to a burning sensation. The third type is commonly pictured as a deep, dull ache. This ache is frequently remote from the causal site and usually is due to the dysfunction of some portion of the viscera. Mountcastle[3] has published in monograph form a very useful review of pain and pain pathways from the sensory physiologist's point of view. It now appears certan that the fast, pricking pain is most often transmitted from the periphery into the central nervous system by delta axons, which are 4 to 6 microns in diameter, whereas the smaller, unmyelinated C fibers normally transmit pain stimuli leading to a burning sensation. It is this latter type of pain with which the physical therapist is most often concerned, pain of slow onset, great persistence, and accompanied by powerful responses, both physiological and psychological. The third general category of pain awareness, visceral or aching pain, is more apt to be a life-threatening indicator and is not often amenable to physical therapy procedures.

Abnormal functioning of local areas of skeletal muscle, circulation, and the nervous system are very much interrelated. Each abnormality can be a cause of pain; each can be the result of noxious stimuli. Each can be a part of the vicious cycle of pain —spasm—more pain—more spasm. Under some circumstances, appropriate administration of the most suitable physical agent can be the best means to interrupt that vicious cycle and thereby achieve cumulative, lasting pain relief.

The psychological aspects of pain are somewhat more elusive and controversial than the physiological components. The psychological aspects can be conveniently considered on the basis of the importance that the subject attaches to his pain. Sternbach[1] expressed these variables quite well when he wrote,

> It is not pain which is mental or physical, functional or organic, psychic or somatic, but our ways of thinking about pain and the systems of terms we use to describe pain which may be so dichotomized. All pain can be described in both languages, the psychological and the physiological. Pain itself is not one or the other. But because pain can be described in both mental or physical terms, pain is a truly psychosomatic concept. From this point of view, all pain is real; and all pain is also psychosomatic since both mental and physical descriptions are possible.

The key to how intense or how minimal is an individual's response to pain is probably previous conditioning plus present distraction. Either can serve to increase or decrease anxiety and thus to increase or decrease pain.

THEORIES OF PAIN AWARENESS

There have been many theories published about possible mechanisms and pathways for pain perception and pain relief. Possibly the one that comes the nearest to affording a reasonable working hypothesis in accounting for all presently known aspects of pain and pain relief is that presented by Melzack and Wall[4] in 1965. Their gate control theory proposed a neural mechanism in the spinal cord which can increase or decrease the flow of pain impulses from the periphery to the brain. When other sensory input is minimal, pain awareness is great. When other sensory input is equal to or greater than pain input, awareness of the latter is diminished. This gate control theory can well account for the concept of counter irritation, which is very useful in attempting to explain why judicious intermittent use of heat, cold, ultrasound, and nerve stimulating currents can relieve pain. By 1974, Melzack[5] was able to state and defend the hypothesis that the neospinothalamic system selects and modulates sensory input in such a fashion as to permit the discriminative dimension of pain. He further stated that activation of reticular and limbic structures through the paramedial ascending system underlies the motivational drive and unpleasant affect that trigger the organism into action. Lastly, Melzack presented evidence that neocortical or higher central nervous system processes (suggestion, anxiety, and attention) exert control over activity in both discriminative and motivational systems (Fig. 1-1).

Figure 1-1. Schema for demonstrating the gate control theory of pain. L — large, fast-transmitting axons. S — small, slow-transmitting axons. T — transmission cephalad from spinal cord after sorting. Motivational processes include central intensity monitoring. Sensory processes include spatiotemporal analysis. From International Symposium on Pain (Advances in Neurology, Volume 4), p. 526. Editor, John J. Bonica. © 1974 by Raven Press, New York.

As physical therapists, our primary concern with pain and pain relief is to add sufficient energy to the patient to provide sufficient increase in nonpainful sensory input to override or counterbalance the painful sensory input, or to transiently diminish the ability of axons to conduct. The problem frequently is how to drive a physiologically acceptable quantity of energy to the needed depth without damaging intervening tissues.

KNOWN EFFECTS OF CLINICALLY APPLICABLE HEAT AND COLD

When cold is applied to a patient for the purpose of relieving pain, the objective is to lower tissue temperature within physiological limits. Fortunately, altering the temperature of cutaneous nerves can do much to reduce hyperactivity of underlying contractile tissue. Miglietta[6] showed that application of cold to the skin can bring about significant reduction of deep muscle spasm within one minute. However, Wolf and Basmajian[7] have demonstrated that even when intense cold is applied to a small area of skin, it takes an application time of at least five minutes before there will be a 1°C reduction in muscle temperature at a depth of 5 cm. In earlier experiments more nearly approaching standard clinical application of cold to a local area, Bierman[8] demonstrated that cold must be applied for thirty minutes before there is a similar drop in deep muscle temperature. Abramson et al.[9] have published evidence that there is always vascoconstriction with a drop in muscle temperature.

Reviews of clinical cryotherapy[10] and of the physiological effects of heat and cold[11] indicate that much of the measurable effect of conductive and/or radiant heating and of conductive cooling is an indirect response due to the stimulation of cutaneous nerves. Effects of these agents on skeletal muscle and subcutaneous circulation are due more to such indirect effects than to primary energy absorption or release by subcutaneous tissues.

Voluminous literature has developed over the years demonstrating that when cutaneous thermal receptors are stimulated by heat, there is an increase in nerve conduction velocity, an increase in cutaneous circulation brought about by local cutaneous release of histamine (a potent vasodilator) or histaminelike substances, and a further increase in cutaneous circulation as warmed blood reaches the vasomotor regulators within the central nervous system. There is also reduction of skeletal muscle tension as motor nerve impulses diminish in number in response to cutaneous thermal stimulation.

When cold is applied to the skin, with techniques suitable for relieving pain, there is reduction in cutaneous nerve conduction velocity, vasodilation followed by vasoconstriction, and reduction in skeletal muscle tension. It is interesting to note that both increase and decrease in sensory nerve conduction velocity, as well as both cutaneous vasodilation and vasoconstriction, can lead to relaxation of underlying muscle. Any standard text on electromyographic techniques[12] will give ample data indicating that both sensory and motor nerve conduction velocity shift in direct proportion to temperature change in those tissues.

When heat is applied locally, one anticipates transient local vasodilation, rise in tissue temperature, and an increase in nerve conduction velocity and muscle relaxation. When cold is applied in a similar fashion, the effects are the opposite, except that cutaneously applied cold, like heat, leads to muscle relaxation. Both heat and cold are effective in relieving pain. Heat appears more useful in the chronic phase of most pathologies, with the notable exception of lesions resulting in central nervous system induced spasticity. Cold appears to be more useful in the acute phase of the pathology and/or where skeletal muscle hyperactivity is quite severe.

Both heat and cold are useful in reduction of edema, with and without concomitant pain. Again, heat is likely to be more useful in the chronic phase, i.e. when residual edema is still present more than forty-eight hours after the trauma resulting in edema has occurred. With any soft tissue or bone trauma, blood vessels are usually disrupted, allowing fluid to leak out. Normal repair processes seal off the torn vessels within minutes. Larger vessels require longer than small vessels. When there is no evidence of any continuing edema formation, heat may be safely applied to increase capillary permeability and thus aid in the resorption of the extravasated fluid and dissolution of the organized hematoma which is a necessary part of the sealing procedure. Heat should not be applied if the local area is still hemorrhaging, since the subsequent increase in capillary permeability will prevent adequate sealing of torn blood vessels.

On the other hand, application of cold induces vasoconstriction, decreases capillary permeability, and so tends to slow continued fluid leakage from ruptured vessels. This is usually desirable for forty-eight to seventy-two hours after trauma.

One must be sure that edema present is due to local trauma rather than due to cardiac, pulmonary, and/or renal pathology before using either heat or cold. Vigorous application of either heat or cold in the presence of any such lesion is hazardous. If both trauma and such major life-threatening lesions are present, use of heat or cold should be much gentler.

Application of short wave or microwave diathermy, or ultrasound, will all cause a greater temperature rise in deeper tissue than will the application of any form of conductive heat (hot packs, paraffin bath, whirlpool) or radiant heat (infrared lamps and bakers).[13] Conversely, the diathermies and ultrasonic energy will not cause as much of a rise in skin temperature or have as much effect on cutaneous nerves or circulation. There is good evidence that when these more deeply penetrating physical agents are properly utilized, the increased depth of penetration is in large part dependent upon the frequency of the energy delivered to the patient.[13,14] The wide range of operating frequencies available to the physical therapist is discussed in some detail in the material dealing specifically with the electromagnetic and acoustic spectra (*see* Chapter 2).

REFERENCES

1. Sternbach, Richard A.: *Pain: A Psychophysiological Approach.* New York, Acad Pr, 1968.
2. *Dorland's Illustrated Medical Dictionary,* 24th ed. Philadelphia, Saunders, 1965.
3. Mountcastle, Vernon B.: Somethesis, a review. Published in Italian in *Enciclopedia Italiana.* Rome, Fondata da Giovanni Trecani.
4. Melzack, R. and Wall, P.D.: Pain mechanisms: a new theory. *Science, 150*:971-79, 1965.
5. Melzack, R.: Control Mechanisms: Psychologal Aspects. In Bonica, J. (Ed.): *Advances in Neurology,* Volume 4. New York, Raven, 1974, pp. 275-80.
6. Miglietta, O.: Action of cold on spasticity. *Am J Phys Med, 52*:198-204, August, 1973.
7. Wolf, S.L. and Basmajian, J.V.: Intramuscular temperatures deep to localized cold stimulation. *Phys Ther, 53*:1284-88, December, 1973.
8. Bierman, W.: Therapeutic use of cold. *JAMA, 157*:189-92, 1955.
9. Abramson, D.I. et al.: Vascular basis for pain due to cold. *Arch Phys Med Rehabil, 47*:300-305, 1966.
10. Alson, J.E. and Stravino, V.D.: A review of cryotherapy. *Phys Ther, 52*: 840-853, 1972.
11. Downey, J.A.: Physiological effects of heat and cold. *Phys Ther, 44*:713-17, 1964.

12. Licht, S. (Ed.): *Electro diagnosis and Electromyography,* 2nd ed. New Haven, Licht, 1965.

13. Licht, S. (Ed.): *Therapeutic Heat and Cold,* 2nd ed. New Haven, Licht, 1965, Chapters 5, 8, 9, 11.

14. Goldman, D.E. and Heuter, T.F.: Tabular data on velocity and absorption of high frequency sound in mammalian tissues. *J Acoust Soc Am, 28:*35-37, 1956.

Chapter 2

INTRODUCTION TO THE ELECTROMAGNETIC AND ACOUSTIC SPECTRA

THE PHYSICAL agents which are the domain of the physical therapist include heat, cold, water, ultrasonic energy, nerve and muscle stimulating currents, ultraviolet light, and massage. Massage is not included in this book because it neither adds to nor takes away a significant amount of energy from the patient. When pain is relieved by any of the other physical agents, a major mechanism of pain relief is absorption or removal of energy, with subsequent effects. There is no question that massage can benefit properly selected patients, but there is more question as to the mechanisms involved than there is with the other physical agents.

INFRARED OR THERMAL ENERGY

Perhaps the most widely used physical agent is some type of energy which causes a local transient tissue temperature rise. The source will usually be producing some form of infrared energy. It is clinically applicable in many convenient forms. Hot packs are probably the most widely used form of infrared energy. They are normally stored in water kept at temperatures of 70° to 88°C. Properly applied hot packs are very efficient at raising skin temperature to the upper limit of safety, 45°C. The paraffin bath is equally efficient. It is frequently used when it is desirable to raise the temperature of skin and subcutaneous tissues of the digits, especially of the upper extremities. The paraffin bath is commonly kept at temperatures of 52° to 57°C for use with the upper extremities. If the bath is intended for use with the lower extremities, the temperature is usually kept lower, at about 42° to 50°C, because even in the normal subject, circulation is less efficient, especially in the distal lower extremity.

Infrared lamps and bakers are another source of infrared energy, now rarely used in the physical therapy clinic. Depending upon the type of heating unit used, the source temperature could range from about 400° to more than 3,000°C. Consequently, the lamp is never placed close to the skin. Depending upon intensity of output, the lamp or baker would be positioned 10 to 65 cm away from the skin. Like the hot pack and the paraffin bath, lamps and bakers can raise skin temperature to the upper limit of safety within a matter of minutes.

The whirlpool and the Hubbard tank are widely used sources of infrared energy. Depending upon whether heating or cooling of the skin is desired, the area to be treated is immersed in water at temperatures ranging from 42° to 30°C, and sometimes lower in selected patients. Normal skin temperature approaches 37°C in the head, neck, and trunk and gradually decreases to about 32° in the distal portion of the extremities. It is then obvious that one would not expect as great a skin temperature rise with the whirlpool or Hubbard tank as compared to the hot pack or paraffin bath. However, hydrotherapy is commonly used to treat much larger segments of the patient.

In both the moist and dry forms of infrared used to raise skin temperature, thermal energy is generated and then transmitted to the patient with the intent of causing a beneficial reaction via the cutaneous nervous system and/or the cutaneous circulation. Body reaction to the absorption of a stimulating quantity of any form of infrared usually includes transient local skeletal muscle relaxation. The relaxation can be measured objectively by use of electromyography before and after treatment[1,2] or subjectively by palpation.

It is well established that no form of infrared energy can have primary penetration deeper than 1 cm.[3] Hence the muscle relaxation is rarely due to direct absorption of the infrared energy but rather to direct effect on cutaneous nerve receptors and on cutaneous blood vessels, with a later reduction of motor nerve impulse flow. If the energy is absorbed over a long enough time, there *may* also be an increase in blood flow to underlying muscle. Any and all of these changes can lead to pain relief if the pain was due to muscle hyperactivity.

The gate control theory of pain and pain relief (*see* Chapter 1) could account for the reduction in motor nerve impulse outflow, since the cutaneous nervous system is now being flooded with less noxious stimuli. If this more pleasant stimulus is kept at a steady state for a period of time (minutes), additional steady-state energy addition may no longer be perceived as stimulus but rather as a new environment, with less need for muscle response. One of the net effects of steady-state stimulus is muscle relaxation.[3] It is also possible, if infrared energy is absorbed over a long period of time and in sufficient quantity, that the thermal receptors, which were originally stimulated by exposure to change in temperature, gradually accomodate to the new temperature and gradually diminish in activity.

Another reaction which is known to take place when skin is absorbing infrared energy or when heat is being withdrawn from the skin is the release of histamine by dermal cells. The histamine release causes capillary dilation. This change is perceived in lightly pigmented skin as hyperemia, a reddening of the skin. This reddening of the skin normally disappears within less than thirty minutes after the intense source of thermal energy has been removed.

At the same time that cutaneous thermal receptors and the skin itself is being stimulated, cutaneous blood temperature is being raised. If blood in the local area is warmed enough so that the temperature of all the circulating blood is raised as little as 0.1°C, the hypothalamus (a major vasomotor regulatory center within the central nervous system) responds by causing vasodilation in deeper tissues underlying the area of exposure to intense heat. Since blood to fill the newly dilated capillaries has to come from somewhere within the body, and since underlying muscle is nearby, there is frequently a small drop in muscle temperature in the local area for the first few minutes.[4] Then, when the hypothalamus is triggered by change in blood temperature, vasodilation may also occur in the underlying muscle. Additional blood to supply the underlying muscle is likely to come from the normal blood reservoirs, i.e. spleen, gut, or muscle not in the area absorbing energy. If energy absorption by the skin continues over a twenty– to thirty-minute period, the underlying muscle temperature may also rise slightly, but never as much as the skin temperature if the source of energy is infrared.[4]

Cold, as used clinically, is also a form of infrared energy, since any object which has a temperature above $0°K$ $(-273°C)$ is radiating thermal energy. Cold is frequently applied to a local area of a patient in the form of cold packs, commonly stored at $0°C \pm 10°C$. Such application causes rapid reduction of skin temperature. Underlying skin temperature will frequently decrease by $5°$ to $10°C$ within the standard ten-minute treatment. When this occurs, skin and deeper lying tissues lose energy (heat) in proportion to the temperature differential between the cold pack and the skin.

In procedures where cold is applied, as was the case with the "hot" form of infrared, there is a marked reaction by the cutaneous nerves and the circulation of the skin. There is a lesser reaction by deeper tissues. If the temperature differential is great and prolonged, the reactions will tend to be extensive. The final effect, as is the case when the "hot" form of infared is applied, is likely to be muscle relaxation, but through different mechanisms. Known mechanisms for responses to application of heat and cold are discussed in Chapter 5.

One should remember that the human eye cannot see infrared wavelengths. In the case of luminous sources of infrared radiation, one does see the visible light that is generated concomitantly.

THE DIATHERMIES

In addition to the various ways of generating clinically useful thermal energy and transmitting it to the patient with the intent of causing a local tissue temperature rise (TTR), the TTR can also be achieved upon absorption of high frequency electric and/or magnetic field energy. Absorbing tissues will convert part of the absorbed energy into heat. Thus, the diathermies may be referred to as conversive heating. The common clinical sources for this technic are designated as short wave and microwave diathermy. With proper application, these wavelengths can penetrate more deeply than any form of infrared. Consequently, the diathermies are frequently referred to as "deep heat." When applied improperly or with lack of consideration for variation in response among the various tissues which lie deep to the skin, absorption of energy of diathermy wavelengths can be hazardous. This is in large part true because there are far fewer thermal receptors beneath the skin until energy penetrates to the periosteum. Hence, it is easy to raise the temperature of subcutaneous fat and muscle to destructive levels (above 45°C) without anyone being aware of it at the time of treatment.

The therapist must be very conscious of how much subcutaneous fat overlies the tissues in which a significant rise in temperature is desired. Almost equally important is the realization of the proximity of bone to the surface where the diathermy is applied. It is easy to cause a pathological tissue temperature rise in either of these tissues when they are exposed to energy of wavelengths classified as diathermy. The mechanisms for hazard are different for fat as compared to bone. These mechanisms are discussed in Chapter 4.

NERVE AND MUSCLE STIMULATING CURRENTS

When electrical energy of frequencies appropriate to stimulate peripheral nerve or muscle is absorbed, the ensuing tissue temperature rise should be insignificant and certainly well below a hazardous level. This is because stimulating currents are not used in continuous modulation for prolonged periods of time, i.e. minutes, but rather with some form of surge or interruption. Hence, energy is transmitted to the patient intermittently. Duration of the individual stimulus is usually less than one second, with a pause of one or more seconds between each stimulus.

Nerve and muscle stimulating currents are not used with the intent of causing a tissue temperature rise. They are used with the intent of causing intermittent skeletal muscle contraction and relaxation. The frequency and other stimulus parameters needed to produce the desired response will vary, depending upon the extent and severity of the lesion and whether the muscle to be stimulated is hypertonic of hypotonic. Reasons for needing wide variation in stimulus characteristics are discussed in Chapter 3.

ULTRAVIOLET LIGHT

When electromagnetic energy of the frequency range classified as "ultraviolet" is used, the intent is not to cause a tissue temperature rise but rather to cause one or more chemical reactions within the absorbing tissue. If the dose is heavy, a readily measurable temperature rise will occur, but only as a delayed reaction. The delay will be on the order of several hours. This temperature rise is secondary to the chemical stimulation. Ultraviolet treatment time is of much shorter duration (seconds) as compared to the usual treatment time when any form of energy is used with the intent of causing a tissue temperature rise. This is because ultraviolet energy does not penetrate. Most of it is absorbed within the first millimeter and all within the second millimeter of absorbing skin or other tissue. Hence, there is essentially no volume absorption as there is with all forms of energy used to cause a tissue temperature rise.

Individual treatment time will depend upon the output characteristics of the source of ultraviolet light and upon the reaction desired. Just as is the case with infrared energy, the human eye does not see ultraviolet wavelengths. What is seen is the visible light that all clinical ultraviolet (UV) sources produce at the same time they are producing the shorter UV wavelengths.

Treatment techniques and rationale for use are discussed in Chapter 6.

ULTRASONIC ENERGY

When ultrasonic energy is utilized, for either thermal or non-thermal effects, treatment time is longer than with ultraviolet light but shorter than when any form of infrared or diathermy is used. Even though it is well established that clinical ultrasonic energy penetrates more deeply than any other form of energy that physical therapists use, the net tissue temperature rise may be greater than that achieved with the diathermies or infrared energy. Presumably this is in large part due to the much greater efficiency of transmission of ultrasonic energy from the source into the patient.

Of special importance is the fact that there is a lesser rise in temperature of subcutaneous fat as compared to that of under-lying muscle and bone. Rise in fat temperature can be a real obstacle to adequate rise in muscle temperature when the dia-thermies are used. There are additional thermal and non-thermal effects of absorption of ultrasonic energy which are unique to ultrasound. This form of energy is discussed in detail in Chapter 7.

RELATIONSHIPS OF WAVELENGTH, FREQUENCY, AND DEPTH OF PENETRATION

When considering which type of energy should be applied to a given patient, the first factor which should be considered is wavelength. Among the energy forms available to physical thera-pists, the longer the wavelength, the deeper the penetration. Wavelength is standardly defined as the distance between the top of one wave and the identical phase of the succeeding wave.[5] Frequency is the reciprocal of wavelength and is standardly de-fined as the number of oscillations or vibrations per second.[5]

Nerve and muscle stimulating currents have the longest wave-lengths, and hence the lowest frequencies, of any energy that physical therapists use. These wavelengths are usually expressed as kilometers. The clinical frequency range is on the order of 0.5 to 2,000 Hertz (Hz) or cycles per second (c.p.s.). Since stimu-lating currents are a part of the electromagnetic spectrum, their velocity approximates that of the speed of light in a vacuum (about 300,000,000 meters per second). At sea level, the speed of light is a little slower, about 296,700,000 m/s. Since velocity equals wavelength times frequency ($c = \lambda \times f$), a current having a frequency of 20 Hertz (Hz) has a wavelength of 15,000,000 in a vacuum and about 14,835,000 m at sea level. These wavelengths are equal to 15,000 and 14,835 kilometers (km) respectively.

Since stimulating currents have the longest wavelengths of any energy that physical therapists use, *if all other factors are equal,* their depth of penetration will be the greatest.

Diathermy wavelengths are usually expressed as meters or centimeters. Shortwave diathermy has a wavelength range of 30 to 3 m since the frequency range is 10 million to 100 million Hertz (MHz). Microwave diathermy has a wavelength range of 3 m to 3 cm since it has a frequency range of 100 to 10,000 MHz. These ranges are based on the velocity of electromagnetic energy in a vacuum. At atmospheric pressure, the wavelengths are a little shorter since the velocity is slightly lower.

Infrared and ultraviolet wavelengths are much shorter and their frequencies much higher than those for stimulating currents or the diathermies. It is well established that their depth of penetration is significantly less. Infrared (IR) and ultraviolet (UV) wavelengths are commonly expressed as nanometers (nm) or Angstrom units (Å). One billion nm = 1 meter. An older term, the millimicron, is equivalent to the nanometer. Both are equal to 10^{-9} meter. One Å $= 10^{-10}$ m. Both the nanometer and the Angstrom are very small units of linear measure. The corresponding frequencies are so high that the only practical way to enumerate them is by use of the powers of ten. When one considers that clinical IR sources may range in temperature from below zero to more than 3,000°C, there is consequently a frequency range of 2×10^{12} to 4×10^{13} Hz. The theoretical IR wavelength range that may be used clinically is 15,000 to 750 nm (150,000 to 7,500 Å) for source temperatures ranging from 0 to 3,000°C, respectively.[3]

IR and UV wavelengths are temperature dependent.[3] Table 2-I lists selected temperatures, corresponding wavelengths, and clinical uses. The lower the temperature, the longer the wavelength. A cold pack stored at 0°C (273°K) will have a wavelength of about 10,570 nm or 105,714 Å. If the temperature of an IR lamp averages 3,000°C, the wavelength average will be about 851 nm or 8,510 Å. When one considers UV frequencies, which are higher than those of the hottest infrared source, their wavelengths are shorter still. The average UV source temperature is on the order of 9,700°C. The average UV frequency is on the order of 7 × 10¹³ to 7 × 10¹⁴ Hz. The wavelength range in clinical use is 320 to 185 nm.

Table 2-II places all of the physical agents which are a part of the electromagnetic spectrum in logical order. The reader should bear in mind that ultrasonic energy is not a part of the electromagnetic spectrum (EMS). The most important thing about the

Table 2-I
CONVERSION TABLE FOR KELVIN, CENTIGRADE, AND FAHRENHEIT
TEMPERATURES AND THEIR WAVELENGTHS IN THE
INFRARED AND ULTRAVIOLET SPECTRA

Kelvin	Centigrade (Celsius)	Fahrenheit (to nearest whole number)	Wavelength (in Angstrom Units)	Clinical Example
190	—83	—118	151,895	Not used clinically — too cold. Is "Far Infrared"
250	—23	—10	115,440	Extreme storage of cold pack
260	—13	8	111,000	Usual storage of cold pack
280	7	45	103,072	Usual storage of cold pack
290	17	63	99,517	Very cold Whirlpool (WP)
300	27	81	96,200	Cold WP & Hubbard Tank (HT)
310	37	99	93,097	Neutral WP & usual HT Upper limit HT is 40°C Upper limit WP is 42°C
320	47	117	90,187	Low temperature paraffin bath
330	57	135	87,455	High temperature paraffin bath
340	67	153	84,882	Usual storage hot pack
350	77	171	82,457	Usual storage hot pack
360	87	189	80,167	Upper limit hot pack
370	97	207	78,000	A few degrees less than boiling point of water
700	427	801	41,229	Low temperature Far IR Lamp
1,000	727	1,341	28,860	Medium temperature Far IR Lamp
2,000	1,727	3,140	14,430	Medium temperature Near IR Lamp
3,000	2,727	4,941	9,620	High temperature Near IR Lamp
4,000	3,727	6,766	7,215	Approaching long wavelengths of visible light
5,000	4,727	8,566	5,772	Approaching short wavelengths of visible light
10,000	9,727	17,566	2,886	Within UV spectrum

EMS for the physical therapist is that wavelengths toward the bottom of this table have progressively less depth of penetration. This may at first thought seem paradoxical inasmuch as it is common knowledge that x-rays are very penetrating and produce a clear picture of bone in the intact individual. X-rays and other electromagnetic energy of still shorter wavelengths have a far greater concentration of energy per unit area within the source than is true for the wavelengths used by physical therapists. Thus, energy radiating from sources below UV in Table 2-II have vastly greater driving forces than the energies used by physical therapists.

Only since the 1950s has it been possible to drive EMS energy of longer wavelengths, i.e. infrared, in a manner similar to x-rays. This has resulted in the ability to form LASER beams (Light Amplification by Stimulated Emission of Radiation). LASER is beyond the scope of this book and is not in use by physical therapists.

All professional personnel concerned with physical medicine need to remember that hot and cold packs, paraffin baths, whirlpools, and Hubbard tanks are just as much sources of infrared radiation as are IR lamps and bakers. The generating source temperatures are quite different. Consequently, wavelengths and frequencies of their radiation are different. A cold pack stored at −10°C (263°K) will have initial radiation with a wavelength of 109,734 Å. If it was stored at 10°C, its initial wavelength will be 101,979 Å.* Practice with calculations of this sort should help in remembering the relationships between wavelength and frequency.

Clinicians are in general agreement, however, that the physiological changes induced by absorption of infrared are the same, regardless of wavelength, if they cause the same temperature rise in a given tissue. Likewise, if energy is withdrawn from the patient (the IR source is of colder temperature than the subject's

---

*It is known that IR at a temperature of 3,000°K has a wavelength of 9,620 Å. If these values are multiplied together, the result is 28,860,000. If this constant is divided by the Kelvin temperature of a source whose wavelength is unknown, the wavelength for that temperature will appear as the quotient, in Angstrom units.

Table 2-II
THE ELECTROMAGNETIC SPECTRUM

Category	Theoretical Frequency Range	Theoretical Wavelength Range	Clinically Utilized Frequencies	Clinically Utilized Wavelengths	Clinical Objective
Nerve and Muscle Stimulating Currents	0 to 10,000 Hz (DC or AC)	Infinity to 30 km	0 to 2,000 Hz	Infinity to 150 km	Muscle Contraction. Ion Transfer (DC only)
Commercial and Military Radio and Television Diathermies	10,000 Hz to 10 MHz	30 km to 30 m			
Short wave	10 MHz to 100 MHz	30 m to 3 m	13.56 or 27.12 MHz	22 or 11 m	Tissue Temperature Rise (TTR)
Microwave	100 MHz to 10,000 MHz	3 m to 3 cm	915 or 2,450 MHz	33 or 12 cm	TTR
Various Sources of Infrared	2×10^{12} to 7×10^{13} Hz	28,860,000 to 7,500 Å	2×10^{13} to 7×10^{13} Hz	105,000 to 10,000 Å	Tissue Temperature Drop or TTR
Visible Light	7×10^{13} Hz	7,500 to 4,000 Å			
Ultraviolet Light	7×10^{13} Hz	4,000 to 136 Å	7×10^{13} Hz	4,000 to 1,850 Å	Tissue Chemical Change
High Energy Ionizing and Penetrating Radiation (X-ray, alpha, beta, gamma, and cosmic radiation)	10^{16} to Infinity	136 to less than 1 Å			

skin temperature), the physiological effects will be the same regardless of wavelength.[3]

DIFFERENCES BETWEEN THE ELECTROMAGNETIC AND ACOUSTIC SPECTRA

Sound and ultrasound are parts of the acoustic spectrum of energies. They are not part of the electromagnetic spectrum. Although previously discussed relationships between wavelength and frequency hold for both spectra, there are numerous physical and biophysical differences.

All EMS wavelengths travel most efficiently through a vacuum, suffer a slight loss of velocity when penetrating a gaseous medium, and exhibit a still greater loss when driven through a liquid. Electromagnetic energy utilized by physical therapists penetrates solids poorly. On the other hand, acoustic (vibrational) energy is not transmitted through a vacuum, travels very poorly through gases, and is transmitted quite well through gas-free liquids. Acoustic energy velocity is greatest when penetrating solids of high density.

Irrespective of the medium for transmission, the velocity of all the energies which comprise the EMS is on the order of 300 million meters per second, whereas the velocity of acoustic energy is on the order of a few hundred to a few thousand m/s. With electromagnetic energy, as the density of the transmitting medium increases, velocity decreases because of interfering collisions with the molecules that make up the transmitting medium. Conversely, with acoustic energy, as the density of the medium increases, velocity rises. In biological liquids and soft tissues, clinical ultrasonic energy has a velocity on the order of 1500 meters per second. In cortical bone, the velocity increases to more than 3000 m/s. Acoustic energy is transmitted directly from molecule to molecule.

That portion of the acoustic spectrum which physical therapists use in the treatment of patients has been designated as ultrasound, indicative that these wavelengths are inaudible. For much the same reason, within the EMS, wavelengths close to but longer than those which stimulate the human eye are designated as *infra*red. Those wavelengths which are slightly shorter than those which stimulate the eye are called *ultra*violet.

The term *supersonic* is equivalent to ultrasonic but by convention has been reserved for reference to airplanes which are capable of moving faster than the speed of audible sound.

Because of the significant difference in velocity between electromagnetic and acoustic waves, the relationship between wavelength and frequency is different, even though the formula for expressing the relationship is the same. Velocity equals wavelength times frequency ($c = \lambda \times f$). Thus, for EMS energy having a frequency of one megacycle (1 MHz), the wavelength would be 300 m in a vacuum and about 297 m in atmosphere at sea level. Ultrasonic energy of the same frequency would have a wavelength of 0.3 mm in atmosphere, about 1.5 mm in soft tissue, and 3.5 mm in cortical bone. Since it takes 1000 mm to equal 1 meter, wavelength differences between EMS and acoustic energy for any given frequency are quite large.

Sound of any wavelength, audible or inaudible, cannot travel through a vacuum. Ultrasound travels very poorly through any gas. However, the human ear can testify thousands of times daily that audible sound travels very well through the atmosphere. The difference between sound and ultrasound in this respect is that the gas molecules which make up the atmosphere, i.e. nitrogen, oxygen, carbon dioxide, absorb almost completely the 1 mm and shorter wavelengths that comprise ultrasound, whereas audible sound (frequencies lower than 20,000 Hz) have wavelengths longer than 1 cm and up to 30 cm. One can only wonder if transmission of vibrational energy is influenced by the ratio of wavelength to molecule size and/or to the relatively vast differences in distance between molecules of a gas as compared to a liquid or a solid.

At any rate, ultrasonic energy, as used clinically, requires the use of a liquid or a semisolid (ointment or gel) coupling agent to achieve significant transmission of this form of energy from source to patient.

The majority of ultrasonic generators in clinical use in this country have an operating frequency of 1 Mc and hence a wavelength of about 1.5 mm when penetrating soft tissues. A few generators are in use with operating frequencies as low as 500 Kc and fewer still with frequencies as high as 4 Mc. Reasons for selection of these different frequencies are discussed in Chapter 7.

NATURAL LAWS PERTINENT TO THE USE
OF PHYSICAL AGENTS

Some of the relationships between velocity, frequency, and wavelength of energy forms that physical therapists utilize have been discussed. It is now necessary to explore the physical laws that control what one can and cannot do when adding or removing energy from living tissues. These laws were discovered in the latter part of the nineteenth century and are immutable for physical innanimate systems. Later, it will become obvious that some modifications are necessary when these same laws are applied to living tissues.

The Law of Grotthus-Draper

Whenever energy emanates from a source, it is either absorbed, transmitted, reflected, or refracted. The most important law is that the energy must be absorbed before it can have any effect. This fact was demonstrated at about the same time by two investigators, Grotthus and Draper working independently. Both were studying ultraviolet light. They both established that if energy is not absorbed, it must be transmitted. It follows that the greater the absorption, the less the transmission and hence the less penetration. Therefore, absorption and penetration are reciprocal. If energy is transmitted, it may be in a relatively straight line, or turned away completely from matter with which it collides (reflection), or the angle of transmission within the object with which it collides may be changed (refraction). The classical example of reflection is that of visible light waves striking a mirror. How much of the energy striking the mirror will be absorbed as compared to how much is reflected will depend in part upon the angle at which the light waves strike the mirror. Those waves which strike at a right angle will be largely absorbed. Those waves which strike at other than a right angle will be reflected. The more planar the surface of the mirror, the greater the reflection and thus the more nearly perfect visible image.

Clinically, reflection is a factor which must be taken into consideration when applying luminous infrared, ultraviolet light, or ultrasonic energy. In the case of luminous IR, as the concomitant visible light either strikes the reflector and is thereby aimed toward the patient or radiates directly from the source, some of these eye-stimulating wavelengths will reach the retina. The intensity may be high enough to be irritating to the retina, in which case the patient is apt to move out of position. This problem can be minimized by draping the lamp so that the visible light does not reach the retina in significant quantity.

Ultraviolet lamps usually have highly efficient reflectors. Hence, reflection of the visible output from the lamp can again reach the retina, along with the UV component. In the case of UV, both the visible and UV output can be irritating, and draping the lamp frequently is not an adequate solution. The usual fabric draping materials may re-reflect especially the UV, and almost any lightly colored fabric will reflect more UV than will any darker colored fabric. Hence, some kind of UV filtering goggles usually are indicated to achieve adequate eye protection. There can also be serious reflection from nearby partition material, onto both the patient and the therapist. To minimize this problem, there should be no cubicle curtains or lightly painted walls within about 150 cm of the UV source.

Reflection of ultrasonic energy becomes a problem when bone is within the limit of penetration of this form of energy. In the standard moving sound head technic, approximately 35 percent of the energy which penetrates to cortical bone will be reflected.[6] Thus, tissues close to absorbing bone are exposed to energy coming from the ultrasonic source plus that reflected by the bone. This will give rise to a greater tissue temperature increase than would otherwise be anticipated. Hence, if bone is close to the surface, source intensity should be less than if there is a large volume of soft tissue in the area under treatment. In part because of reflection of ultrasonic energy by bone, direct contact sonation of skin over bony prominences should be avoided. Painful "hot spots" are apt to occur. Fortunately, the periosteum is richly supplied with thermal sensors. Perception of this thermal pain will cause the patient to move away from the energy source before serious damage occurs. Areas with irregular contour can be treated with other ultrasonic technics. These are discussed in Chapter 7.

Refraction may be considered as a lesser case of reflection. In refraction, the penetrating energy is not turned away completely from the surface of the tissue with which it collides but is partially absorbed and partially transmitted. That portion which is transmitted will change direction of penetration within the transmitting medium. Clinically, refraction is of importance only when ultrasonic energy is being utilized. As long as the tissue which is being penetrated is homogenous, there is no significant refraction. Subcutaneous fat is the most nearly homogenous tissue in the intact human. Neglible refraction takes place here. As the transmitted energy penetrates to underlying muscle, nerve, and blood vessels and other structures of highly varying density, some refraction is inevitable. The more dense the tissue being penetrated, the greater the refraction. Thus, exposure of tendon or ligament will cause more refraction than exposure of muscle or fascia. As the energy penetrates from a more dense to a less dense tissue, dispersion of energy will occur. If penetration is from less dense to more dense tissue, there will be shear wave formation. Shear wave formation can lead to concentration of energy in a small volume of tissue and hence to "hot spot" formation. Refraction within tendon plus reflection from adjacent bone can become a major problem in concentration of the ultrasonic energy. If the patient's perception of pain is within normal limits, when this occurs the patient will instinctively move away from the energy source and no harm will be done. If, for whatever reason, the patient's pain perception is not normal, real damage can be done. If any tissue has its temperature raised above 45°C, a burn can occur.

The Arndt-Schultz Principle

The next basic law to be considered is usually referred to as the Arndt-Schultz Principle. It states that (a) if the quantity of energy absorbed is too small to stimulate the absorbing tissue, no significant reaction will take place; (b) if the quantity of energy absorbed per unit of time is adequate to stimulate, the absorbing unit of matter will perform its normal function; and (c) if the quantity of energy absorbed per unit time is too great, the absorbing unit of matter will be disrupted and cannot perform its normal function. Such disruption can be reversible or irreversible, depending both on the quantity of energy absorbed and the rate at which it is absorbed.

The physical therapist's objective within the framework of the Arndt-Schultz Principle is to add (or, with application of cold, to withdraw) enough energy to stimulate the absorbing tissues to normal function. In the case of physical agents known to cause a tissue temperature rise, i.e. most of the sources of infrared, the diathermies, and ultrasound, the local tissue temperature should not be elevated to more than 45°C, since tissue destruction is likely to occur if the temperature of that tissue goes higher. When stimulating currents are utilized, the most common objective is to cause intermittent contraction of skeletal muscle. The stimulation should not be so intense that it causes pain, nor should it cause abnormal muscle hyperactivity. When ultraviolet light is applied, an observable reaction is always delayed, on the order of hours. Hence, testing for an individual's reaction to the UV source prior to treatment is almost mandatory. The desired objective is chemical change within the absorbing tissues.

Maxwell's Precept

There is a third general law which has no precise label. It has evolved from Maxwell's work in electrostatics and can be stated as follows: For any unit of matter at rest, there will be a balance of charge between the inside and outside of the limiting membrane; when that unit of matter absorbs energy, there will be an alteration of charge and the unit of matter will not be at rest until the charge balance is restored.

For the purposes of the physical therapist, this law is quite important when considering actions and reactions of excitable membranes, i.e. nerve and muscle, but physiologists are becoming increasingly aware of the importance of charge shift during intracellular metabolism[7] and in living bone reorientation.[8] For the physical therapist, awareness of potential difference (separation of dissimilar charge) between the inside and outside of excitable membranes is important in choosing the best current type and other electrical parameters when applying nerve and muscle stimulating currents in neurological and other disorders.

Other physical laws, not germane to *all* portions of the electromagnetic and acoustic spectra, are discussed in other chapters as needed.

REFERENCES

1. Licht, S. (Ed.): *Electrodiagnosis and Electromyography,* 3rd ed. New Haven, Licht, 1971, Chapters 10 and 18.
2. Goodgold, Joseph and Eberstein, Arthur: *Electrodiagnosis of Neuromuscular Diseases.* Baltimore, Williams & Wilkins, 1972.
3. Licht, S. (Ed.): *Therapeutic Heat and Cold,* 2nd ed. New Haven, Licht, 1965, Chapters 1, 9, and 17.
4. Abramson, D.I.: *Circulation in the Extremities.* New York, Acad Pr, 1967, Chapters 6, 7, 11, and 12.
5. *Dorland's Illustrated Medical Dictionary,* 24th ed. Philadelphia, Saunders, 1965.
6. Lehmann, J.F. and Guy, A.W.: Ultrasound therapy. *Proc Workshop on Interaction of Ultrasound and Biological Tissues.* Washington, D.C., HEW Pub. (FDA 73:8008), Sept., 1972.
7. Jehle, H.: Charge fluctuation forces in biological systems. *Ann NY Acad Sci, 158:*240-55, May 16, 1969.
8. Bourne, G. (Ed.): *The Biochemistry and Physiology of Bone,* Volume III, 2nd ed. New York, Acad Pr, 1971, Chapter 1.

Chapter 3

NERVE AND MUSCLE
STIMULATING CURRENTS

NERVE and muscle stimulating currents can be useful in any disorder in which the patient has lost, or never had (i.e. congenital lesion), adequate voluntary control over skeletal muscle. The lesion may have been the result of trauma or a disease process, or it may have an emotional basis. The deficit may be orthopedic, neurological, vascular, or psychogenic in origin. There is little question that as soon as the patient regains voluntary control over his muscles to a functional degree, active exercise will be both physiologically and psychologically superior to externally applied nerve and muscle stimulating current (NMSC). But until such time as the patient has achieved useful control, it is better to make use of NMSC rather than do nothing or to use only passive exercise. A host of problems secondary to skeletal muscle hyper– or hypoactivity can be minimized with judicious use of NMSC.

Within the last several decades, as improved apparatus has resulted in greater patient comfort and in increased portability, new uses for NMSC have opened up, including benefits for the cerebral palsied and hemiplegics,[2-4] in pain relief,[5] and in the classical peripheral nervous system lesions.[6,7]

THE LAW OF DUBOIS REYMOND

There is one law which governs nerve and muscle response to externally applied low frequency, low voltage electromagnetic energy, namely the Law of DuBois Reymond. In its simplest form, the law states that it is the variation in current density rather than absolute density at any given instant which acts as a stimulus to nerve or muscle.[8,9]

To restate this law in a way more useful to the physical therapist, one may say that three criteria must be met in order to stimulate an excitable membrane to normal response:

1. The amplitude of the individual stimulus must be high enough so that depolarization of the membrane will take place.
2. The rate of change of voltage must be sufficiently rapid so that accommodation does not occur.
3. The duration of the individual stimulus must be long enough, i.e. energy must flow long enough in one direction, so that the time course of latent period, action potential, and recovery can take place.

All excitable membranes have a resting potential (separation of charge between the inside and the outside of the membrane), measurable in millivolts.[9] The membrane requires a decrease in potential (depolarization) or an increase (hyperpolarization) before an action potential can occur. Normal human axons require a 15 to 20 mv depolarization before formation of an action potential. An axon will not propagate impulses, nor will a muscle fiber contract, until the action potential is generated by a stimulus.

An excitable membrane is a capacitor. In other words, when the membrane is in its resting state, there is a potential difference between the inside and outside of the membrane, with the membrane itself acting as the dielectric. The capacitance of a normal axon is on the order of 1 to 1.3 microfarads/cm^2. The capacitance of a normal muscle fiber is on the order of 4.5 to 6 mf/cm^2.[9] The larger the capacitance, the *less frequently* a capacitor can discharge. A useful physical analogy is to consider two capacitors, one having plates the size of a dime, the other with plates the size of a half dollar. If equal DC voltages are applied separately to each capacitor, the smaller unit will have reached the limit of its ability to store electrons sooner than the bigger unit. When a capacitor can no longer store incoming energy, it discharges.

Hence, if equal quantities of energy are added at an equal rate, the unit with a lesser capacitance will discharge more often.

All normal nerve fibers have a smaller capacitance than any muscle fiber. Variation in the fastest possible rate of discharge is inherent in the individual membrane. The electrical and chemical events within the membrane which are responsible for the variation in rate of discharge are not known at this time. The clinical effect of the difference in capacity between nerve and muscle is that since nerve can respond to a greater number of stimuli per unit time, muscle with an intact nerve supply can respond to a higher frequency (60 Hz and higher) of stimulus than can denervated muscle. Denervated muscle requires frequencies of 40 Hz or lower before it can respond to each stimulus.[10]

The clinical picture is complicated by the fact that in the patient exposed to NMSC, a single axon or muscle fiber is never stimulated, but rather hundreds of axons and thousands of muscle fibers respond to the stimulus. Within a muscle mass, i.e. biceps brachii, some of the muscle fibers may have a normal nerve supply, others a hyperactive nerve supply, and still others a hypoactive nerve supply. Thus, a single stimulus can produce a wide variety of responses, and serial stimulation can cause major change in the mass response.

In general, but with many exceptions, large diameter axons have a small capacity and therefore are capable of responding to each of 1,000 or more stimuli per second. Axons of small diameter and large capacity may not respond to stimuli at a rate of more than fifty per second. If the stimulus amplitude is held constant at a threshold or higher level, the visible response is continuing muscle contraction (tetanic response) until the series of stimuli is stopped, providing the stimulus frequency is approximately 50 Hz or higher. If the stimulus frequency is appreciably lower (40 Hz or less), the visible response takes on the appearance of intermittent contraction and relaxation, even though the peak intensity is constant. If DC with continuous modulation is applied, there will be a visible response only at the time of make and, rarely, break of the patient circuit, even though the amplitude is held constant for a matter of seconds. This is termed a twitch response. The reason for the difference in response to this truly constant current is that as long as energy is flowing at a constant amplitude *in one direction,* the excitable membrane cannot recover from its depolarized (or hyperpolarized) state. Having once contracted and relaxed, the muscle cannot contract again until the normal resting potential of the stimulated excitable membranes has been restored. After the single twitch, the muscle remains flaccid until energy flow in one direction has ceased.

A completely denervated muscle mass often requires a stimulus rate as low as $\frac{1}{2}$ to 20 Hz in order to be able to respond to each stimulus. At 20 Hz, the peak (stimulating) amplitude can occur no more than fifty times in one second ($1000 \div 20 = 50$). Hence, the membrane will have at least 20 ms to restore normal resting potential.[10] Axons of smallest capacity require a stimulus of about 0.1 ms duration in order to become depolarized and thus to propagate impulses.

If the intensity is high and current must flow for more than 1 ms before there is an observable muscle response, there is a significant lesion affecting motor nerve supply.[10] Modern clinical apparatus can provide a wide range of stimulus duration and other stimulus parameters with an adequate degree of precision. Since in general the shorter the duration of the individual stimulus, the greater the patient comfort, a part of the therapist's task is to determine what frequency will give the best compromise between desired muscle response and patient comfort. This compromise frequency may vary as the degree of neurological damage fluctuates for better or worse. Hence, it is wise to have available apparatus which permits easy variation in stimulus duration, frequency, and other stimulating current parameters.

CLINICAL SIGNIFICANCE OF THE LAW OF DUBOIS REYMOND

If the time, in milliseconds, required to go from zero to peak amplitude is too slow, an excitable membrane will adjust its ion flow (calcium, sodium, potassium, chloride) across the membrane so as to maintain its resting potential rather than depolarize. This adjustment is called accommodation. No action potential is generated. There is no propagation of impulse and no muscle contraction. Clinically, no axon will depolarize if the time to go from zero to peak amplitude is more than about 10 ms.[10] Consequently, if the stimulus frequency is lower than 40 to 50 Hz, any response is likely to be due to direct stimulation of muscle because axons supplying the muscle will accommodate to the more slowly rising peak amplitudes. The smaller the capacity of the axon, the greater the likelihood that accommodation will take place.

Clinically, the fact of accommodation can be very useful if denervated muscle lies deep to normally innervated muscle. If the rate of rise from zero to peak amplitude is slow, the more superficial but normally functioning axons will not respond, but underlying denervated muscle, having a greater capacitance (greater ability to store energy before discharge), will respond to the slower change in amplitude by depolarization, formation of muscle action potential, and, finally, fiber contraction. Patients with such incomplete denervation patterns usually tolerate slowly rising current peaks better than rapidly rising peaks, since the normally innervated muscle is not likely to contract. The fewer the number of muscle fibers which contract in response to a given stimulus, the greater the patient comfort. This is especially true if the patient's sensory nervous system has remained intact, since sensory as well as motor axons respond by depolarization if stimulus parameters are suitable for axon stimulation.

If a continuous modulation direct current (DC) of threshold or higher intensity is applied to a normally innervated muscle mass, there will be a contractile response only at the instant of completion of the externally applied electrical circuit. While DC is flowing at a uniform rate (no significant voltage rise or fall), there can be *no* nerve or muscle response after the single contraction (immediately followed by relaxation) even though the DC flows for seconds or minutes. Depolarization will have occurred at the instant of circuit completion, *and it is maintained* in axons stimulated by the negative (−) pole. Hyperpolarization will have occurred at the positive pole at that same time, and it likewise is maintained as long as DC flows. The single muscle response which occurs with this type of stimulus is called a twitch response.

On the other hand, if a current of equal intensity but with a frequency of 60 Hz is applied for a matter of seconds to a normally innervated muscle mass, the muscle will contract upon completion of the circuit *and stay contracted* until the circuit is opened. This is called a tetanic response. Obviously, the 60 Hz current has caused a much greater stimulus response in the normally innervated muscle. The greater response is due to the fact that the voltage fluctuated from zero to peak amplitude 120 times each second.

Conversely, if an identical stimulus was applied to a completely denervated muscle, no response would occur. Change in voltage level 120 times per second does not cause depolarization of the higher capacity muscle membrane. If a 10 to 20 Hz stimulus was applied for several seconds to a denervated muscle, a series of twitches would occur. Voltage fluctuations less than about 40 times per second permit energy to flow long enough in one direction so that the denervated muscle membrane can depolarize, generate a muscle action potential, and lead to muscle contraction.

In general, axons require current flow in one direction for 0.1 to 1 ms for depolarization to occur. Muscle fibers, in the absence of a normal motor nerve, must have similar current flow for 2.5 to 3 ms for depolarization to occur.[10] When the muscle has been deprived of its nerve supply for weeks, the necessary duration of current flow increases markedly, so that flow in one direction for up to 10 ms may be needed. The difference in time required of current flow in one direction depends largely on the difference in capacity of the different types of excitable membranes.

SKIN IMPEDANCE

Another major clinical variable is the skin impedance (resistance) to the externally applied stimulus. Sea water has a resistivity of about 20 ohm-cm. Normal skin has an impedance of not less than 200 ohm-cm to all frequencies in clinical use.[11]   In various lesions, especially those involving cutaneous nerves, impedance can be many times higher. This is also true for some skin diseases, even though the skin where the electrodes are applied gives no evidence of disease. Patients with psoriasis are the prime example.

The higher the impedance of the skin, the greater the strength of stimulus needed in order that a threshold intensity will reach the underlying motor nerve. It is generally accepted that no muscle with a normal nerve supply should require more than 50 volts AC or 80 v DC to elicit a contractile response. Skin impedance to DC is usually higher than that for AC. Electron flow in one direction only (DC) leads to chemical reactions in the skin that transiently increase impedance. About 10 percent of patients with a normal nerve supply will have a skin chemistry which permits equivalent response with a lower intensity of DC as compared to AC.

VARIATION IN STIMULUS–RESPONSE IN THE CLINIC VERSUS THE LABORATORY

If the motor nerve supply to a muscle is intact and skin impedance is within normal limits, but the patient does not have voluntary control over skeletal muscle for other reasons, use of stimulating currents at or above 1000 Hz will usually cause muscle contraction with less discomfort than when lower frequencies are used.

A single motor nerve will supply anywhere from one or two hundred to several thousands of muscle fibers. Furthermore, in ordinary volitional contraction, not all fibers within the muscle mass are contracting simultaneously, even though the mass has developed considerable tension and has undergone shortening in length in response to internal stimulus. If an external stimulus of 50 to 250 Hz is applied, many more muscle fibers may contract simultaneously than if voluntary contraction takes place. The more fibers that contract simultaneously, the more painful the tetanic response will be. Cutaneous axons are also stimulated by the external stimulus. For any given intensity, they are stimulated more than the underlying motor nerves because cutaneous receptors and axons are closer to the source of stimulus; hence, they receive more of a stimulus.

In the laboratory, as opposed to the clinic, anesthetized or isolated denervated muscle preparations can be studied. Under these circumstances, it may be more convenient to increase intensity rather than alter frequency of the stimulating current. Where stimulus intensity can be unlimited, denervated muscle can be stimulated with a 60 Hz or higher current. Patients with intact skin and sensory nervous systems, however, would not tolerate such intensities. In the laboratory, nerve or muscle can be stimulated directly rather than through intervening skin and subcutaneous fat. Therefore, the intensity required for a contractile response will be far less—on the order of one volt—whereas, as stated before, clinically one may need up to 50 v AC or 80 v DC for eliciting a contractile response.

If the therapist is using a stimulating current on a patient with an intact peripheral nervous system, the muscle response *always* occurs as a result of depolarization of motor nerves rather than from direct depolarization of the muscle membrane. The smaller the capacity of the membrane the less amplitude of stimulus required to cause the depolarization.

INFLUENCE OF THE LAW OF DUBOIS REYMOND ON STIMULATOR DESIGN

Many models of nerve and muscle stimulating apparatus have the capability of delivering current to the patient in continuous, or surge, or interrupted modulation. Also, the frequency of the stimulus (AC or DC) can be varied anywhere from zero (DC only) to $\frac{1}{2}$ to 3,000 Hz (AC or DC). The surge or interrupted modulation can be varied in rate from five to sixty times *per minute*. Sophisticated stimulators may also have DC with automatically reversing polarity, with full or half wave rectification, and the capability of simultaneous use of up to ten electrodes. Justification for this wide range of variation in stimulus parameters is the wide variety of peripheral and central neurological lesions, vascular and orthopedic problems, as well as the great range of skin impedance, depending upon the effect of the lesion on axons, receptors, and circulation of the skin in the area to be stimulated. With a wide choice of parameters to draw upon, the therapist should always be able to elicit a contractile response, unless the lesion has been of such long duration that muscle fiber has been replaced by fatty or fibrous tissue. If this has occurred, no stimulus can cause contraction.

The designation *continuous modulation* indicates that the stimulus amplitude does not fluctuate. Figure 3-1a is representative of a continuous AC sine wave. Figure 3-1b illustrates continuous modulation DC. It is clear that continuous modulation DC has no waveform and no rise or fall of voltage at any given intensity, whereas AC sine wave continuous modulation has a constantly fluctuating voltage with a symmetrical pattern. Both are correctly called continuous modulation, but the induced muscle contraction will appear totally different.

Figure 3-1. (a) Alternating Current (AC), sine waveform, continuous modulation. Note the regular rise and fall in amplitude, with reversal of direction of electron flow once each cycle.

(b) Direct Current (DC), continuous modulation. There is no waveform. Note that the amplitude, at any given intensity, is constant, and that there is no reversal of direction of electron flow.

An AC sine wave *surge modulation* is pictured in Figure 3-2a. Figure 3-2b diagrams DC *surge modulation*. It can be seen in both cases that there is a gradual fluctuation of amplitude. With an *interrupted modulation* (Figs. 3-3a and 3-3b), there are repeating periods of energy flow and no flow, with *abrupt* shift from zero to a constant peak amplitude. The induced contractile response will vary depending upon current type (AC or DC), modulation used (continuous, surge, interrupted), and, of course,

Figure 3-2. (a) AC, sine waveform, surging modulation. Note the regular fluctuation in amplitude over and above the regular rise and fall of voltage within a cycle, as well as the regular reversal of direction of electron flow once each cycle.

(b) DC, surging modulation. There is a gradual rise and fall in amplitude but no reversal of direction of electron flow.

Figure 3-3. (a) AC, interrupted modulation. When current is flowing, it is at a uniform amplitude. There are regular intervals of current flow and no flow. As is *always* the case with AC, there is reversal of direction of electron flow once each cycle.

(b) DC, interrupted modulation. When current is flowing, it is at a uniform amplitude. There are regular intervals of current flow and no flow. As is usually the case with DC, there is no reversal of direction of electron flow. Apparatus with automatically reversing polarity is available, but such sophisticated apparatus is not in common clinical use.

whether or not the peripheral nervous system (motor and/or sensory) is intact.

When applied to a normally innervated muscle, a stimulus having a frequency of about 50 Hz or higher will cause muscle contraction if the intensity of stimulus is great enough to cause membrane depolarization. Continuous modulation at threshold or greater intensity will cause a tetanic contraction of the muscle.

Enough individual muscle fibers are stimulated, through their motor nerves, each cycle per second so that the muscle mass maintains tension development to an approximately uniform degree as long as energy is flowing through the muscle, even though the individual muscle fibers *do not* maintain their shortened state throughout the entire time course of several seconds or more that the stimulus is applied. If the same intensity is used, but with a surging rather than continuous stimulus, intermittent muscle contraction and relaxation will occur. There will be a *gradual* rise and fall in tension development occurring several times *per minute*. If all parameters are the same except that an interrupted modulation is used, there will again be intermittent tetanic contraction and relaxation. This time, the rise and fall in muscle tension will be much more abrupt.

As the frequency of stimulus is decreased from 50 Hz and approaches $\frac{1}{2}$ Hz, fewer and fewer motor nerves will be stimulated by each energy peak. More and more of the nerve fibers will accommodate to the more gradual rise and fall in the applied voltage. Consequently, the muscle response will be less tetanic and more like a twitch.

When a stimulating current is applied in similar fashion to a denervated muscle, the energy must flow *in one direction* for a longer period of time (milli-seconds) before membrane depolarization can occur, with subsequent contractile response. In a denervated muscle, the motor nerve is no longer functioning and the muscle membrane has a larger capacitance than its axon membrane. Hence, current must flow for a longer period of time, in one direction, before denervated muscle will contract.

When a stimulating current of adequate duration is applied to a denervated muscle at a uniform rate, there will be only a single, brief twitch response regardless of whether the current flows at that rate for milliseconds or for seconds. The twitch response results whenever either AC or DC having a stimulus frequency of $\frac{1}{2}$ to 20 Hz is applied. If intensity is raised from zero to peak too slowly, accommodation will occur and no contraction will take place. If these same frequencies are used, but with a surging modulation, there will be a single muscle mass contraction with each surge. If an interrupted modulation is used, but all other factors are the same, the contractile response will be stronger. The more abrupt the change in intensity, the greater the number of muscle fibers which will respond at the same instant.

There can be widely varying degrees of deficit in motor nerve supply to a muscle mass. Trauma or disease anywhere in the peripheral nervous system commonly will result in loss of ability to conduct impulses by some, but not by all, of the motor nerve fibers supplying that muscle mass. The greater the number of malfunctioning axons, the lower the stimulus frequency necessary to elicit a contractile response. When nearly all axons are unable to conduct, the stimulus frequency must be 20 Hz or less (AC or DC) in order to have current flow in one direction long enough to bring about adequate depolarization. If a muscle mass is completely denervated, sometimes DC with a low interrupted modulation rate is the only feasible means of causing muscle membrane depolarization. A DC interruption rate of five times *per minute* can give rise to a current flow in one direction with nearly uniform intensity for over *one second* each time the current is flowing. If the rest period between interruptions is long enough, there is ample time for recovery of membrane potential to its resting level.

Variable *frequency* controls can be used to reduce the risk of injury (chemical burn of the skin) or discomfort to the patient. Such problems are less when AC is applied, at any frequency, as compared to DC at any frequency. The chances of abnormal chemical buildup in the skin are negligible with AC. Electron and then ion flow reverse in direction each half cycle with AC. The net effect is no residual acidic or alkaline buildup under either electrode. Such buildup is inevitable with application of DC because there is no periodic reversal of direction of electron or ion flow.

Even though present-day stimulating apparatus permits use of DC at almost any frequency that is used with AC, high frequency DC is usually less comfortable to persons whose sensory nervous system is intact. Although ion flow with 60 Hz DC is clearly intermittent, it is still ion flow in one direction only, rather than ion flow with periodically reversing direction, as is the case for AC. When DC is applied to the skin, free oxygen and acid are formed at the anode and free hydrogen at the cathode. This results in cauterization of tissues closest to the electrodes if the concentration becomes high enough.[29] Visible hyperemia is an anticipated reaction, even when current density is insufficient to cause skin damage. Hyperemia is rare when the stimulating current is AC.

SAFETY STANDARDS FOR CLINICAL ELECTRICAL STIMULATING APPARATUS

It is obvious that any device which is applied to a patient should at least do no harm. Federal regulatory agencies establish, revise, and enforce safety standards, after consultation with physicians, bioengineers, biophysicists, and manufacturers of equipment. Two federal agencies which have major responsibility over equipment which physical therapists use are the Bureau of Radiological Health, with its Acoustic and Electromagnetic Divisions, and the Federal Communications Commission.

Ultimately, it is the physical therapist's responsibility to see to it that the devices used cannot harm the patient. This is especially important in applying electrical energy directly to the patient's skin. This occurs when nerve and muscle stimulating apparatus is used, as well as in the diathermies, where high frequency electrical and magnetic energy is directed toward the patient, and in ultrasonic energy, wherein electrical energy is converted into acoustic energy, which is then transmitted directly through the skin and into the patient. In the latter case, both electrical and acoustic energy are sometimes transmitted simultaneously.

It is simple to perceive macroshock, which can occur from defective equipment. It is more difficult to be aware when microshock occurs.* Both can be fatal. Patients with cardiac lesions, especially those who are wearing pacemakers, are particularly susceptible to microshock. Current leakage is most apt to occur

---

*The American Association for the Advancement of Medical Instrumentation defines microshock as current leakage of less than one milliampere. Macroshock is current leakage greater than one ma. (AMI: *Seven Steps to Electrical Safety,* 1970).

when there is improper grounding of the apparatus. This can be due to poor quality control on the part of the manufacturer, to deterioration of electrical or electronic circuitry after extensive use, or to a defect in the institution's provision for grounding through line outlets.

Microshock testing of all apparatus from which there is any possibility of uncontrolled low or high frequency electrical energy reaching the patient should be done at least annually by persons trained in these technics. Adequate maintenance of all stimulating current, diathermy, and ultrasonic apparatus more than justifies the costs when the alternative is improper treatment or possible physiological or psychological harm to the patient.

EQUIPMENT CONTROLS

All nerve and muscle stimulating current apparatus (NMSC) is designed to modify standard house (wall outlet) current. The standard current is 110 v, 60 cycle, sine wave alternating current. Current delivered to the patient may be AC or DC, or a simultaneous combination through two or more circuits. The voltage range to the patient may be from 0 to 50 v (AC) or to 100 v (DC). The amperage range may be from 0 to 100 milliamperes. The waveform may be sine, square, faraic, pulse, or exponential. Modulation may be continuous, surging, or interrupted. In modern equipment, all modification is electronic rather than mechanical. The general principles involved in such modification of line current are outlined in Chapter 8.

The more kinds of modification available with any single piece of apparatus, the better the chances of being able to achieve the desired contractile response with maximum patient comfort. It also follows that the more modifications available, the greater the cost of the unit. Very few NMSC generators will have all of the above modification capabilities available. The most elaborate models are intended for teaching or research rather than clinical use.

Many stimulators will have one or more electrical meters which measure the amperage, voltage, or wattage delivered to the patient with an acceptable degree of precision. Such meters can be used by the therapist to provide an objective record of energy needed to produce the desired response through a series of treatments. This kind of record can indicate improvement or deterioration of a patient's condition.

Regardless of size or cost of the apparatus, all stimulators will have provision for the following:

1. on-off control
2. intensity control
3. waveform and/or modulation selection
4. polarity control (DC only)

The intensity control should be at zero (no energy in the patient circuit) when electrodes are being applied to the patient or whenever any change is to be made in the parameters of the energy to be delivered to the patient. Also, any change in intensity should be made slowly, over a period of several seconds, rather than going up or down as rapidly as possible. The Law of DuBois Reymond is operative whenever the patient circuit is complete. If change in intensity is too rapid, so many muscle fibers will contract simultaneously that the contraction will be unnecessarily painful.

CURRENT TYPE

Some stimulators will deliver to the patient only AC, others only DC. Most units in clinical use can deliver either current type to the patient. Patients with peripheral nervous system involvement may respond to low frequency AC (20 to 60 Hz) or may need DC (0 to 20 Hz), depending upon the stage of degeneration or regeneration of peripheral axons. Patients whose primary problem is some form of organic occlusive peripheral vascular disease usually will respond to AC, although if their circulatory inadequacy is accompanied by long-standing diabetes mellitus, low frequency AC, or DC, may be needed. The patient with chronic diabetes may have a peripheral neuropathy. The individual whose loss of voluntary control over joint motion is related to psychosomatic rather than neurological deficit should always respond to AC. If the loss of voluntary control over joint motion is due to a central nervous system defect but the peripheral motor axons are intact, an AC stimulus should be effective. If there is concomitant peripheral nerve deficit, low frequency AC (less than 60 Hz) may be needed.

With the advent of circuit design which permits transmission of slowly cycling AC ($\frac{1}{2}$ to 60 Hz), there is less and less need for stimulators to deliver DC. The key to muscle or nerve response to externally applied stimulating current is whether current flows long enough *in one direction* to cause depolarization of the membrane that is being stimulated. The less excitable the membrane, i.e. the greater the capacitance, the longer the stimulus must flow in one direction before adequate depolarization will take place. Normal nerve is *always* much more easily depolarized than is denervated muscle.

Furthermore, it has been this author's clinical experience that more than 90 percent of all patients prefer AC to DC from the comfort standpoint. Presumably, this is due to neglible alteration of acidity or alkalinity on the skin when AC is used.

If current flows in one direction for more than a few seconds, an unnecessary and painful chemical irritation of the skin is likely to occur. This does not occur with AC at any frequency because of the automatic reversal of direction of current flow each cycle. This can and does occur whenever DC is applied to the skin and occurs to the greatest degree when the modulation is continuous (zero frequency). The preceding can be easily demonstrated. Apply two pad electrodes (5 × 5 cm or a little larger are convenient) to any area of the body. The electrodes may be close together or far apart. Attach each electrode to a lead cord. Attach the lead cord to the machine circuit. The patient circuit is now complete. Use AC of 60 Hz or higher, with continuous modulation. Turn up intensity to the subject's tolerance. A muscle contraction is not necessary. Let the current flow for at least two minutes, with a flow for five minutes being better. Adjust the intensity to the subject's comfort if necessary. Observe and record the percent of available power used, or voltage and amperage if such meters are available. When five minutes are up, turn the intensity down to zero. Remove the electrodes, and inspect the skin. There will be little or no hyperemia. Replace the electrodes at the same or adjacent areas. Switch the current type to DC, continuous modulation. Turn up the intensity to the same level as with AC. If the subject will tolerate this intensity let the DC flow for the same time interval as with AC. Adjust intensity to the subject's comfort as needed. Turn the intensity to zero, remove the electrodes, and inspect the skin. There will be a strong hyperemia under one or both electrodes. This may not appear for a minute or two after electrode removal if treatment time was less than two minutes. Very likely, the hyperemia will become steadily stronger during the next five to ten minutes and will remain plainly visible for several hours.

The hyperemia is due to the local release of histamine or a histaminelike compound by cutaneous cells in response to a significant change in their environment. If voltage, amperage, and wattage were identical for AC and DC treatment, then the experimental variable has to be duration of current flow *in one direction*. With a five-minute treatment with DC, electrons and then ions have been flowing in one direction infinitely longer as compared to electron and ion flow induced by AC.

If the DC had been pulsed at the same rate as AC, the DC-induced hyperemia would be less intense than if the DC had an infinite wavelength, but it would still be visibly greater than that seen with AC at any pulse rate. Thus, whenever DC is used, regardless of modulation or other parameters, there is a greater chemical irritation of the skin. The same events take place with AC, but during each AC cycle there is a regular reversal of electron and ion flow so that there is insufficient time for a significant irritation of the skin. Hence, occurrence of pain or numbness is extremely rare when AC is used but common when DC is applied.

Another way to demonstrate the fundamental difference between AC and DC is to fill any transparent container with tap water. One to two hundred ml is a convenient volume. Place the bare metal terminals from two lead cords in the water, keeping them separate. Plug the other lead cord terminals into appropriate terminals of any NMSC generator that can deliver either

AC or DC. Start with intensity at zero. Turn up intensity to any desired level, and observe the terminals in the water. When DC is transmitted by the lead cords, bubbles will appear at both terminals, always in greater quantity at the negative pole. Turn intensity down, reverse polarity of the leads, and note the rapid shift in quantity of bubbles at each terminal. The bubble formation is due to the partial dissociation of water into H^+ and O^- ions. Since approximately twice as many hydrogen ions are formed as compared to oxygen ions, and since $(+)$ ions are attracted to the $(-)$ pole, more bubbles appear at the $(-)$ pole. This reaction does not take place to any significant extent when AC is delivered to the lead cords. Since the DC-induced chemical reaction is *not necessary* for the formation of action potentials in nerve or muscle, usually AC of some frequency can be used as an adequate and more comfortable stimulus to cause muscle contraction. This is true regardless of the cause of denervation, and there is far less risk of skin damage.

Occasionally, a patient's skin chemistry will be such that DC is tolerated better than AC. Once in a great while, the degeneration-regeneration process will be such that DC of continuous modulation and uniform amplitude will be needed to elicit a contractile response. In most cases, however, the desired response can be achieved with some variety of AC.

WAVEFORMS

The therapist may have need of the sine, pulse, square, faradic, or exponential waveform to obtain the desired contractile response. Figure 3-4 shows a schematic representation of these waveforms. The sine wave has a gradual buildup and a gradual decline of intensity two times each cycle, with reversal of direction of electron flow once each cycle. The pulse wave has an abrupt increase and decrease in amplitude, along with reversal of direction of electron flow. The square wave has an abrupt increase in intensity, followed by a plateau, followed by a much larger change in intensity simultaneous with reversal of direction of electron flow.

With one exception, if DC is converted into similar wave-

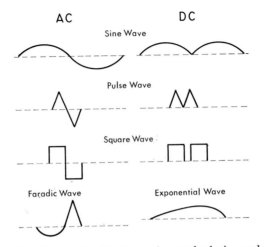

Figure 3-4. (a) *Sine Wave.* (1) AC—Note the gradual rise and fall of amplitude twice in each cycle, with reversal of direction of electron flow once each cycle (2) DC — Note the gradual rise and fall of amplitude once each cycle, with no reversal of direction of electron flow.

   (b) *Pulse Wave.* (1) AC—Note the rapid rise and fall of amplitude twice in each cycle, with reversal of direction of electron flow once each cycle. (2) DC—note the rapid rise and fall of amplitude once each cycle. Unless the apparatus has automatically reversing polarity, there is no reversal of direction of electron flow.

   (c) *Square Wave.* (1) AC—Note the abrupt rise and fall of amplitude twice each cycle. There is a plateau wherein the intensity is uniform twice each cycle. There is reversal of direction of electron flow once each cycle. (2) DC—Note the abrupt rise and fall of amplitude, with a plateau occurring once each cycle. There is no reversal of direction of electron flow.

   (d) *Faradic Wave.* This waveform *always* has reversal of direction of electron flow once each cycle and hence is always AC. However, the net effect is that of a rapid DC pulse because of the significant difference in amplitude of the two segments of the waveform. Whether this waveform stimulates nerve or muscle depends on its frequency. If the frequency is 60 Hz or higher, only nerve will be stimulated. If the frequency is lower, nerve or muscle will be stimulated.

   (e) *Exponential Wave.* (Also called the triangular or sawtooth forms, there is no reversal of direction of electron flow. The exception is DC with automatically reversing polarity, which physiologically becomes identical to AC.

The true faradic waveform is obsolete. Equipment with waveform selection that is labeled faradic (derived from standard wall outlet current) is actually producing a pulse wave. The amplitude of the first segment of the true faradic wave is small in proportion to the amplitude of the second segment. If the peak of the second segment is clinically tolerable, the peak of the first segment is not of sufficient amplitude to cause depolarization. Frequently, what the manufacturer labels "Faradic" will be of higher frequency (100 to 250 Hz) than that which is labeled "Sine" or "Pulse" (50 to 100 Hz). The faradic waveform derived from a house current source is physiologically the same as the pulse waveform. The most effective way to determine what waveform and frequency is actually being delivered to the patient is to display the patient circuit output on an oscilloscope. It is recommended that the derived data be permanently attached to each device.

The exponential waveform features a slowly rising amplitude, followed by an abrupt decline. It is sometimes referred to as a saw-tooth or triangular rather than exponential waveform. In theory at least, this waveform permits stimulation of denervated muscle that lies deep to normally innervated muscle without painful massive contraction of the superficial muscle. The muscle with a functioning motor nerve supply tends to accommodate to the slowly rising ion flow, and hence depolarization is less apt to occur.

It is obvious that as frequency is increased, with any of the

---

wave). This waveform was developed in the 1940s specifically for stimulation of denervated skeletal muscle. Note its slow amplitude rise time and rapid amplitude decline. This waveform is not commonly available on apparatus used in this country. It is always DC. Selective stimulation of denervated muscle without stimulation of intervening normally innervated muscle is possible with this waveform as well as with other waveforms of slowly rising amplitude.

above waveforms, all will tend to appear more and more like the pulse waveform. In part for this reason, fewer and fewer manufacturers are providing any choice in waveform. When the waveform is limited to one, it usually approximates the ideal pulse form.

The waveforms as drawn (Fig. 3-4) are theoretical or ideal. They are rarely generated exactly as shown. Only oscilloscopic display will reveal what is actually delivered to the patient circuit. Periodic recheck of the display is a useful means of determining whether the generator is undergoing electronic deterioration, in which case repair or replacement may be indicated.

The house current modification of sine wave into other waveforms, other frequencies, and other current types requires a number of steps. Filtering of electron flow through various circuit components is perhaps the most important for patient comfort, especially for the rectification of AC into DC. The better the filtering, the less discomfort. The better the filtering, the greater the cost. Chapter 8 discusses in detail house current modification for nerve and muscle current stimulators as well as for all other equipment that physical therapists use.

CURRENT MODULATION

Most modern stimulators offer a choice of continuous, surge, or interrupted modulation for AC or DC or both. The term *continuous modulation* can be difficult to grasp. In terms of NMSC, continuous modulation means that the amplitude is uniform and nonvarying for a prolonged period of time, i.e. seconds to minutes. Yet continuous modulation DC (Fig. 3-5a) is obviously physically different from continuous modulation AC (Fig. 3-5b). From the viewpoint of neurophysiology, if the stimulus repeats itself more than fifty to sixty times per second, with equal peak amplitude for each cycle, enough motor nerves, and the muscles they supply, will be stimulated by each cycle to give rise to a sustained contraction. Note that if the stimulus repeats itself less than about fifty times per second, an incomplete alternate contraction and relaxation of the muscle mass will occur. This response is sometimes called an intermittent tetanic contraction in order to distinguish it from the twitch response which is invariably produced by true continuous modulation DC, irrespective of whether the muscle is innervated or denervated.

When DC is pulsed rather than being truly continuous (Fig. 3-5c) at a rate of less than fifty times per second, it too will produce an intermittent contraction and relaxation, i.e. an intermittent tetanic response. This will hold true for any DC waveform. DC pulsed at a rate of greater than about fifty times per second will cause a true tetanic response. Because of concomitant skin

Figure 3-5. (a) DC continuous modulation. For any given intensity, the rate of electron flow is uniform. There is no reversal of direction of electron flow. The stimulated muscle responds only with a twitch and only upon rise or fall of amplitude (make or break of circuit).

(b) AC continuous modulation. For any given intensity, there is constant variation in rate of electron flow. There is reversal of direction of electron flow once each cycle. If the frequency is high enough, the stimulated muscle mass maintains a level of tension development which is clinically designated as a tetanic response. If the frequency is lower than about 50 Hz, there will be intermittent muscle mass contraction and relaxation.

(c) DC, *pulse wave*, continuous modulation. If the pulses occur at 50 Hz or higher, the muscle mass response is designated as tetanic because of a maintained level of tension development within the stimulated mass. If the pulse rate is lower, there will be intermittent mass contraction and relaxation because there is significant fluctuation in amplitude.

chemical changes, it is usually less comfortable and usually requires a higher voltage to produce an equivalent response.

Placement of a voltmeter and a milliamperemeter in the patient circuit will confirm this fact. Stimulate a muscle on one side of the body, obtain a palpable response, and note both the volt and ma readings *at the time of stimulation,* using either AC or DC. Replace the electrodes in the contralateral position and repeat, using the other current type, and obtain an equivalent palpable response. Again, record the meter readings at the time of stimulation. In normal subjects, the voltage will always be higher when DC is used (5 to 10 v). The ma reading may be higher, the same, or very slightly less when DC is used. Since watts equals volts times amperes, the milliwattage will always be higher when DC is used.

It should now be clear that the key to understanding variation in contractile response to continuous modulation is knowing what is the frequency of stimulation (per second) as well as what is the modulation, as much or more than being aware of the current type (AC or DC).

Contractile responses to other available modulations are easier to understand. The term *surging modulation* means there are alternate periods of current flow and no flow, with a gradual buildup and decline in intensity (*see* Figs. 3-2a and 3-2b). Most stimulators will permit a choice of surges through a range of about five to sixty times *per minute.* Oscilloscopic monitoring of the various surge rates will show that the control systems for variation in surge rates tend to be rather imprecise.

Some stimulators also permit variation in ratio of surge to the rest period between surges, irrespective of surge rate. This can be useful when the lesion is such that the stimulated muscle is slow to relax after the stimulus has ceased. In this case, the rest interval needs to be long. Also, if the patient has a chronic arterial insufficiency, the surge rate may need to be low and the rest interval long so that the impaired arterial flow can adequately meet the demand for increased blood supply as the muscle is regularly contracting and relaxing.

The term *interrupted modulation* means periodic current flow and cessation of current flow. The difference between interrupted and surging modulation is that with interrupted modulation, the shift from energy flow to no flow is abrupt rather than gradual. The net effect is that when a muscle is stimulated with an interrupted modulation, more fibers contract simultaneously because stimulus adequate to cause depolarization occurs in a shorter period of time. This obviously can be less comfortable, but it may be needed when skin impedance is high or many muscle fibers are denervated.

Perhaps the most important modulation of house current (110 v, 60 cycle AC) is that of frequency. Most stimulators that give the operator a choice will do so for AC only. If the unit will deliver only DC, variation in frequency rate is often not available. In sophisticated apparatus, one may select either AC or DC through a wide range of frequencies ($\frac{1}{2}$ to 3000 Hz) as well as DC with automatically reversing polarity. Where variation in frequency rate is permitted, it may be for only a few fixed frequencies, or stepless, or for many fixed frequencies. An AC frequency range of 20 to 1000 Hz with four or five choices within that range is probably adequate for the department that uses NMSC on only one or two patients a day. For the teaching hospital with an active neurological service, a wider choice of frequencies can be justified. The greater the capability of choice of both AC and DC frequencies, the greater the likelihood of being able to obtain the desired contractile response with minimum discomfort to the patient.

THE PATIENT CIRCUIT

The patient circuit consists of lead cords which connect the stimulator to the electrodes, the electrodes themselves, and the patient. The circuit must have a minimum of two lead cords and two electrodes to be complete. When AC is delivered to the patient, each electrode is carrying energy to the patient for one half of the cycle and returning energy to the apparatus for the other half at precisely opposite times. Hence, each electrode is both stimulating and dispersive during each complete cycle.

When DC is delivered to the patient, the situation is different:

one electrode is always active (stimulating) and the other is always inactive (dispersive). Usually, it is advisable to have the active electrode be of negative and the inactive electrode be of positive polarity because the negative pole electrode is almost always more stimulating than the positive pole. This is in part due to the fact that chemical changes on the skin exposed to the negative pole tend to be irritating whereas changes at the positive pole tend to be sedative. Also, the charge separation between the inside and outside of excitable membranes is normally $(+)$ on the outside and $(-)$ on the inside. If the stimulating electrode is $(-)$, the requisite depolarization is readily achieved. If the stimulating electrode is $(+)$, hyperpolarization will occur and a greater intensity is needed to produce equivalent response. This point can be simply confirmed.

Use any apparatus that delivers DC of continuous modulation and has a built-in voltmeter and an ammeter. Select any muscle mass to be stimulated and do so, noting the voltage and milliamperage needed to produce a palpable response. Reverse polarity, and stimulate the contralateral muscle, keeping all other factors equal. In the normal individual, it will invariably require at least 10 volts more when the stimulating electrode is $(+)$ than when it is $(-)$ because the excitable membrane is being hyperpolarized rather than depolarized.

Connecting the Patient to the Stimulator

It is advisable to check that the components of the patient circuit are in good order before attaching them to the patient. After making sure that the lead cord terminals are tightly connected to their lead cords, plug the appropriate cord terminal into one of the apparatus terminals. Do this for each of two lead cords. Then place the distal lead cord terminals together and turn up the intensity part way. The ma meter should give a reading. If not, either the lead cord terminals are not fitting tightly in the machine terminal sockets, one of the lead cords itself has a short circuit (broken wire underneath its insulation), or the connecting terminal between lead cord and electrode is loose. If the ma meter does read when the intensity is above zero, turn the intensity down and attach a tap water soaked electrode to each of the two lead cords. Hold them firmly together. Turn up the intensity control, and again the ma meter should rise above zero, indicating that the metallic part of the patient circuit is ready for use. If the meter does not read after connecting the electrodes, either the electrodes have not been adequately soaked or an electrode plate is corroded or broken and should be discarded. If the electrode was completely dry prior to use, it may need to be soaked for at least one half hour in warm water before it will conduct safely and effectively. If the electrode was in use within the last twenty-four hours, soaking it for five to ten minutes will usually be adequate.

If the NMSC apparatus does not have an ammeter, the procedure outlined above can be followed with substitution of moistened fingers when checking the lead cords themselves; for electrodes plus lead cords, place the electrodes firmly on any skin surface. In both cases, as intensity is turned up slowly, the subject should perceive a gentle tingling. If such a sensation is not achieved when the intensity control reads 50 percent of available power, something is defective in the patient circuit.

If the apparatus has both a voltmeter and an ammeter, the voltmeter will indicate whether the instrument circuit (*not patient circuit*) is in good condition. One does not need to have the patient circuit attached for this test. Being sure that the on-off control is set at zero and that the apparatus is plugged in, proceed to turn up the intensity. The voltmeter should rise above its zero reading. If it does not, the chances are that the line cord (not lead cord) is defective, a machine circuit fuse has blown, or the line current supply has been interrupted. If the line current is on, as indicated by the wall panel fuse or circuit breaker, trouble-shooting of a possibly defective machine circuit may be done by the institution's electrician. All NMSC apparatus will have a machine circuit fuse. Most often this fuse is readily accessible, but in some units, one or more chassis panels must be removed to locate the fuse. Spare fuses of appropriate type and size should be kept on hand, as this is the most common component failure. Fuses are designed to be safety valves and to be the weakest link in any electrical circuit. The most common cause of fuse failure is a brief surge in line current. Line current circuit fuses (or circuit breakers) commonly have a rate capacity of 20 to 30 amperes. Machine circuit fuse capacity is usually 2 to 5 amperes. Patient circuit fuses, which are integral parts of many NMSC units, will have a capacity of $1/16$ to $1/4$ ampere. Thus, a small, uncontrolled current surge will cause only the patient circuit to fail. A much larger surge is needed to interrupt the line current supply.

One word of caution: Before attempting to check any fuse, always unplug the apparatus from the line current supply. Many times a defect in a fuse is not visible. Fuses are cheap. If after replacing a suspect fuse the apparatus still does not work, the chances are good that the fuse was functioning and that the problem is in another circuit component. If the replacement fuse blows on attempt to test the apparatus, the problem is more serious and professional servicing is needed.

ELECTRODES

Down through the years, many electrodes have been designed. Those in widespread use have some sort of connector for attachment to the lead cord on one side and the surface to be in contact with the patient on the other. The connection for the lead cord should always be tight for efficient conduction of electricity from cord to electrode. Hence, a spring-loaded snap fit or a spring clip is commonly used. The connector is permanently attached to a slightly flexible metal plate or screen mesh. On the terminal connecting side, the plate or screen is covered by an insulating material, usually a synthetic rubber or an insulating plastic. Loosely attached to the other side of the plate or screen is a layer of orthopedic felt or layers of asbestos paper to a thickness of about 1 cm. This in turn is covered with a loosely woven fabric, commonly cotton, which is sewn to the insulating cover. The fabric is porous and will admit any liquid into the felt or asbestos paper. Tap water is ordinarily used in the clinic as the electrical conducting link between the metal plate and the patient. When this kind of electrode is dry, the electrical circuit cannot be completed. If the felt is not thoroughly soaked, current may be concentrated in a small area since current always follows the path of least resistance. The purpose of the electrode is to spread or diffuse the current delivered by the lead cord. For patient comfort, the current should be diffused uniformly throughout the electrode. Soaking in warm (37° to 40°C) water will always add to patient comfort.

Since the same electrode will be used on many patients (unless the patient is known to have a communicable disease which could be transferred by the electrode), most therapists prefer to insert a disposable cover between the electrode patient surface and the skin. Any soft, absorbent paper toweling is the most readily available and cheapest disposable cover. It should be cut to fit the patient surface of the electrode rather than left with a wide margin. Roller bandage gauze or a thin layer of cotton can also be used. The disposable cover must also be thoroughly wet, or there can be conduction problems.

The above described electrodes are available in many sizes, ranging from about 5 × 5 cm to about 20 × 25 cm. The smaller the electrode, the greater the stimulus for any given intensity. When selecting one large and one small electrode, the smaller will be the active electrode and the larger will be the inactive or dispersive electrode.

Some therapists prefer using bare metal electrodes with a layer of electrode paste or jelly placed between the electrode and skin. Lead cords are then attached with alligator clips to a turned-up corner of the metal plate.

Electrodes need to be securely fixed to the skin to assure uniformity of contact. Body weight, of either trunk or extremity, is frequently used to insure good uniform contact. Elastic bandages or sandbags are also adequate.

When stimulating a single muscle, a different type of electrode may be useful. The contact surface is much smaller, ranging from 1 to 3 cm in diameter. This is always the active electrode, and it is commonly referred to as the tap-key stimulator or diagnostic handle. It is always held in place by the therapist's hand and so can be readily moved from one muscle to another within a treatment period.   The usual design includes a flat spring attached to an insulated handle the size of a pencil, adjusted so that when no pressure is applied to the spring, the circuit is open and no current can flow.   Thumb or finger pressure will close the contact and complete the circuit.   Some tap-key electrodes are designed so that they may be used as above, or if the lead cord is attached at a different terminal, the circuit is made upon contact of the patient surface with skin and the circuit is broken when the electrode is lifted away.   When the electrode offers this choice one needs to be aware of which terminal is attached to the lead cord.   In both cases, the patient surface contact consists of a small metal disc covered with $\frac{1}{2}$ to 1 cm of felt and then the usual thin layer of fabric.   The therapist should add a disposable cover for use with each patient.   A small piece of roller bandage gauze is adequate and easily held in place with a rubber band.   The tap-key electrode does not require prolonged soaking in water.   Five minutes is adequate, but because the volume of felt is small, it needs to be rewet every few minutes during a treatment session.

MONOPOLAR VERSUS BIPOLAR STIMULATION

The term *monopolar stimulation* indicates that only one electrode is placed on or near a muscle mass which is to be stimulated. The other electrode is remote from that area and should be placed on the skin overlying any muscle which is not an antagonist to the muscle to be stimulated.   When electrodes are far apart, a relatively small amount of energy reaches the intervening motor nerves.   The smaller the amount of current per unit volume of tissue, the more comfortable the patient will be, and, as long as the desired contractile response is obtained, this approach constitutes the most effective treatment.   The monopolar technic can be used in individual muscle stimulation (IMS) problems if degeneration is not severe, but frequently IMS problems will require a bipolar technic.

On occasion, bipolar technics are also necessary in CNS and vascular problems.   Once in a while, one of the effects of a CNS lesion will be to cause impairment of peripheral motor nerve's ability to propagate impulses.   An example would be a lesion in the spinal cord resulting in continuing edema formation in the cord. Pressure from the edema in the ventral horn area of the cord could give rise to dysfunction of the motor neurons in the edematous area. A major cause of organic occlusive peripheral vascular impairment is diabetes mellitus of long-standing duration. This can lead to a peripheral neuropathy which can affect both sensory and motor peripheral axons.

In the bipolar technic, one electrode is placed at each end of a muscle or muscle group. When the current is flowing, the concentration of energy is much higher per unit of volume of tissue than is the case when only one electrode overlies the muscle. Consequently, for a given intensity of stimulus, more energy is reaching the muscle that needs to be stimulated. The bipolar technic may be necessary when skin impedance is unusually high, when massive edema is present in the area to be stimulated, and/ or when a majority of the nerve supply to a muscle has been physiologically or anatomically interrupted. Any of these complicating factors may occur in any of the categories of disease that have been discussed, except that of impaired motor nerve conduction, which does not often occur unless there has been a PNS lesion.

The bipolar technic can create a problem of overflow of energy into normally innervated synergistic or antagonistic muscles. The problem is usually solvable by careful replacement of electrodes, by lowering of skin impedance, or by alteration of stimulus parameters. The same adjustments can be used if this problem arises with monopolar stimulation.

TECHNIQUES FOR REDUCING SKIN IMPEDANCE

Patients with central (CNS) or peripheral (PNS) neurological deficits, as well as those with peripheral circulatory or emotional disturbances, are apt to have a significantly higher skin resistance than normal individuals. Washing the area to be stimulated with soap or detergent and then rinsing thoroughly with water is usually adequate to remove skin debris and any excess oil. The washing will very likely cause sufficient hydration of the skin to adequately lower the impedance. If that does not permit the desired response with reasonable comfort, a five– to ten-minute application of a hot pack or an infrared lamp should be helpful. This will increase skin hydration and electrolyte content. When neither of these methods are successful, soaking the electrodes in tea or in a fresh "Sine-Solution"* before use will be highly effective in lowering skin resistance. The tannic acid in tea and the lactic acid in the "Sine-Solution" are very effective at dissolving the waxy coating which may accumulate on the epidermis. However, tea will permanently stain the electrode and may transiently darken the skin. Occasionally, the patient will develop a dermatitis after exposure to the "Sine-Solution." This irritation will disappear within a few days after exposure to lactic acid ceases. The use of continuous modulation DC (−) pole is also effective in dissolving the outermost dead portion of the epidermis but is apt to be painful when used for the necessary three– to five-minute period, even though intensity is kept low enough so that there is no significant motor nerve depolarization.

GROUP VERSUS INDIVIDUAL MUSCLE STIMULATION

Positioning of the inactive or dispersive electrode will vary according to the type and severity of the disorder being treated, as well as in accordance with complicating factors such as scars, cuts, or other skin lesions, and cardiac status. Two general technics of stimulation are in use, namely group muscle stimulation (GMS) and individual muscle stimulation (IMS).

Group Muscle Stimulation

Stimulation of groups of muscles will be most often used with patients with disorders other than peripheral nerve lesions (PNS). In GMS, two or more pad electrodes are used. Choice of size is dependent on the area of application. If the electrodes are of equal size and AC is delivered to the patient, each electrode will be equally stimulating. If the electrodes are of different size, the

---

*"Sine-Solution" consists of 2½ oz. lactic acid in 95% ethanol to make one quart. Enough distilled water is then added to dilute to one gallon. This solution was developed by Frank H. Krusen, M.D., at the Mayo Clinic in 1956. It is not stable and must be made up fresh at least once a month.

smallest will be more stimulating. If DC (but not AC—at $\frac{1}{2}$ to 20 Hz) is used, the $(-)$ electrode will be more stimulating unless the $(-)$ electrode is significantly larger than the $(+)$ electrode.

Since in all lesions other than those involving the motor division of the PNS the axons supplying the muscles are functioning normally, a vast number of muscle fibers within several muscle masses can be adequately stimulated simultaneously with a relatively small concentration of current. Thus, for a CNS lesion, it is possible to apply one electrode to the skin over the posterior midshaft of the humerus and the other to the skin of the middorsal forearm and stimulate the elbow, wrist, and finger extensor muscles simultaneously. In the case of generalized arteriosclerosis, one electrode can be applied to each posterior calf and adequately stimulate ankle plantar flexor muscles bilaterally.

If the patient has any known cardiac pathology, bilateral upper extremity stimulation should be avoided. A small amount of the applied current inevitably will pass through the cardiac muscle or its motor nerve supply. This can be hazardous in any cardiac condition, especially if the patient uses a cardiac pacemaker.

There also may be a slight risk of causing irritation of the coughing reflex with bilateral upper extremity stimulation. The chances of this occurring, in this author's experience, is somewhat greater if DC is used. The reasons for this difference between AC and DC are not known. For the same reasons, it is better to avoid placing one electrode on the anterior and the other on the posterior thorax. Risk from positioning one electrode on the anterior and the other on the posterior abdomen is neglible, except in the case of major unstable cardiac disease.

A useful contractile response would not occur if the dispersive electrode were to be placed on the antagonist of the muscle to be stimulated. Thus, if elbow extension is desired, one electrode should be placed over the extensor muscles and the other on almost any group except the elbow flexors. The dispersive electrode would be much more effective and comfortable on the posterior thorax, lumbar area, or dorsal forearm.

CHRONIC CENTRAL NERVOUS SYSTEM LESIONS

Lesions within the telencephalon, diencephalon, mesencephalon, or spinal cord may give rise to loss of voluntary control over some of the patient's skeletal muscles. In the acute stage of the lesion, the most common clinical picture is a reduction of normal resting muscle tension plus inability to increase tension on attempt to cause joint motion. Clinically, this picture of loss of control is called flaccidity. The flaccidity may persist for days to weeks (moderate lesion) to months (severe lesion). The flaccidity may continue indefinitely. As time goes on, frequently the flaccidity will disappear, being replaced by an abnormal increase in skeletal muscle tension, especially on attempt at motion or in response to external stimuli. Clinically, such an abnormal increase in tension is usually designated as spasticity.

In addition to causing loss of volitional control over skeletal muscle, if the lesion is within the cranial vault it may cause disruption of awareness of body image. The patient may not even be aware that the paralyzed segments are a part of his body, as well as having either an increased or decreased awareness of pain or other normal sensory input. The patient's ability to comprehend written and/or spoken language or his ability to express himself verbally or in writing may be altered.

If the lesion is within the spinal cord, usually the sensation normally present in the trunk or extremities is diminished or absent distal to the level of the lesion. Thus, the sensations of pain, touch, heat or cold, and proprioception are lost. Most commonly, this loss is permanent. More rarely, sensation may be heightened after onset of lesion, especially the sensation of pain.

The pattern of loss of volitional control over skeletal muscle and of altered sensation will vary with the individual patient. Even though a hundred patients may be labeled as hemiplegic (or paraplegic) on the basis of their gross motor deficits, the individual pattern of motor and/or sensory disruption is likely to be demonstrably different. The pattern of deficit within an individual patient will vary in accordance with location and severity of the lesion.

If the lesion is congenital rather than with onset later in life, any and all problems with sensory and/or motor deficits may be compounded because the child has never known normal sensation and has never had a chance to feel what it is like to move his joints in the normal sequence. There is increasing speculation, at least in that category of congenital lesions clinically labeled as the cerebral palsies, that sensory nervous system input, such as proprioception, is misinterpreted rather than not being transmitted supraspinally.[12] The misinterpretation could add to the abnormal motor response to external stimuli.

Nerve and muscle stimulating currents can be used to help the patient gain or regain sensory awareness and to gain or regain volitional control over skeletal muscle, although the NMSC cannot be regarded as a solution to the problem since they will not alter the CNS pathology.

It has been this author's experience that a majority of patients with CNS deficits as described will tolerate application of NMSC better than will patients with PNS lesions or those with no known neurological lesion as a basis for loss of voluntary control over their skeletal muscles. There are at least two reasons for this impression. Patients with CNS lesions will usually require far less intensity of stimulus to their affected muscles as compared to their unaffected muscles in achieving equivalent response, regardless of whether the affected muscle is flaccid or spastic. Presumably, this is because the affected motor neurons have been largely released from normal CNS inhibition and they tend to be hyperactive in response to any stimulus. Also, since the motor nerves are intact, there is only rarely need to use either DC or AC of less than 60 Hz. For reasons detailed earlier in this chapter, AC at a frequency of 1,000 Hz or better is usually more comfortable than either AC or DC of lower frequencies and is entirely adequate to obtain muscle contraction. The major exception is where there is massive chronic edema between the skin and muscle to be stimulated. When this occurs, it will usually be in the distal extremity. Modification of standard stimulation technics to insure adequate localization of stimulus through edema is discussed in the technic section of this chapter.

In both flaccid and spastic states, there may be circulatory impairment in the involved extremities, even in the absence of vascular disease. The impairment is in large part related to the loss of intermittent skeletal muscle contraction. Such contraction is normally a major factor in the return of venous blood to the heart. Daily use of NMSC to cause regular intermittent muscle contraction can be helpful in maintaining more nearly normal circulation in the extremities, especially in the presence of flaccidity and while the patient is confined to bed. The benefit of such treatment can be objectively monitored by regular digital skin temperature recording.

Many patients who have suffered upper motor neuron lesions resulting in paralysis will undergo an eventual shift from flaccidity towards spasticity. A factor in this shift may be the resorption of the cranial and/or spinal cord edema that accompanies the acute phase of many CNS lesions. When large numbers of neuron cell bodies and their processes are subjected to an abnormal increase in intra- or extracellular pressure, the affected nerves can no longer function. As the excess fluid is gradually resorbed, the nerve may return to erratic or to normal function, depending upon the degree of residual damage. When upper motor neurons are not functioning, the clinical picture is flaccidity. If large numbers of these neurons suffer residual damage and/or chronic impairment of function but have regained some capability to function, the clinical picture may be that of spasticity.

Many CNS lesions are vascular in origin. Some common vascular lesions are a plug of a blood vessel because of a thrombus or an embolus or a hemorrhage out of a vessel at a weak point in the vessel wall at a time when the blood pressure is transiently high. Any of these lesions will cause edema, which may take weeks to months to be resorbed. If the pressure on the neuron cell body or its processes is great, metabolism may be impaired and the cell dies. If the volume of edema is not too great, cells in the periphery of the edematous area may gradually return to some level of function. Neurons so affected tend to become hyperirritable. The clinical result, when areas affecting motor divisions of the CNS are involved, is inappropriate reaction to a given stimulus. This phenomenon is often described clinically as release from normal CNS inhibition. There is often an inappropriate skeletal muscle response to voluntary attempts at change in muscle tension. Vascular lesions within the cranial vault commonly affect the motor areas of the brain and give rise to that collection of symptoms clinically labeled as hemiplegia. Frequently, on one side, the facial muscles will be paralyzed. On the other, some of the muscles of the trunk, arm, and leg will suffer equal or greater loss of voluntary control.

In addition to the problem of circulatory stagnation, loss of ability to move joints at will can rapidly lead to muscle shortening, which can become permanent and lead to contracture formation. This can evolve into soft tissue and eventually bony ankylosis, in extreme cases. Rapidity of onset and the severity of these common sequelae to the loss of voluntary control over joint motion can be minimized by regular use of passive motion and regular use of NMSC to cause intermittent muscle contraction and relaxation. Appropriate application of NMSC can be useful when one muscle group, i.e. knee flexors, becomes hyperactive in response to any stimulus while its antagonist (knee extensors) has lost its ability to respond to normal stimulus. Such imbalance in response can lead to contracture formation. Careful application of NMSC to the antagonistic muscle group (knee extensors) can do much to prevent contracture formation and/or ankylosis.[13-16]

Stimulus parameters and other details are critical for successful application of NMSC to patients with either acquired or congenital lesions within the CNS. Many therapists are reluctant to take the time required for effective utilization of these procedures. In the author's opinion, it is usually time well spent with properly selected patients.

GROUP MUSCLE STIMULATION FOR THE PATIENT WITH HEMIPLEGIA

In the acute and subacute phases of cerebral vascular insults, even though the patient may be conscious, he frequently is not aware that the involved arm and leg are part of his body. This lack of awareness may be retained for weeks to months after his vital signs are stable. If the patient is not aware that these limbs are a part of his body, it is difficult to encourage him to try to use them. Appropriate use of nerve and muscle stimulating currents can be useful in helping the patient regain this awareness. Such treatment is best started as soon as the vital signs are stable and should be discontinued as soon as the patient exhibits ability to assist the stimulating current in tension development on command.

It must be recognized that if the patient is not verbally encouraged to work along with the intermittently stimulating current and perceive that the current is causing contraction which the patient could not voluntarily induce, he will often develop the attitude that the current alone will restore control of joint motion. After the therapist is satisfied that the patient is aware that the intermittent current flow is causing alternate muscle contraction and relaxation, he should ask the patient to try to help perform the movement when the current comes on. Palpation by the therapist will tell whether there is an increase in tension development with the patient's attempts at assistance. If not, the NMSC should be used passively a few more days, and then another attempt should be made for patient assistance. As soon as the patient can assist in tension development, the intensity of the electrical stimulus should be decreased. Once the patient can assist the use of NMSC for that muscle group, treatment with NMSC in that area can usually be discontinued within a week or two. If the patient cannot comprehend instruction, then the NMSC utilization must be entirely passive. However, within any time period, NMSC will be capable of causing a greater number of intermittent contractions and relaxations than any therapeutic exercise technic, with the net result of better maintenance of muscle elasticity, with minimal energy expenditure on the part of the therapist.

When attempting to stimulate *extensors* in the presence of either spastic or flaccid flexors, the patient with a stroke commonly will have a flexion reaction first, especially when stimulus is at low intensity. If the surge or interrupted current modulation is at a sufficiently low rate, the flexion reaction will be followed by contraction of the extensor group. As *intensity* is increased, the flexion reaction will diminish and the extensor response increase. A modulation rate of five to fifteen surges per minute will usually be effective in management of this problem. Although there has been much speculation as to why attempts at extension often lead to flexion, with and without application of NMSC, the reasons for this reaction in the stroke patient are not known. Perhaps it is because nerves supplying flexor musculature respond faster, or the flexor muscles themselves have the capacity for faster response to equal stimulus, or because the ratio of flexor nerves (gamma as well as alpha) to flexor muscles is different from that of extensor nerves to extensor muscles. Although not entirely comparable because of difference in type of stimulus, Bishop's recent discussions of vibratory stimulation[17] amply point up the complexity of the neurophysiology involved in stimulus through the skin.

The first response to NMSC applied to extensors or abductors is likely to be flexion or adduction, respectively, in the patient with a CNS lesion. However, if the modulation rate is low and the intensity is high enough, the unwanted response will be over-ridden by the slower-appearing desired response. The dual response usually disappears within a few treatments, leaving only the desired response.

Increase in intensity must be slow when using NMSC on patients with spasticity. Otherwise, a massive, whole-body flexor-adductor response is likely to occur with the first few surges of current, regardless of location of electrodes.

Consider a chronic severely involved hemiplegic patient, one who has deltoid atrophy leading to subluxation, loss of both active and passive range in shoulder flexion and abduction, spasticity in elbow flexors with elbow flexion contracture, marked forearm pronation, wrist and finger flexor contracture with spasticity, and wrist ulnar deviation. The hand and fingers are edematous. How can NMSC be best utilized? The starting point should be with the proximal muscle groups. Something must be done to minimize the shoulder muscle atrophy and pain or the patient will not make any attempt to use his shoulder.

Until such time as the patient regains capability of voluntary deltoid contraction, an effective physical therapy approach is application of one small pad electrode to the posterior and another to the anterior deltoid, followed by stimulation with a high frequency (1000 Hz or higher) slowly surging AC for five to ten minutes several times daily. This can be done safely with the patient supine or semireclining. This treatment will cause far more intermittent muscle contraction and relaxation of the entire deltoid than any amount or type of therapeutic exercise that can be given manually in an equal time span. The therapist should not forget to instruct the patient, as soon as he can comprehend such instruction, to attempt to try to aid contraction when he feels the current come on; stimulus intensity should be decreased as soon as he can voluntarily increase contraction on command. As soon as active motion toward shoulder flexion and abduction is possible, the electrical stimulation can be discontinued. The therapist should not expect significant return of deltoid bulk. This will rarely occur. Return of a functional degree of strength is considerably more important as well as more common.

Similar treatment may be applied to the elbow and wrist extensors, with either a monopolar or bipolar technic, depending upon how responsive the extensors are to electrical stimulus. Usually, this can be done during the same treatment period in which the deltoid is stimulated, but not simultaneously. When the monopolar technic can be used, one electrode should be positioned over the midposterior humerus, the other on the middorsal forearm.

If this sort of treatment accomplishes nothing else, it minimizes the circulatory stasis that is so common in long-standing flaccidity or spasticity. The reduction of circulatory stasis will be due to the induced intermittent contraction and relaxation of paralyzed skeletal muscle.

The wrist and fingers are commonly more severely involved than the more proximal musculature, so that with initial treatment, the bipolar technic is often mandatory. One electrode should be placed on the proximal dorsal forearm and the other on the distal dorsal forearm. This can be conveniently done with the patient supine or sitting. When sitting, it is easier to have the forearm supported in pronation with the elbow and wrist in comfortable flexion, and frequently it is easier for the patient to see as well as feel what is happening when the current flows. If overflow to antagonists is a problem which has not responded to variation in current parameters or to previously discussed methods for reduction of skin impedance, then smaller electrodes can be used. Sometimes it is necessary to use two tap-key electrodes, connected for automatic rather than manual make and break of the patient circuit. The tap-key electrodes are held in place by hand rather than with bandages. Use of two tap-key electrodes is especially valuable when grossly visible edema is present. The smaller the electrode, the greater the concentration of current immediately deep to the electrode. The high electrolyte content and volume of gross edema tends to diffuse or dilute the current.

Similar procedures can be used throughout the lower extremities. Such treatment can be very effective in helping the patient regain awareness of sensation generated by intermittent contraction in hip and knee extensors. Again, as soon as the patient can comprehend instruction to attempt to assist contraction, he should be asked to do so. As soon as he can significantly increase tension on command, the electrical stimulus intensity can be decreased and then discontinued.

Since ankle dorsiflexor muscles are small and weak in comparison with plantar flexor bulk and strength, bipolar stimulation is almost mandatory. As soon as the patient can walk with any degree of safety, if ankle dorsiflexion during the swing phase of his step is a problem, a battery-powered patient foot switch device can be used.[2,3] There appears to be reasonable carryover after training with such devices. Evidence is accumulating that male patients benefit more than female from use of such devices.[18,19] Reasons for this are not known at this time.

It cannot be stressed too strongly that use of NMSC in hemiplegic lesions will not restore function to normal. The same can be said for any other procedure the physical therapist may use. However, when used as outlined above, it can be very useful in increasing rate of return to whatever level of function the residual deficit will permit. Active patient cooperation in assisting intermittent muscle contraction and relaxation is essential. Without it, it is all too easy for the patient to sit back and believe the magic black box is going to "cure" him.

SPINAL CORD LESIONS

Similar technics can be used for the para– and quadriplegic patient. In traumatic lesions resulting in such paralyses, there is usually less expectation of partial return of function as compared with the hemiplegic patient. Benefits will be largely in minimizing circulatory inadequacy, slowing onset of contractures, and possibly in decreasing rate of onset of osteoporosis. Once the patient is able to stand or walk, by whatever means, the intermittent spasticity usually produced by these activities will probably do as much to minimize the common sequelae as would regular use of NMSC. However, if the patient must be confined to bed because of intercurrent disease or other malfunction, regular use of NMSC is indicated, as outlined for the hemiplegic patient, until the cord lesion patient can be mobile again. The setback in rehabilitation progress will be minimized by such treatment. Treatment can be easily done in the patient's room.

CHRONIC PERIPHERAL NERVOUS SYSTEM LESIONS

Peripheral nervous system (PNS) lesions may involve sensory, motor, or autonomic nerves or any combination of these three functional types of nerves. The patient most likely to be seen by the physical therapist will be the one who has some motor deficit. This may be a result of trauma or a disease process within the anterior (ventral) horn area of the spinal cord or anywhere peripherally, including malfunction of the myoneural junction. The chronic stage of any peripheral motor deficit invariably results in muscle flaccidity because of loss of ability of the motor nerve to conduct the stimulus needed to generate the muscle action potential.

Peripheral nerves, unlike those within the central nervous system, do have a capacity for regeneration. Where the sheath of Schwann remains intact, the prognosis for regeneration is good, but by no means does regeneration always occur, and it will never occur if the cell body (the anterior horn cell) has been killed by the lesion. If the sheath of Schwann has been damaged, the likelihood of regeneration is much less, but chances of regeneration are improved with appropriate surgical repair.

The usual sequelae of skeletal muscle flaccidity, namely circulatory stasis, edema, muscle shortening, contracture formation, fibrous ankylosis, and bony ankylosis, can and do occur. This is especially likely if most of the nerve supply to a major muscle mass controlling a joint motion is lost while the motor nerve supply to its principal antagonist remains intact and functional.

The physical therapy procedures available, including the use of NMSC, do nothing to alter the nerve lesion per se, but hopefully, adequate use of NMSC will help to maintain denervated muscle elasticity—the capability to contract and relax. Intermittent muscle contraction and relaxation will help to minimize circulatory stasis, thus maintaining better nutrition and more adequate removal of waste products while waiting to see how much, if any, regeneration is going to take place. If regeneration is to occur, it will be no faster than at the rate of one millimeter per day. If an axon has been anatomically severed at the level of the midshaft of the humerus and was supplying an intrinsic muscle of the hand, for an average size adult this would mean that the distal axon must grow more than 450 mm. Functional regeneration over distances such as this do occur, with subsequent return to useful function of the denervated muscle,[20] but it may take two to three years. If all other factors are equal, the shorter the distance between site of start of degeneration and the point of the myoneural junction, the better the chances for regeneration.

In considering a muscle mass, i.e. biceps brachii, which is denervated, if enough of its motor nerve axons do not regenerate, eventually the denervated muscle fibers will atrophy. These muscle fibers may be infiltrated by noncontractile components such as fibrous connective tissue. Such deterioration of the muscle fibers usually does not take place until eighteen months to two years after denervation. When such deterioration has taken place, there can be no contractile response to any kind of stimulus. Use of NMSC will not prevent this process from occurring but can delay the rate at which it occurs.

The person who has suffered a peripheral motor nerve lesion but whose peripheral sensory nervous system has not been impaired will as a general rule have more acute sensation of any externally supplied electrical stimulus than either the individual whose entire nervous system is intact or the patient who has suffered both sensory and motor nerve malfunction. The classical example is the patient with anterior poliomyelitis, which is a disease process which involves anterior horn (motor nerve cell bodies) but not the dorsal ganglia (sensory nerve cell bodies) or dorsal horn cell bodies. Fortunately, this formerly common epidemic disease is rarely seen in this country now, subsequent to wide utilization of appropriate vaccines. For patients with an intact sensory nervous system but with a nonfunctioning or partially functioning motor nervous system, it is difficult to provide adequate electrical stimulation to cause denervated muscle contraction using intensities that the patient can tolerate.

Stimulation of denervated muscle requires a longer duration current flow in one direction to generate a muscle action potential.[10,20] One of the skin's reactions to this longer duration flow appears to be accumulation of abnormal and painfully irritating substances on or within the skin. The differences in skin reaction to DC as compared to AC are discussed in this chapter's section on current type.

Depending upon the number of axons involved, a PNS lesion may affect some or all muscle fibers within a muscle mass, or some fibers in each of several muscles. If more than one muscle is affected, it is more likely than not that they will be affected in varying degrees. For these reasons, in PNS lesions, individual muscle stimulation is indicated far more often than is group muscle stimulation. The standard procedure in IMS is to use one large (5 × 5 cm or bigger) dispersive pad electrode plus a tap-key electrode for stimulation of only one muscle or segment of that muscle. When the monopolar technic will produce the desired contractile response, there is less chance of an overflow problem than if the bipolar technic must be used. If the bipolar procedure is necessary, it is usually, but not always, more effective when the stimulating electrode can be distal to the dispersive electrode. If AC can produce the desired response, even if its frequency must be lower than 20 Hz, there is less risk of skin damage than when DC must be used.

When DC must be used, Erb's Polar Formula should be kept in mind. This formula states that in the normal individual, a cathode closing contraction (CCC) will be more stimulating than an anode closing contraction (ACC). Next in order of stimulus strength will be an anode opening contraction (AOC), and finally, a cathode opening contraction (COC) may produce the desired muscle contraction.[20] In the individual with a PNS lesion, anodal stimulation may give a response at a much lower intensity. With rare exception, contraction on opening the circuit requires far more intensity (five to ten times as much) so that neither COC or AOC will cause muscle contraction with a clinically tolerable intensity. An ACC will be more effective than a CCC only when degeneration of the axon has resulted in reversal of charge separation such that the outside of the membrane has an excess of negatively charged ions relative to the ionic charge on the inside of the membrane.

Care must be taken to avoid fatigue when using IMS technics. A muscle with deficit in its nerve supply will tire far more easily than a muscle with a normal nerve supply. The net result may be that for a few stimuli there may be a good contractile response, but then the response weakens, even though the intensity is gradually increased. As intensity rises, nearby synergistic or antagonistic muscle may start to contract. If stimulation is continued to a fatiguing muscle, there is some evidence that nerve regeneration may be delayed or arrested.[21,22] Clinical literature on poliomyelitis in the 1940s and early 1950s stressed that any kind of stimulus evoking a contractile response and repeated too often could cause a recovering axon to fail permanently. Laboratory experiments on denervated rat muscle[23] indicate that the hazard of regeneration retardation is minimized if the denervated muscle is stimulated with short bouts (five to ten contractile responses) of stimulation four or five times each day rather than providing twenty to one hundred stimuli within a single twenty-minute period. In the presence of a PNS lesion, if stimulation is to be beneficial treatment should be given *at least* once a day until signs of fatigue appear.[20] It is better to give the stimulation twice a day if possible. The need for short but frequent sessions of electrical stimulation is critical and may explain the poor results obtained when stimulation is given only two or three times per week.

Motor Points

When IMS is indicated, the therapist must be able to locate one or more motor points over the muscle to be stimulated. A motor point may be defined as that area on the skin which overlies a point where many single terminal nerve branches connect to the muscle fibers they supply. Most skeletal muscles are ovoid in mass, and the greater number of muscle fibers are at the center rather than at either end of the mass. Hence, the primary motor point will be on the skin overlying the greatest bulk of that muscle. Since some muscles are deep to others, it is fortunate that all muscles have secondary motor points. Thus, it is easy to find motor points of muscles like the biceps brachii or the gastrocnemius, since they are superficial, but much harder to find motor points for the brachialis or soleus, which lie deep. A motor point can be identified because far less intensity is required to elicit an equivalent response at that point than anywhere else on the skin over that muscle mass. This is because a greater number of axons supplying a single muscle mass are collected in a small volume of tissue. Appendix A at the end of this chapter gives the location and result of stimulation of motor points throughout the body. Location of these points will become very easy for the therapist who works with patients with PNS lesions on a regular basis.

In general, motor point stimulation is more comfortable in muscles that are remote from bone. Stimulation of shoulder or hip musculature is not as disagreeable as stimulation of intrinsic hand or foot muscles, or most of all, the facial muscles. At least part of the reason for this difference is that when muscle lies close to bone an appreciable amount of energy reaches the sensory receptors in the underlying periosteum, as well as the cutaneous receptors. The more the sensory stimulation, the greater the discomfort.

Obesity and Hirsute Skin

The more obese or hirsute the subject (insofar as location of electrodes is concerned), the more uncomfortable is any electrical stimulation. The more obese the individual, the thicker the sub-cutaneous fat layer. Hydrated skin is a good conductor of electricity since there are many openings on the surface—hair follicles, sweat glands, etc.—all of which have a high electrolyte content and thus easily transmit electrical energy through the skin. Sub-cutaneous fat is a poor conductor. It has a low water content as well as a poor blood and lymph supply, and hence a low electrolyte content. Since NMSC penetrate fatty layers largely via the blood vessel and lymph channels, the thicker the fat layer, the more trouble the electrical energy has in reaching the motor axons. Therefore, the more subcutaneous fat overlying the muscle to be stimulated, the higher the intensity needed. The normal overlying fat layer is a major reason why it can be difficult to find motor points of muscles such as the gluteus maximus or gluteus medius.

Hair follicles transmit NMSC readily because of their high electrolyte content. If the hair is dense and stiff, however, it is difficult to insure uniform contact of the patient surface of the electrode with the skin. This can lead to concentration of the current in an irregular manner and cause the stimulation to be more painful than it need be. If feasible, the easiest solution is to place the electrodes in areas where hair is sparse. If this is not possible, shaving the area may be necessary. An electric razor is preferable since even the slightest nick or cut in the skin will lower the skin resistance dramatically, leading to undesirable irregular current concentration.

Scar Tissue

It is not wise to place electrodes on either old or new scar tissue. Old scars (in Caucasians, more pale than surrounding skin) have a poor blood supply. They have no openings into subcutaneous tissue and a very high resistance to current flow since electrolyte concentration is low. All of the above is equally true for old acne scars. On the other hand, new scar tissue and active acne or other eruptive skin lesions usually have an excellent blood supply. In the case of new scars, exposure to significant quantities of NMSC, especially DC, can arrest completion of wound repair. In all cases where there has been eruptive skin damage, current concentration is apt to be irregular and consequently more painful than it would be if it is feasible to apply electrodes elsewhere.

There are also skin lesions wherein, even though the skin may appear completely normal in the area where one wishes to place an electrode, the skin impedance will remain continuously high.[24] The patient with psoriasis is a prime example.

CHRONIC ORGANIC OCCLUSIVE PERIPHERAL VASCULAR DISEASES

As more and more of the population is living well beyond retirement age, more and more people are faced with the pain and other handicaps which are a direct result of increasingly impaired circulation. While the various chronic organic occlusive peripheral vascular diseases are usually systemic rather than local in effect, the fact that blood has a longer way to go to return from the lower extremities to the heart than from elsewhere in the body means that circulatory insufficiency is apt to be more of a problem in the legs than in the arms, even though the effects of equivalent impairment in cerebral or coronary vessels may be more life threatening. The major reason why the chronic vascular diseases are more severe in the lower extremities is the stronger effect of gravity on the return of blood to the heart. More work must be done both by venous valves and skeletal muscle. The weight of the much longer column of blood on the valves frequently leads to a need for additional intermittent skeletal muscle contraction and relaxation, especially by the calf musculature. If there is arterial insufficiency due to intimal deposition and consequent decrease in lumen size, there is apt to be an instinctive decrease in ambulation. The net result is often a marked venous stasis. Clinically, valvular venous incompetency is frequently seen as a factor in varicose veins.

In all of the organic occlusive vascular diseases, there is a gradual deposition of minerals (chiefly calcium salts) or lipid complexes on the inside lining of the walls of arterial vessels. There may or may not be significant mural irritation and thrombus formation. As the deposits accumulate over the years, the lumen of the arterial vessels gradually decrease in diameter. This increases resistance to blood flow. At first, the vasoregulatory system compensates for this increased resistance by raising the blood pressure, thus insuring adequate circulation. In time, this may lead to other problems, such as cardiac enlargement or vascular aneurysm formation. All of these and many more vascular changes make treatment more complex as the pathology progresses. This is especially true since the early and potentially reversible changes are relatively pain free. By the time the pain is persistent and severe enough for the subject to seek medical attention, the impairment is often quite severe and largely irreversible. Two very useful books detailing these problems are the volumes by Shepard[25] and Abramson.[26]

When the patient cannot or will not engage in enough ambulatory activity to make enough intermittent use of calf musculature to keep the circulatory insufficiency within tolerable limits, regular use of NMSC can be a useful adjunct in overall management of the patient. A major reason why NMSC can be useful in chronic circulatory impairment is that intermittent skeletal muscle contraction with the patient prone puts less demand on circulation than does ambulation but more demand than if the patient is confined at rest in a bed or wheelchair. It is generally accepted that when a patient with a chronic occlusive peripheral vascular disease must be confined, the rate of increase in circulatory stasis goes up sharply. As the degree of diminution of blood flow goes up, the risk of thrombus formation increases. Wakim[27] and Martella[28] were among the first to demonstrate that regular use of NMSC can be helpful in combatting this kind of circulatory inadequacy.

Just as is the case when using NMSC in the presence of central or peripheral nervous system deficits, here again the physical agent does not get at the cause of the disorder, but it can help to delay or arrest further damage. If it can delay or arrest the progression of circulatory impairment so that amputation does not become necessary, the time and effort involved in the procedure is certainly worthwhile. There are other physical therapy procedures which can and should be used concurrently with treatment by NMSC, but they are not within the scope of this book.

In most cases of chronic arteriosclerosis or atherosclerotic peripheral vascular disease, the simplest use of NMSC is to position the patient prone (or supine with the lower extremities elevated 10 to 20 degrees with pillows) and apply one electrode to each posterior midcalf. Surging AC of 60 Hz or higher frequency will produce adequate intermittent tetanic contraction and relaxation of the ankle plantar flexors. Ideally, the treatment would be given twice daily, for twenty to thirty minutes each time. The modulation rate would be adjusted so that there would be five to ten contractions per minute. Digital skin temperature measurement before and after treatment and/or weekly checking of distance which can be walked before onset of intermittent claudication will provide an objective record of effectiveness of treatment.

If the patient has chronic diabetes mellitus, with a resultant peripheral neuropathy, a bipolar technic may be necessary. In this case, each calf should have two electrodes applied, one proximal and the other distal. If the neuropathy is far advanced, it may be necessary to use an interrupted modulation DC, but the skin should be carefully inspected before and after each treatment because of the greater risk of skin damage with DC as well as the fact that the neuropathy may involve sensory as well as motor nerves. If there is a marked difference in severity of involvement in the two extremities, it may be necessary to treat them separately because of the difference in current intensity and other electrical parameters necessary to elicit the desired response. However, if the intermittent contraction and relaxation is approximately equal in the two extremities, they can be treated simultaneously. Many models of NMSC have provision for simultaneous use of two or more circuits.

If this type of treatment is effective for a given patient, it will produce a transient rise in toe skin temperature on the order of 5° to 10°C as well as an increase in pain-free walking distance of better than 10 percent within three weeks of daily use. If such results have not occurred within a three– to four-week period, there is little reason to continue this type of treatment.

PSYCHOSOMATIC DISORDERS

Patients who suffer from apparent skeletal muscle weakness or from other loss of volitional control despite apparently intact nervous and circulatory systems may benefit from NMSC. The procedure may help the neurologist or psychiatrist decide whether there is neurological damage or whether the apparent paralysis is the result of extreme emotional conflict. If the loss of voluntary control is entirely related to a nonneurological crisis, the quantity of energy required to induce a contractile response is likely to be significantly greater as compared to that needed for response in the patient's contralateral uninvolved muscles. There are at least two reasons for this. The skin impedance is usually much higher in the apparently paralyzed area, and the circulation, both cutaneous and deep, is apt to be diminished, as compared to the contralateral muscles. Earlier in this chapter, the hyperirritability of motor nerves in patients with central nervous system lesions was pointed out. This rarely occurs in patients whose nervous system is intact. In the patient where emotional conflict has led to loss of control over skeletal muscle, the skin is frequently very dry, and significant vasospasm is likely to be present in the paralyzed area. Hence, the quantity of energy necessary to elicit a contractile response is likely to be higher than it is for uninvolved areas. If the paralysis is actually the result of a peripheral motor nerve deficit, involved muscles would not respond to current flow of short duration in one direction, i.e. 60 Hz or higher AC, but would respond to low frequency AC or to DC. The patient whose apparent paralysis is related to an emotional crisis will always respond to 60 Hz or higher AC. Hence, it is easy to rule out nervous system lesions as the cause of the paralysis.

At the conscious level, the patient may be firmly convinced

that he cannot voluntarily move the affected joint (s). It is frequently helpful to the patient's attempts when he can see and feel the controlling muscle contract.

There is another category of patient who may quite sincerely believe that he can no longer move an apparently paralyzed body segment—the individual who was injured while at work and who stands to be awarded greater compensation for the injury the more severe the permanent damage appears to be. Again, appropriate use of NMSC can go far to demonstrate to all concerned whether the lesion is as damaging as it may appear to be.

Finally, there may be patients with no demonstrable neurological or other lesion who have a low grade chronic pain and muscle spasm which is usually worse on attempts at either active or passive motion. If the more usual procedures of intermittent application of heat or cold in whatever form do not bring lasting relief, frequently a different use of NMSC will help. The gate control theory of pain, discussed in Chapter 1, states that awareness of pain is likely to be diminished when the sensory nervous system is flooded with less painful stimuli. A special form of NMSC can be used to produce such flooding. This can result in palpable relaxation of chronic low grade muscle spasm and can, with a short series of treatments, produce lasting pain relief.

In this situation, the stimulator is not used to produce a contractile response but is used at an intensity that the patient can feel without the intensity being high enough to cause appreciable excitable membrane depolarization. Alternating current at 1000 Hz or higher, *with continuous modulation,* for ten to twenty minutes per treatment seems very effective. Some therapists advocate a more sophisticated technic using two circuits simultaneously, each at a slightly different frequency. Certainly this could increase the counterirritation of the sensory nervous system more than either frequency alone. In the author's experience, this treatment has been useful in chronic low back pain and has worked when other procedures have failed.

There is a simple experiment that will demonstrate reduction of cutaneous sensation by use of high frequency AC with continuous modulation. Run a thumbnail with moderate uniform pressure on the skin over an area about 30 cm in length. Instruct the subject to fix in his mind the sensation produced. Then place two pad electrodes, 5 × 5 cm or a little larger, 15 to 20 cm apart, in the area subjected to the thumbnail test. Apply AC at a frequency of 60 Hz or higher, continuous modulation, to the level where the patient reports feeling muscles tighten, then lower the intensity until the subject says he does not feel tension, and let the current flow for ten minutes. Immediately after removal of the electrodes, repeat the thumbnail test, striving to insure the same pressure and rate of movement, to the same area as before. The chances are excellent that the subject will report considerable decrease in sensation. The decrease will be most marked under the area of each electrode but still significant in the area between electrodes. A retest one-half hour later will usually indicate residual decrease in sensation.

ION TRANSFER

Ion transfer is a technic which utilizes NMSC with continuous modulation DC only, where the objective is to drive topically applied medication into the epidermis for slow release (hours to days) or, in the case of selected medication, into systemic circulation. Ion transfer has also been variously called iontophoresis, electro-osmosis, electrophoresis, and dielectrolysis. Use of this technic has been largely abandoned in this country because of major hazards, controversy of efficacy, and improved management of many of the lesions for which it was previously prescribed.[20]

The medication to be introduced is topically applied. It may be in liquid or ointment form. No advantage is gained through medication strength greater than 1% or 2%.[20,29-31] In the late 1920s, it was demonstrated that inorganic ions rarely penetrate deep to the epidermis. This is in large part due to the difference in rate of mobility of ions upon exposure to DC. The H^+ ion is the lightest in weight and hence moves the fastest, about twice as fast as $(OH)^-$ and approximately five times faster than K^+, Cl^- and Cu^{++}.[29] Since hydrogen, in one form or another, is normally occurring and in plentiful supply in the human body, excitation into H^+ utilizes much of the DC which passes through the epidermis, leaving relatively little energy to mobilize the heavier atoms. When compounds such as KI, NaCl, $ZnCl_2$, or Cu_2SO_4 are used, their major effect is to liquify (I^-, Cl^-) or to dehydrate (Zn^{++}, Cu^{++}) the skin.

Organic compounds react differently when ionized by DC and do penetrate rapidly into systemic circulation.[30,32] However, careful preparation of the medication, with particular attention to pH, is essential. Then, primary penetration through intact skin and to a depth of 1 cm is possible.[30-33]

For both inorganic and organic compounds, the manner in which the specific compound ionizes must be known, as well as whether the effective ingredient will be repelled from the positive or the negative pole. If a medication can be ionized by DC, one or more of the component atoms will be dissociated from the others. Some will become deficient in electrons (H^+, K^+, Zn^{++}, Ca^{++} and thus are driven into the skin from the positive pole. Other ions will acquire an excess of electrons [Cl^-, I^-, $(SO_4)^{--}$] and hence are driven in from the negative pole. When the component atoms are dissociated by exposure to DC, the primary reaction is the formation of chemical active atoms; second, there will be chemical recombination of these atoms with electrolytes within the living tissue through which they are being driven (and with the electrode metal); third there will be a reaction of the living tissue to the newly formed chemicals.[29] All of the above reactions will almost always be rapidly attenuated as soon as the driving force is removed.

Electrodes to be used for ion transfer should be separated from those used to cause a contractile response. Some of the inorganic compounds used, i.e. NaCl, will be corrosive to the conducting metal plate. Other compounds will tend to dissolve the felt and/ or fabric which normally intervenes between the skin and the metal. Furthermore, it is difficult to rinse out traces of medication from pad electrodes. Thus, if later used for muscle stimulation, an ion transfer treatment may be inadvertently done simultaneously. For these reasons, when medication is in liquid form, many therapists use bare metal electrodes, with care being taken to avoid direct contact with the skin or mucosal surface undergoing treatment.

If the electrodes are of equal size, current density will be equal under each. If they are of different sizes, current density will always be greater under the smaller electrode. If one wishes to treat a large area, or one of irregular contour, i.e. distal forearm, wrist, and hand, an immersion technic is convenient. The contralateral body segment can function as the dispersive area. With an immersion technic, the active and the dispersive electrode should *not* be placed in the same bath. More than 99 percent of the current would then flow through the conducting medication and bypass penetration into the body, thus serving no useful purpose.[15] With the immersion technic, care should also be taken to avoid direct electrode-skin contact.

When treatment is by ion transfer, a major hazard is burn of the exposed tissue. This is due to the use of continuous modulation DC, not the medication. Normal skin will not tolerate an intensity higher than 1 ma/cm^2 of skin surface exposed to this form of DC.[20,29] If the current is applied to scar tissue or to an area where the skin is abraded or lacerated, the risk of damage is great since impedance is dramatically lower in such areas. Because of the numbing effect of continuous modulation DC (flooding of the cutaneous receptors), neither the therapist nor the patient may be aware of skin damage until the electrodes are removed.

For all of these reasons, it is recommended that the current density used never exceed 1 ma/cm^2 and that the initial treatment duration not exceed ten minutes. The standard treatment is ten to twenty minutes. Hyperemia is to be expected as skin reaction (capillary dilation) to DC, both poles, irrespective of the medication used.[20]

At this time, at least insofar as complex organic compounds are concerned, when introduction of medication by topical application is indicated, the technic of phonophoresis would appear simpler as compared to iontophoresis.[34] This technic is discussed in Chapter 7.

CONTRAINDICATIONS OF USE OF NERVE AND MUSCLE STIMULATING CURRENTS

There are three major contraindications for the use of stimulating currents. The most important is the patient with significant unstable cardiac pathology, especially if the lesion requires use of a pacemaker. Most of the externally applied energy will flow from electrode to electrode in the patient circuit, but inevitably some of the energy will reach the cardiac motor nerve supply, the cardiac muscle, and/or the pacemaker leads. This can interfere with normal function of the pacemaker and hence cause cardiac arrest. Even if the patient is not wearing a pacemaker, if he has an uncontrolled arrhythmia, the stimulus could cause further irregularity in heartbeat. Obviously, the risks would be greater if one or both electrodes were applied anywhere on the thorax, or one on each upper extremity, but it is recommended that nerve and muscle stimulating currents not be used anywhere on the body if there is significant cardiac pathology. Patient selection is the responsibility of the referring physician.

It is also important to realize that if there is clinical evidence of phlebothrombosis or thrombophlebitis, stimulating currents should not be applied adjacent to or distal to the area of mural irritation. There is a definite risk of the induced skeletal muscle intermittent contraction and relaxation causing a fragment of a thrombus to be converted into an embolus. Phlebothrombosis and thrombophlebitis are far more common in the lower extremities than elsewhere in the body.

Lastly, electrodes should not be applied in an area of abnormal skin. The skin impedance may be abnormally high (psoriasis) or low (abrasion or laceration). If impedance is high, high intensity must be used, increasing the risk of skin damage, especially with DC. If impedance is low, this will raise current concentration in a small volume of tissue and can lead to burn, especially with DC.

SUMMARY

Use of nerve and muscle stimulating currents (NMSC) should be considered whenever dealing with disease or injury which results in partial or complete loss of voluntary control over skeletal muscle contraction. This is true whether the loss of control has lead to pain, flaccidity, or spasticity, and whether the primary lesion is a chronic central or peripheral nervous system lesion, a chronic peripheral vascular disease, or a psychosomatic problem.

Almost always, NMSC should be used prior to or in conjunction with attempts at utilizing some form of therapeutic exercise. Rationale and techniques are given in some detail.

The major contraindications for use of NMSC are the presence of cardiac pacemakers or an active phlebitis or thrombophlebosis at or proximal to the area to be stimulated.

Improvement in equipment over the years now makes it possible to use alternating current of less than 60 Hz frequency in many cases where formerly DC had to be used. Advantages of AC over DC are discussed at some length. Known reasons for the greater likelihood of skin damage and of patient discomfort upon exposure to DC are examined.

APPENDIX A

EASILY LOCATED MOTOR POINTS – THEIR APPROXIMATE LOCATION AND RESPONSE TO STIMULUS

A. Neck and Trunk

Muscle	Location	Action
1. Sternocleidomastoid	Anterolateral neck, midway between the mastoid process and the sternal notch	Acting separately, the muscle laterally flexes the neck toward the shoulder on that side or, if neck is fully rotated, flexes the neck toward the thorax
2. Upper Trapezius	Superior border of the shoulder, midway between the spinous and acromion processes	Elevation of the scapula with slight lateral rotation of the inferior angle
3. Middle Trapezius	On the posterior scapula, near the vertebral border and slightly inferior or to the spine of the scapula	Adduction of the scapula toward the spinous processes
4. Lower Trapezius	3 to 5 cm lateral to spinous processes T9 or T10	Diagonal pull between spinous processes and acromion, resulting in medial rotation of the inferior angle and depression of the scapula

	Muscle	Location	Action
5.	Rhomboids	Between the spinous processes and the vertebral border of the scapula and inferior to the spine of the scapula	Diagonal pull of the inferior angle of the scapula up and toward the spinous processes
6.	Latissimus Dorsi	Posterolateral aspect of trunk, inferior or to the scapula but usually on the thorax	Shoulder depression
7.	Serratus Anterior	Lateral aspect of thorax and on (*not* between) ribs 6 through 9	Scapular abduction
8.	Pectoralis Major	Anterolateral thorax, 3 to 5 cm superior to the nipple	Humeral adduction

B. Upper Extremity

	Muscle	Location	Action
1.	Anterior Deltoid	Anterior proximal third of humerus, midway between the acromion process and the deltoid insertion	Flexion of the humerus
2.	Middle Deltoid	Lateral proximal third of humerus, midway between the acromion process and the deltoid insertion	Abduction of the humerus
3.	Posterior Deltoid	Posterior proximal third of humerus, midway between the acromion process and deltoid insertion	Extension of the humerus

Appendix A con't.

B. *Upper Extremity*

Muscle	Location	Action
4. Coracobrachialis	Medial proximal third of humerus, best found when humerus is in 90° abduction and full external rotation. Caution — median and ulnar nerves are close and if stimulated will cause strong wrist and finger response	Adduction of the humerus
5. Biceps Brachii	Anterior middle third of humerus	Flexion of elbow
6. Brachialis	Lateral (usually) or medial distal third of humerus	Flexion of elbow
7. Triceps Brachii	Posterior middle third of humerus	Extension of elbow
8. Extensor Carpi Radialis Longus	Dorsal proximal third of forearm, toward the thumb side	Dorsiflexion and radial deviation of the hand
9. Extensor Carpi Radialis Brevis	Dorsal forearm at junction of upper and middle thirds, toward the thumb side	Dorsiflexion of the hand without radial deviation
10. Extensor Digitorum	Dorsal forearm distal third, toward the thumb side	Extension of the metacarpal phalangeal of the four lesser digits. Rarely will stimulation of the motor point cause all digits to respond

11. Extensor Carpi Ulnaris	Proximal third dorsal forearm, toward the ulnar side	Dorsiflexion of hand with ulnar deviation
12. Extensor Indicis Proprius	Dorsal middle third of forearm, midway between radius and ulna	Extension of all joints of the index finger
13. Abductor Pollicis Longus	Dorsal distal third of forearm, toward thumb side	Abduction of the metacarpal phalangeal joint in the plane of the forearm along with extension of the distal phalanx
14. Extensor Pollicis Longus	Dorsal distal third of forearm, toward thumb side – usually more distal and more lateral than the abductor	Extension of the distal phalanx of the thumb
15. Dorsal Interossei	Dorsal aspect of hand, 2 to 3 cm proximal to the metacarpal phalangeal joints and between them	Abduction of the metacarpal phalangeal joints individually
16. Lumbricales	Usually found on dorsal aspect of hand 1 to 2 cm proximal to metacarpal phalangeal joints. If palmar fat pads or callous is not thick, may be found on volar hand at this level	Flexion of metacarpal phalangeal joint plus extension of distal phalanx
17. Volar Interossei	Dorsal hand between motor point for dorsal interossei and lumbricales	Adduction of the metacarpal phalangeal joints individually

Appendix A con't.

B. Upper Extremity

Muscle	Location	Action
18. Brachioradialis	Proximal third anterior (volar) forearm, toward the thumb side	Elbow flexion plus forearm rotation toward neutral
19. Pronator Teres	Proximal third anteromedial forearm	Forearm pronation with slight elbow flexion
20. Flexor Carpi Radialis	Proximal third anterolateral forearm	Flexion and radial deviation of hand
21. Flexor Carpi Ulnaris	Proximal third anteromedial forearm	Flexion and ulnar deviation of hand
22. Flexor Digitorum Sublimis	Middle third anterior (volar) forearm midway between radius and ulna	Flexion of metacarpal phalangeal joints
23. Flexor Digitorum Profundus	Distal third anterior forearm, toward little finger side	Flexion of distal phalanges of fingers
24. Flexor Pollicis Longus	Distal third anterior forearm, toward thumb side	Flexion of the distal phalanx of thumb
25. Abductor Pollicis Brevis	Proximal thenar eminence, close to carpo metacarpal joint	Radial (anterior) abduction of the carpo-metacarpal joint of thumb
26. Opponens Pollicis	Anterolateral thenar eminence midway between carpometacarpal and metacarpophalangeal joints	Rotation of thumb so that thumbnail rotates from lateral toward anterior

Muscle	Location	Action
27. Flexor Pollicis Brevis	Medial thenar eminence	Flexion and adduction of the carpometacarpal joint of the thumb
28. Adductor Pollicis Brevis	Distal thenar eminence	Adduction and slight flexion of the carpometacarpal joint of the thumb
29. Flexor Digiti Minimi	Anteromedial hypothenar eminence at the midpoint of the fifth metacarpal bone	Flexion of the metacarpophalangeal joint
30. Abductor Digiti Minimi	Medial aspect of hypothenar eminence either distal or proximal to the motor point of the flexor	Abduction of the metacarpophalangeal joint

C. Lower Extremity

Muscle	Location	Action
1. Gluteus Medius	Lateral Pelvis, 2 to 5 cm posterior to a line between the anterior superior iliac spine and the greater trochanter	Abduction of the femur
2. Gluteus Maximus	On the buttock within a circle of 2 cm radius surrounding the ischial tuberosity	Extension of the femur
3. Semimembranosus	Posteromedial thigh, midway between knee and hip joints	Knee flexion

Appendix A con't.

C. Lower Extremity

	Muscle	Location	Action
4.	Semitendinosus	Posterior distal third of femur, slightly towards medial	Knee flexion
5.	Biceps Femoris, Long Head	Posterior thigh at junction of upper and middle third	Knee flexion
6.	Biceps Femoris, Short Head	Distal third of posterolateral femur	Knee flexion
7.	Rectus Femoris (Quadriceps)	Anterior thigh, midway between hip and knee	Knee extension
8.	Vastus Medialis (Quadriceps)	Anterior femur, distal third, slightly medial	Knee extension
9.	Vastus Lateralis (Quadriceps)	Anterolateral femur, distal third	Knee extension
10.	Sartorius	Anterior proximal femur, on a line between the anterior superior iliac spine and the medial condyle of the tibia	Hip and knee flexion
11.	Adductor Longus	Medial thigh at junction of proximal and middle third	Adduction of the femur
12.	Gracilis	Medial middle third of femur	Adduction of the femur
13.	Adductor Magnus	Medial distal third of femur	Adduction of the femur

14. Tibialis Anterior	Slightly lateral to crest of tibia, 5 to 10 cm inferior to head of fibula	Ankle dorsiflexion with inversion of the foot
15. Extensor Digitorum Longus	Lateral calf, 5 to 10 cm distal to head of fibula, on a line between head of fibula and the lateral malleolus	Extension of the distal phalanx of the lesser toes
16. Peroneus Longus	Lateral aspect of calf, slightly posterior to a line from the head of the fibula to the lateral malleolus, 10 to 15 cm inferior to the head of the fibula	Ankle plantar flexion with eversion of the foot
17. Peroneus Brevis	Lateral aspect of calf, 15 to 20 cm inferior to the head of the fibula	Eversion of the foot
18. Extensor Hallucis Longus	Distal third of tibia, slightly lateral to the crest of the tibia	Extension of the distal phalanx of the great toe
19. Extensor Digitorum Brevis	Dorsal aspect of foot, midway between ankle and tarsometatarsal joints	Extension of the proximal phalanx of the toes
20. Gastrocnemius (lateral head)	Posterolateral aspect of proximal third of tibia, 5 to 10 cm distal to head of fibula	Ankle plantar flexion
21. Gastrocnemius (medial head)	Posteromedial aspect of tibia 15 to 20 cm distal to the popliteal space	Ankle plantar flexion

Appendix A con't.

C. Lower Extremity

Muscle	Location	Action
22. Soleus	Posterior calf, 10 to 15 cm proximal to either the lateral or medial malleolus	Ankle plantar flexion
23. Flexor Hallucis Longus	Posterior to the lateral malleolus	Flexion of the distal phalanx of the great toe
24. Flexor Digitorum Longus	Posterior to the medial malleolus	Flexion of the distal phalanx of the four lesser toes

D. Facial Muscles

Muscle	Location	Action
1. Frontalis	3 to 5 cm superior to the medial third of the eyebrow	Horizontal wrinkling of forehead skin
2. Corrugator	1 cm superior to medial border of eyebrow	Draws eyebrow toward midline and causes vertical wrinkling of forehead skin
3. Orbicularis Oculi Superioris	1 cm superior and slightly lateral to lateral corner of eyelid	Raises upper eyelid
4. Orbicularis Oculi Inferioris	1 cm inferior to midline of lower eyelid	Opens lower eyelid

5.	Nasalis	At junction of nostril and face	Nostril flares
6.	Zygomaticus	1 to 2 cm inferior and medial to angle of mandible with the zygomatic arch when mouth is closed	Upper lip moves laterally and superiorly
7.	Quadratus Labii Superioris	Midway between nostril and upper lip	Upper lip closes
8.	Quadratus Labii Inferioris	1 cm inferior to lower lip, closer to corner than to midpoint of mouth	Lower lip closes
9.	Orbicularis Oris	1 to 2 cm lateral to corner of mouth	Upper and lower lips close simultaneously
10.	Mentalis	1 cm lateral to point of chin	Vertical wrinkling of skin of chin

APPENDIX B

MOTOR POINT AND DERMATOME CHARTS

*　　　*　　　*

As there are many anatomical variations, the charts are standardized in reasonable manner.

Segmental innervation of muscles is taken from Gray's Anatomy published by Lea and Febiger.

The following abbreviations are used:

> M — Muscle
> N — Nerve
> B — Branch of Nerve
> C — Cervical Nerve Roots
> T — Thoracic Nerve Roots
> L — Lumbar Nerve Roots

*　　　*　　　*

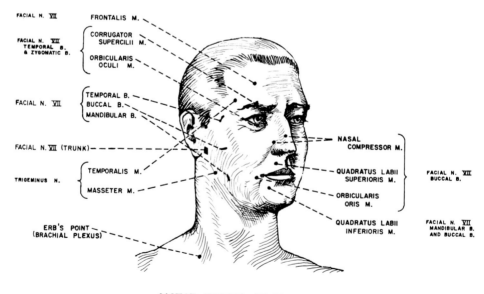

MOTOR POINTS OF FACE

Structure 1.

MOTOR POINTS OF ANTERIOR ASPECT OF UPPER EXTREMITY

Structure 2.

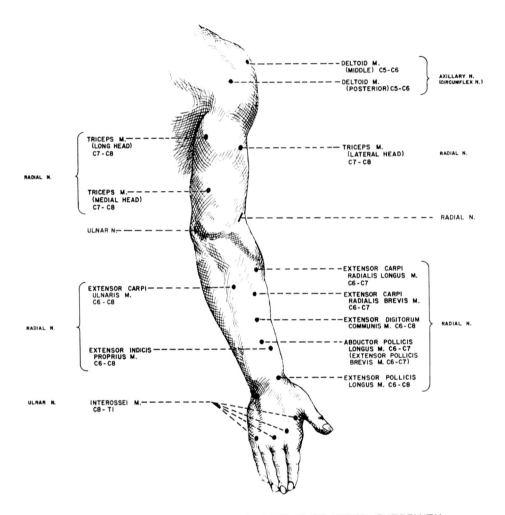

MOTOR POINTS OF POSTERIOR ASPECT OF UPPER EXTREMITY

Structure 3.

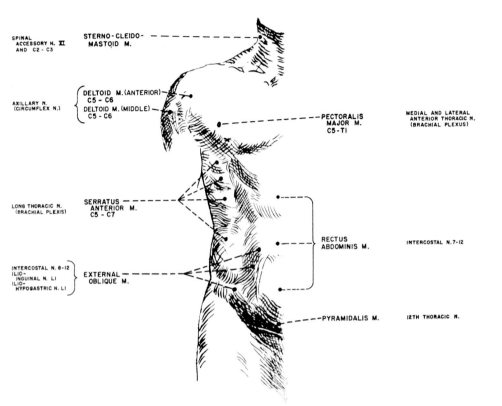

MOTOR POINTS OF ANTERIOR ASPECT OF TRUNK

Structure 4.

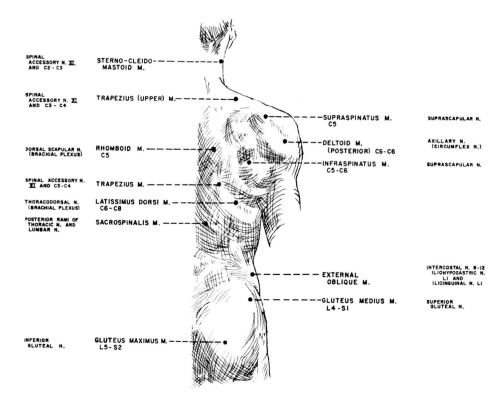

MOTOR POINTS OF POSTERIOR ASPECT OF TRUNK

Structure 5.

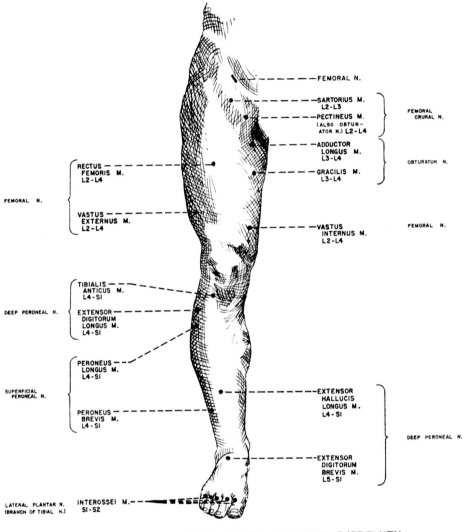

MOTOR POINTS OF ANTERIOR ASPECT OF LOWER EXTREMITY

Structure 6.

MOTOR POINTS OF POSTERIOR ASPECT OF LOWER EXTREMITY

Structure 7.

Diagram to show distribution of spinal cutaneous nerves on the ventral surface of the body. The position and course of the nerves are shown on the
left side of the body and the segmental distribution of each as numbered
is shown on the right side. By Permission from Morris' Human Anatomy, by
J. Parsons Schaeffer, M.D. Copyright, 1953, McGraw-Hill Book Co., Inc.

Structure 8.

Diagram to show distribution of spinal cutaneous nerves on the dorsal sur
face of the body. The position and course of the nerves are shown on the
left side of the body and the segmental distribution of each as numbered is
shown on the right side. By permission from Morris' Human Anatomy, by
J. Parsons Schaeffer, M.D. Copyright, 1953, McGraw-Hill Book Co., Inc.

Structure 9.

Medial supraclavicular
Intermediate supraclavicular
Lateral supraclavicular
Medial antibrachial cutaneous
Lateral brachial cutaneous
Intercosto-brachial cutaneous
Lower lateral brachial cutaneous
Medial brachial cutaneous
Medial antibrachial cutaneous
Lateral antibrachial cutaneous
Lateral cutaneous of intercostal 12
Lateral femoral cutaneous, posterior branch
Ulnar cutaneous
Median digital branches
Ulnar digital branches
Ilio-inguinal
Lumbo-inguinal
Lateral femoral cutaneous
Obturator cutaneous
Anterior femoral cutaneous
Anterior medial cutaneous
Infrapatellar branch of saphenous
Saphenous
Sural branches of peroneal
Superficial peroneal
Lateral dorsal cutaneous
Medial dorsal cutaneous
Deep peroneal

C 2,3
C 3,4
C 5,6
T 2
C 5,6
C 5,6
C 8 T1
C 5,6 7,8 C8 T1
6,7,8
T 2
3
4
5
6
7
8
9
10
11
12
L 1
L 1,2
L,S 2,3,4
L 2
3
L 2,3
L 2,3
L 2,3
L 3,4
L 5, S 1,2
L 4,5, S 1
L 4,5, S1

Lateral cutaneous branches
Anterior cutaneous branches

Structure 8.

Great occipital

Small occipital
Great auricular

Posterior
supraclavicular

Lateral brachial
cutaneous
Posterior brachial
cutaneous
Intercosto-brachial
cutaneous
Lateral brachial
cutaneous
Medial brachial
cutaneous
Dorsal antibrachial
cutaneous
Lateral antibrachial
cutaneous
Medial antibrachial
cutaneous
Thoracic 12
Iliohypogastric
Radial
Ulnar
Medial
cluneal

Long pudendal
Lateral femoral
cutaneous

Obturator cutaneous

Posterior femoral
cutaneous

Posterior branch of
medial cutaneous

Posterior femoral
cutaneous
Saphenous

Common peroneal

Anastomotic branch
of peroneal

Sural

Twigs from saphenous

Sural

Lateral calcaneal
branches

Medial calcaneal
Medial plantar
Lateral plantar

C 2 3

C 3

C 3,4

C 5,6

Posterior-cutaneous branches
Lateral cutaneous branches

C 5,6,7,8

C 8
T 1

C 8
T 1

C 6,7,8

S 1,2,3

L 2
3

S 1,2,3

L 2
3

L 4 5
S 1

L 3
4

L 5
S 1

S 1,
2

S 1,2

S 1
2

L 4,5

Structure 9.

REFERENCES

1. Harris, F.A. et al.: Electronic sensory aids as treatment for cerebral palsy children. *Phys Ther, 54:*354-65, 1974.

2. Liberson, W. et al.: Functional electrotherapy in cerebrovascular accidents. *Arch Phys Med Rehabil, 42:*101-5, 1961.

3. Glanville, H.J.: Electrical control of paralysis. *Proc R Soc Med, 65:*233-35, 1972.

4. Rebersek, S. and Vodovnik, L.: Proportionally controlled functional electrical stimulation of the hand. *Arch Phys Med Rehabil, 54:*378-82, 1973.

5. Fordyce, W. et al.: Operant conditioning for pain. *Arch Phys Med Rehabil, 54:*399-408, 1973.

6. Farmer, W.C.: Electrophysiological bracing in radial nerve compression injury. *Phys Ther, 46:*857-61, 1966.

7. Stanwood, J.E. et al.: Diagnosis and management of brachial plexus injuries. *Arch Phys Med Rehabil, 52:*52-60, 1971.

8. *Dorland's Illustrated Medical Dictionary,* 24th ed. Philadelphia, Saunders, 1965.

9. Davson, Hugh: *A Textbook of General Physiology,* 4th ed. Baltimore, Williams & Wilkins, 1970, pp. 1041-44.

10. Bouman, H.D. and Shaffer, K.J.: Psychological basis of electrical stimulation of human muscle and its clinical application. *Phys Ther, 37:*207-23, 1957.

11. Kinnen, E.: Electrical impedance of human skin. *Med Electron Biol Eng, 3:*67-70, 1965.

12. Harris, F.A.: Inapproprioception — a possible sensory basis for athetoid movements. *Phys Ther, 51:*761-70, 1971.

13. Levine, M. et al.: Relaxation of spasticity by electrical stimulation of antagonistic muscles. *Arch Phys Med Rehabil, 33:*668-73, 1952.

14. Vogel, M. et al.: Use of tetanizing current for spasticity. *Phys Ther, 35:*435-37, 1955.

15. Covalt, N.K. and Griffin, J.E.: The place of low volt currents in hydrotherapy. *Phys Ther, 36:*99-105, 1956.

16. Vodovnik, L. et al.: Pain response to tetanizing currents. *Arch Phys Med Rehabil, 46:*187-92, 1965.

17. Bishop, B.: Vibratory stimulation. III. Possible applications of vibration in treatment of motor dysfunctions. *Phys Ther, 55:*139-43, 1975.

18. Woo-Sam, J. et al.: Sex differences in adaptation to peripheral electrostimulating surgical implants. *Arch Phys Med Rehabil, 53:*425-9, 1972.

19. *Clinical Evaluation of the Ljubljana Functional Electrical Peroneal Brace.* Report E-7, National Academy of Sciences, 1973.

20. Shriber, W.: *A Manual of Electrotherapy,* 4th ed. Philadelphia, Lea & Febiger, 1975.

21. Thomson, J.D.: Effects of electrical stimulation on denervated muscle.

*Am J Phys Med, 36:*16-20, 1957.

22. Stillwell, G.K. and Wakim, K.G.: Electrical stimulation of muscle. *Arch Phys Med Rehabil, 43:*95-8, 1962.

23. Smith, E. and Steinberger, W.: Direct electrical stimulation of denervated rabbit muscle. *Arch Phys Med Rehabil, 49:*566-73, 1968.

24. Reed, J. and Jarrett, A.: Enzymatic and histological effects of a standard stimulus to the skin of normals and the clinically normal skin of psoriatic patients. *Arch Dermatol, 95:*632-41, 1967.

25. Shepard, J.T.: *Physiology of the Circulation in Human Limbs in Health and Disease.* Philadelphia, Saunders, 1963.

26. Abramson, D.I.: *Circulation in the Extremities.* New York, Acad Pr, 1967.

27. Wakim, K.: Influence of frequency of electrical stimulation on circulation. *Arch Phys Med Rehabil, 34:*291-5, 1953.

28. Martella, J. et al.: Prevention of thromboembolic disease by electrical stimulation of leg muscles. *Arch Phys Med Rehabil, 35:*24-9, 1954.

29. Abramowitsch, D. and Neousskine, B.: *Treatment by Ion Transfer.* New York, Grune, 1946.

30. O'Malley, E. and Oester, Y.: Influence of some physical chemical factors on iontophoresis using radio-isotopes. *Arch Phys Med Rehabil, 36:*310-6, 1955.

31. Murray, W. et al.: The iontophoresis of C_{21} esterified glucocorticoids: preliminary report. *Phys Ther, 43:*579-83, 1963.

32. Wedekind, W.H.: Research on electrical full and part current baths (Stanger system): a contribution on the effectiveness of the hydro-electric bath. *Z Gesamt Physik Ther, 43:*183-213, 1932.

33. Gordon, A. and Weinstein, M.: Sodium salicylate iontophoresis in treatment of plantar warts. *Phys Ther, 49:*869-70, 1969.

34. Griffin, J. et al.: Patients treated with ultrasonic driven hydrocortisone and ultrasound alone. *Phys Ther, 47:*595-601, 1967.

Chapter 4

THE DIATHERMIES

INTRODUCTION

DIATHERMY MAY BE DEFINED as the generation of heat in the body tissues due to the resistance offered by the tissues to the passage of high frequency electric currents. There is medical diathermy, wherein the anticipated tissue temperature rise is within physiological limits, and surgical diathermy, wherein the anticipated tissue temperature rise is destructive.[1] This volume is concerned only with medical diathermy.

Any device which generates an electric current will simultaneously generate an electric field and a magnetic field.[2] Tissues will selectively absorb more of the electric or more of the magnetic field depending upon their chemical composition. Tissues with a high fat content will tend to act as insulators and resist the passage of electric field energy. In the process of resisting the penetration of the electric field, the tissue temperature will rise.

Fat does not resist the passage of the magnetic field. Tissues of high electrolyte content will tend to oscillate in the presence of a high frequency magnetic field. The degree of oscillation, at the intraatomic level, will be in direct proportion to the polarity of the absorbing molecule. Water is the most polar molecule present in tissues in large quantity and is the major constituent of normally occurring electrolytes. Thus, it is the reaction of absorbing tissues to both the electric and magnetic field which causes the tissue temperature rise (TTR). The objective of treatment by medical diathermy is to cause vasodilation and/or skeletal muscle relaxation, with subsequent pain relief.

HISTORICAL BACKGROUND

In the early twentieth century, as the then infant science of electronics developed practical ways to generate high frequency oscillating currents (f > 1 Mc), radio came into existence. It was soon discovered that if living tissue was exposed to practical quantities of this high frequency energy, their resistance to penetration of the energy caused the absorbing tissue to get hot. This form of energy caused less rise in skin temperature and more rise in subcutaneous fat and underlying muscle as compared to infrared lamps, bakers, and whirlpools.

The first commercially available clinical diathermy units appeared in the late 1910s and early 1920s. The high frequency energy was generated by multiple spark gaps. The frequencies were unstable but within the range of 1 to 10 million Hertz (MHz). The electrodes were flexible bare metal plates. A layer of conducting jelly was placed between the plate and the skin. Electrical burns were a frequent occurrence, especially when the electrodes were applied to a surface of irregular contour. Maintenance of adequately functioning spark gaps was a nuisance. As radio came into widespread use, the spark gap diathermies caused many problems, particularly because of generation of an unfilterable static in both nearby and remote radios, but these diathermy machines were capable of causing a deeper TTR than any form of conductive heating.

In the late 1920s and the 1930s, advances in electronics permitted generation of still higher frequencies on a practical scale. Most importantly, spark gap generation of high frequencies became obsolete, and frequency control on the order of $\pm$ 1 percent became possible. To distinguish between the older and newer diathermy machines, the older was designated as long wave and the newer as short wave (SWD) diathermy. Reasonably close frequency tolerance became possible in the 10 to 100 MHz range. Because radio broadcasting was playing an ever-increasing role in society, with the number of broadcasting stations steadily increasing, authority to regulate the frequency and power output of each station was granted to the Federal Communications Commission (F.C.C.) along with the capability and resources to closely monitor the airwaves.

Any medical diathermy unit is actually a radio transmitter. Although the power output of such units rarely exceeds 200 watts, this is sufficient to cause nearby radio and television reception to be garbled, because of frequency interference. In the late 1930s, the Federal Communications Commission assigned certain short wave frequencies for medical diathermy. Medical use of long wave diathermy was banned, since adequate frequency control was not feasible at competitive cost. To give manufacturers time to adjust production to the new standards and to give purchasers of the older style of equipment a reasonable chance to recover their investment, 1947 was set as the year when long wave diathermy could no longer be used. Under the F.C.C. regulations, SWD design had to be tested and approved for frequency stability and other performance characteristics before the unit could go into production. The F.C.C. assigned as primary frequency 27.12 MHz $\pm$ 0.6 percent. Allowable secondary frequencies were 13.56 and 40.68 MHz, each with a permitted fluctuation of $\pm$ 0.05 percent.[4] Calculations based on frequency and wavelength relationships discussed in Chapter 2 yield a wavelength of 11 m for the primary frequency, 22 m for the lower frequency and 7 m for the highest allowed frequency. No American manufacturer uses the high frequency, since it cannot be manufactured competively. Only one uses the lower allowed frequency.* since frequency toleration of $\pm$ 0.6 percent is easier to design than toleration of $\pm$ 0.05 percent.

Further advances in electronic circuitry, especially the development of the multiple cavity anode, permitted generation of frequencies called microwave. These are in the range of 100 to 10,000 MHz. Microwave diathermy came into clinical use in the late 1940s. Until 1972, the only microwave frequency allowed for medical use was that of 2,456 MHz, a 2 percent tolerance. Yet early in the 1950s, it was clearly demonstrated that lower microwave frequencies would be much more effective in causing a significant TTR in soft tissues at a depth of 3 to 5 cm.[3] The wavelength of electromagnetic energy having a frequency of 2,456 MHz is approximately 12 cm. For a frequency of 900 MHz, the wavelength is about 33 cm.[5,6]

Neither short wave or microwave diathermy is in as widespread

*The Birtcher Crystal Bandmaster, Model 800. The Birtcher Corporation, Los Angeles, California.

demand now as it was in the 1950s. A major factor in the decline of use is that, in the presence of a subcutaneous fat layer more than 1 cm thick, the fat temperature is likely to rise to dangerous levels (above 45°C) while the underlying muscle temperature rise is insignificant or may even drop.[7,8] Subcutaneous fat is an excellent resistor to the penetration of an electric field, because of its low electrolyte content, and is not stimulated by penetration of the magnetic field. Both these factors, coupled with the low specific heat of fat (approximately 0.5, compared to 1.0 for water) can give rise to a serious burn in fat even though there is little visible evidence of temperature rise in skin.

Furthermore, efficient and effective electrode placement takes time, and selection of the right type of electrode for the area to be treated can make the difference between a placebo and a physiologically effective treatment. Lastly, evolution of the use of ultrasonic energy, which does produce a significant deep tissue temperature rise without the danger of overheating of subcutaneous fat, and within in a much shorter treatment time, has diminished demand for utilization of the diathermies.

SHORT WAVE DIATHERMY ELECTRODES

The 1930s saw the development of four types of short wave diathermy (SWD) electrodes. In order of development, they are as follows:

1. pads and cuffs
2. air-spaced plates
3. the drum
4. the induction field cable

Pad Electrodes

Two pad electrodes are required to complete the electrical circuit. The patient becomes a part of the electrical circuit. The pad electrode is nearly equal in length and width. It consists of a flexible metal plate about 1 mm thick, covered with rubber or other insulating material several millimeters thick, on all surfaces. For uniform distribution of energy transfer from electrode to patient, contact pressure should be uniform throughout the electrode surface. Consequently, in standard application, a 1 to 2 cm layer of soft insulating material is placed between the electrode and the skin. Frequently, the electrode is supplied with a loose cotton sack plus soft felt pads having an area slightly larger than the metal plate. This padding is held in place by the loose sack and serves to minimize small areas of firm versus light pressure when the pad is held in place by body weight or a sandbag. Such dielectric spacing helps to insure that the skin temperature will not rise to injurious levels even though enough energy is used to raise subcutaneous tissue temperature.

The pad electrodes should not be placed closer together than about 5 cm and may be positioned a meter or more away from each other. If too close together, most of the energy will travel from pad to pad through air or across skin surface rather than from one pad into the patient and then to other pad. This will not cause a deep tissue temperature rise.

The cuff electrode is similar in construction and use to the pad electrode, except its length is much greater than its width. It is intended for use as a "wrap-around" electrode. Two are required to complete the electrical circuit. When the electrical insulation covering the cuff is in good condition the ends of the metal plate may be overlapped with safety, but for longer cuff electrode life it is recommended that several layers of toweling or felt be inserted between the overlapping ends.

Neither the pad or the cuff electrode will cause a significant deep tissue temperature rise unless contact pressure is uniform throughout the electrode surface. For this reason, their use when a deep TTR is desired was banned by the Council on Physical Therapy equipment of the American Medical Association in 1952.[3] They are as effective as hot packs or other sources of infrared energy for causing a superficial TTR, and since the diathermy generator with its electrodes can be awesome in appearance, some patients will undoubtedly perceive more pain relief from a TTR caused by this form of diathermy as compared to relief gained from exposure to hot packs.

Air-Spaced Plate Electrodes

The next development in short wave diathermy electrodes was the air-spaced plate. Two are needed to complete the electrical circuit. The patient becomes a part of the electrical circuit. All these electrodes have a rigid metal plate. In older designs, this was covered on all surfaces with a layer of bakelite, several millimeters thick. This is a good electrical insulator. The plate is surrounded by an adjustable plate guard, one surface of which is placed in contact with a single layer of bath toweling which should always be on the skin. The guard adjustment permits the plate to be placed 1 to 6 cm from the skin, thus permitting variation in depth of penetration of energy.

Newer designs consist of a bare metal plate enclosed in a transparent electrical insulator. The insulator (guard) is not adjustable, but the plate is adjustable within the guard, through a range of 1 to 3 cm. Figure 4-1 illustrates the arrangements of the essential components of an air-spaced plate electrode. The purpose of the plate guard is to prevent touching of the electrode plate when the patient circuit is energized. A severe electrical burn could result, especially if the contacting skin is moist.

Figure 4-1. A typical air-spaced plate designed in the 1950s.

A. Bare metal plate about 15 cm in diameter and 2 mm thick.
B. Clear plastic plate guard, allowing adjustment of plate through a range of 3 cm.
C. Adjusting handle, with a pin lock so that electrode will not change position while in use.
D. Lead cord from plate to apparatus terminal. One lead is required for each plate.

Depth of penetration of energy from air-spaced plate electrodes is *inversely proportional to the distance from plate to skin, as long as the plate guard is in contact with the single layer of toweling on the skin.* Conversely, the sensation of heat produced within the absorbing tissues is in *direct proportion* to the distance from the plate to the skin.

There are far more thermal receptors in the skin than in subcutaneous fat or muscle. Hence, it is simple to demonstrate the relationships between sensation and penetration with use of air-spaced plates. With a subject sitting on a wooden or plastic stool *(not* metal), expose a shoulder. Place a small towel roll in the axilla to absorb perspiration. Place a single layer of toweling over all surfaces of the shoulder. Place one plate anterior and the other posterior to the shoulder. Each plate *guard* should be in firm contact with the toweling. Adjust the plates within their guards so that they are visually equidistant from the skin. Turn up the intensity until the subject reports a gentle sensation of warmth. This will usually require an intensity of 30 to 50 percent of available power. Treat for five minutes. It is anticipated that the subject will report equal sensation of warmth posteriorly and anteriorly. If either the clavicle or the spine of the scapula has minimal soft tissue covering, the subject may report more warmth on one side or the other, as the case may be. Turn the intensity of zero. Adjust the distance of *one* of the plates so that it is different from the other by one or more centimeters. Return the intensity to the previous level. In two or three minutes, the subject will volunteer that the sensation of heat is now different on the anterior as compared to the posterior aspect of the shoulder. If the plate was moved away, *sensation* of heat will have decreased in that area. If the plate was moved closer, the *sensation* will have increased.

The closer a plate is to the skin, the greater the chances that more energy will be directed perpendicularly toward the skin. Hence, there will be more absorption and less reflection. If more than 700 to 800 microwatts per cm^2 per second are absorbed by the skin, hyperemia or erythema and finally skin destruction (burn) will occur.[9] When the plate is further away, the chances are increased for reflection of energy from the skin. However, the chances of that reflected energy hitting the plate and being redirected back toward the skin are less. Hence, the closer the plate, the greater the chances for absorption. If the plate *guard* is not in contact with the toweling and the plate is at maximum distance from the guard, then there is so much reflection and scattering that an insignificant quantity of energy is absorbed, and little or no temperature rise will occur in the skin or underlying tissues.

Air-spaced plates function much like a capacitor. A capacitor by definition consists of conducting plates separated by a dielectric. The opposing plates are oppositely charged by a source of voltage, and the electrical energy of the charged system is stored in the polarized dielectric.[1,2] For clinical purposes, a dielectric is any material, including dry air, which is an electrical insulator. The presence of such an insulator between plates of opposite charge forces transfer of energy by induction rather than conduction. In normal clinical usage, a part of the patient is placed between the two plates. The skin acts as a dielectric, since dry skin is a poor conductor. High voltage (3,000 to 15,000 volts), low amperage (microamperes) current is passed by the high frequency oscillating circuit to each plate millions of times per second. When the plate that is storing energy is filled to capacity, it discharges, transferring energy through and around the patient to the plate of low potential, which returns much of the energy to the apparatus. The net effect of the resistance to passage and absorption by intervening tissue is a rise in tissue temperature.

Certain precautions must be exercised in the use of air-spaced electrodes or there will be insignificant penetration of energy through the skin and hence no deep temperature rise. Thus, if 10 cm diameter plates are used, one on the anterior and the other on the posterior forearm, the plates will need to be at least 10 cm apart to achieve significant penetration. Otherwise, 90 percent or more of the energy will go directly from plate to plate or across the skin. This is especially true on a humid day. However, if one plate is placed on the distal volar forearm and the other on the proximal posterior forearm, the distance between the plates will be more than 10 cm and good deep heating would occur.

Most plates presently in use have a diameter more on the order of 20 cm. This limits the areas of the body which may be treated by this type of electrode. The usual procedure is to center the area to be treated between the electrodes. Thus, if a TTR is desired among tissues in and around the knee, one electrode could be applied to the medial or anterior midthigh and the other to the posterior midcalf. When the patient circuit is energized, for the first few minutes he will have a greater sensation of heat under one of the electrodes. Then he will note this sensation gradually moving toward the knee. Within ten minutes of treatment, he will note a greater sensation at the knee than on the skin under either of the plates. Skin temperature measurements before and after treatment will confirm this point.

As a general rule, when using air-spaced plates, the area to be treated should be centered between the plates in order to assure that the distance between the plates is greater than their diameter. If the distance is significantly less, there will be little deep tissue temperature rise, even though the sensation of heat is great.

Because air-spaced plates can function when they are 75 to 100 cm apart, the resultant thermal effect is superior to that of other SWD electrodes and to other forms of energy available to the physical therapist when a mild TTR is desired in a large volume of tissue. Thus, in the early stages of a chronic organic occlusive peripheral vascular disorder, when vasospasm is a larger factor than actual decrease in arterial lumen, air-spaced plates can be more effective, and safer, than multiple hot packs or infrared lamps. When the electrodes are far apart, the quantity of energy available for absorption per volume of tissue is lower than it would be for an equivalent energy source covering a smaller area, such as a hot pack or whirlpool.

The Drum Electrode

The drum electrode consists of one or more monoplanar coils of thick (3 to 4 mm) single strand copper wire which is rigidly positioned inside a bakelite housing (Fig. 4-2). The housing has a dead-air space of 1 to 2 cm in all directions from the coil. For treatment of small, flat areas, a single coil drum may be used. For treatment of larger areas, two or three coils are linked together in series, with hinged sections so that some attempt may be made to follow contour. Still other types of drums are intended only for use on extremities. These will have a fixed curve built into the coils and their housings to accommodate the roughly cylindrical circumstance of a segment of an extremity.

Figure 4-2. A typical drum electrode. Two or three drums, with hinge joints between each unit, are usually linked in series.

A. A single strand of copper wire, 3 or 4 mm thick, shaped into a rectangle of approximately 5 × 15 cm.

B. Dead air space of about 1 cm in all directions.

C. Bakelite housing 2 to 3 mm thick.

D. Lead cord from plate to apparatus terminal. One lead is required for woven copper, with a diamter of 4 to 5 mm, covered by a loosely fitting rubber or plastic insulation several millimeters thick. Two leads are required, irrespective of whether one or more than one drum is linked together.

When a drum electrode is utilized, the patient is *not* a part of an electrical circuit as is the case with air-spaced plates. When the drum is energized, the nearby body segment is within the magnetic field but much less within the electric field created by the diathermy generator. Tissues of high electrolyte content, i.e. tissues with a good blood supply, respond to the presence of a strong magnetic field with the formation of "eddy currents" through intramolecular oscillation. This attempt to follow the rise and fall of the magnetic field millions of times per second causes rise in tissue temperature. When the subject feels a gentle sensation of warmth (skin temperature rise), a significant quantity of magnetic field energy has penetrated to a depth of 2 to 3 cm, providing the skin is no more than 1 to 2 cm distant from the coil. Good technic requires that the coil *housing* be in light contact with the single layer of bath toweling which should always cover the skin in the area of the electrode.

Subcutaneous fat has a poor blood supply and hence a low electrolyte content. Thus, it is not stimulated by passage of the magnetic field. It does respond, however, to the concomitant electric field which also radiates from the coil. When the drum electrode is efficiently applied, it can be anticipated that approximately 50 percent of the absorbing tissue response will be due to the electric field and 50 percent due to the magnetic field.[3,4] With poor drum positioning, the magnetic field effect will be diminished. Then the patient will perceive a stronger *sensation* of warmth but is likely to have an insignificant temperature rise except in the skin and subcutaneous fat.

The coil is fixed within a rigid housing. The patient surface of the housing should be as close to the single layer of toweling as possible without indenting the skin. If a corner of the housing actually does indent the skin, a "hot-spot" may occur. The electric field does not radiate strongly as far as the magnetic field. If the housing is too close to the skin, fat temperature may rise enough to cause enough perspiration formation to concentrate the electric field at that point, since the electric field will always follow the path of least resistance.

When the drum is energized, the patient is actually absorbing both electric and magnetic field energy. Any high voltage, high frequency current flow through a metallic conductor will generate a substantial electrical field in the area close to the conductor and a significant magnetic field through a greater distance. With the frequencies and voltages used in short wave and microwave diathermy, the magnetic field will be significant up to 5 cm away from the metallic conductor. The magnetic field actually extends much farther, but it is only strong enough to cause a substantial TTR a few centimeters away at patient circuit power levels that the skin can tolerate without damage.[3]

It is the living tissue reaction to the magnetic field which causes the beneficial temperature rise when the drum electrode is used. The magnetic field penetrates the subcutaneous fat without causing a significant fat temperature rise. The magnetic field is absorbed by the deeper tissues with a high electrolyte content. Blood has the highest electrolyte content (approximately 154 mEq/liter) of all normal body tissues. Although not classified as a tissue, urine can have a much higher, the same, or a much lower electrolyte content as compared to blood, depending upon the concentration of the urine at any given time.

Penetration of the electric field is resisted by the subcutaneous fat because fat is an electrical (but not magnetic) insulator. Fat has a low water and salt content. The net result is that the temperature of the subcutaneous fat is raised rapidly by exposure to an electric field. Because fat has a lower specific heat than water (about 0.5 to 1.0), it is very easy to cause a dangerous fat temperature rise with little or no rise in temperature of underlying tissues.

In contrast with the drum electrode, the air-spaced plate electrode system generates a much stronger electric field and weaker magnetic field. This is in large part due to the fact that there is a stronger dielectric inherent in the capacitor system.[3,4,10,11]

The drum electrode, whether it consists of one or more than one coil linked in series, cannot cause a TTR in as large a volume of tissue as can widely separated air-spaced plates, but it can cause a deeper TTR because of its greater magnetic field generation.[4,10]

In almost all clinical usage, the drum is the easiest electrode to apply. However, if the subcutaneous fat is more than about 2 cm thick, there will be no TTR of any consequence in any underlying tissue at any intensity the subcutaneous fat will tolerate. Only in unusual circumstances can one anticipate a useful TTR more than

3 cm deep to the skin with short wave diathermy, regardless of the type of electrode used.[3,7,8,10,11]

There is one recent development in short wave generator design which permits generation of a magnetic field stronger than the accompanying electric field. This has become possible only with the development of solid state circuitry. All the patents on this design are the property of a single company.*

> The drum applicator of the *Auto-Therm* produces an extremely high current at low voltages, and it is a well-known fact that the high currents from an electromagnetic field produces deeper heat than pad applicators, which develop a very high voltage. This is why the old Council on Physical Therapy Equipment of the American Medical Association never would approve the use of pad applicators. In the case of other drum applicators, so much voltage is developed within the patient that his entire body becomes a short wave antenna. This is why the entire drum section and support arm in other short wave generators are made of insulating materials.
>
> *Autotherm* deep heat tests were recently conducted by a highly qualified independent group. After a twenty-minute treatment, three large normal subjects showed an average temperature of 105°F at an average depth of two inches, next to the thigh bone. Unlike other tests, these were run at a comfortable patient tolerance, proving *Autotherm's* effectiveness for deep heating. Please note the final temperature in the subcutaneous tissues is approximately the same as in deep muscle next to the bone. Naturally, the temperature rise was greater in the subcutaneous fat, which would be expected. The reason the power in watts can be so low for these excellent temperature rises is that the patient's body and cable connections are not operating as short wave antennas as is the case with all units in the past.**

This SWD unit is supplied only with a single fixed coil drum electrode, which limits its possible areas of application, with no provision for following contour of a body segment. However, it is the easiest of all diathermy units to operate, in the authors' clinical experience.

---

*Mettler Electronics Corporation, Anaheim, California.

**These tests were conducted at the Loma Linda School of Medicine, Loma Linda, California, 1969.

The Cable Electrode

The cable electrode consists of a multistranded woven copper wire cable about 1 cm in diameter and varying in length from 2.5 to 4.5 m as supplied for different short wave generator units. The cable is covered, except at its terminals, by a flexible rubber insulating material 3 to 5 mm in thickness (Fig. 4-3).

Figure 4-3. A typical cable electrode.

A. Solid metal tip 5 to 10 mm in diameter and 3 to 5 cm in length.

B. Rigid plastic or ceramic hollow insulator 10 to 15 mm in diameter and 5 to 10 cm in length.

C. Multistranded woven copper wire about 5 mm in diameter and 2.5 to 4.5 m in length.

D. Flexible rubber or plastic insulation, 2 to 5 mm thick, throughout the length of the cable.

The cable is much more flexible than either the air-spaced plate or the drum electrode. It can follow the contour of any body segment readily and hence can be used to cause a relatively deep TTR in more areas of the body. However, there is no question that it takes more time, skill, and linen to apply the cable electrode safely and effectively.

Since the cable is not enclosed within a plate guard (air-spaced plate) or in a rigid housing (drum), the therapist must place a dielectric material between the patient and the cable to insure an adequate dielectric space between skin and cable. Bath toweling should always be placed next to the skin, as the toweling is a good absorber of perspiration. The layer of toweling should be followed by more toweling or other standard linen. If the cable is to lie on the patient, the total dielectric space should be approximately 1 cm. If the patient is to lie on the cable, his body or extremity weight will compress the dielecric material so that an additional 1 to 2 cm of soft insulating material must be added. The hazard of an electrical burn increases markedly when the dielectric space is less than 1 cm, especially on a humid day.

It is imperative that turns of the cable never touch each other when the patient circuit is energized. If cable surfaces touch, a short circuit can result, which can ruin the cable. More seriously, the short circuit can cause nearby linen to catch on fire. Rubber sleeves or other insulating material should be placed between turns where they must cross. Stiff spacers of any insulating material should be used to establish and maintain a uniform distance between turns when the cable is wound as either a two- or a three-dimensional coil. All winding and other preparations should be completed and not modified while the patient circuit is energized.

After each treatment, the cable should be unwound and stored as nearly linearly as possible. If the cable is left wound in a pattern for a prolonged period of time, it will be more difficult to adjust it for a different coil size or shape. The time and care needed to prepare a cable electrode for safe and effective use is a major reason why it is no longer commonly used.

When properly applied, the cable produces as much magnetic field as the drum electrode. It has the added advantage that it can cause a TTR deep to *all* surfaces of an extremity simultaneously and with great uniformity, since it follows contours readily. The monoplanar drum can add energy to only one surface at a time. When the drum is applied in a biplanar fashion, as many as three surfaces can be treated simultaneously, but the drum is hard to position for uniform energy absorption because few body segments are of a regular contour.

When the cable is improperly applied (turns too close together), both the electric and magnetic fields are apt to jump from turn to turn of the cable. This will shorten the useful life of the cable. More importantly, if turns are too close, there will be only superficial heating of the patient. In apparatus designed specifically for the cable electrode, the turns can be 10 cm or more apart and still add enough magnetic field energy to the patient to cause a significant deep TTR. The cable then becomes the ideal electrode to generate a mild tissue temperature rise throughout an extremity with greater uniformity of energy absorption than with any other SWD electrode.

GENERAL PRECAUTIONS WITH
SHORT WAVE ELECTRODES

There are several points about use of SWD electrodes which, if followed faithfully, will minimize the risk of burning the patient and increase the life expectancy of the electrode.

Whenever diathermy is applied, there will be accumulation of perspiration on the skin. Perspiration is composed largely of water and various salts. It is an excellent conductor of electricity. Hence, a single layer of bath toweling should always cover the skin in the area being treated. Bath toweling is an excellent absorber of perspiration and will prevent its pooling in skin hollows or where skin surfaces ordinarily touch one another. Its regular and faithful use will make the risk of the patient receiving a severe and painful electrical burn negligible.

The lead cables from the generator to the electrode should never be allowed to touch each other when the unit is in operation. High voltage, high frequency electrical energy is being put into the metallic circuit. If the lead cables touch, a short circuit is likely. In the case of the cable electrode, the entire cable is the "lead" as well as the electrode. Therefore, the physical therapist should utilize spacing of any insulating material as indicated when inspecting the set-up prior to energizing the circuit. A 1 to 2 cm separation is adequate.

Living tissue should never be permitted to touch either the lead cable or the electrode when the patient circuit is energized. This can result in a severe electrical burn, especially if the contacting skin is moist.

Three demonstration experiments are outlined at the end of this chapter. These procedures will simply and readily confirm the differences in heating patterns with the air-spaced plates, the drum, and the cable electrodes.

MICROWAVE DIATHERMY ELECTRODES

With *short wave* diathermy generators, much of the energy is lost within the machine circuit and/or patient circuit before there can be energy transfer to the patient. This is because the oscillating circuit which converts line current into the requisite high frequency radiates energy in all directions and because the lead cables which carry energy from the machine circuit to the electrodes are not shielded against loss of electric field energy. At any given intensity, at least one third of the generated high frequency energy never comes close to the area to be treated.

With *microwave* transmission, essentially no energy is lost between the oscillating circuit and the transmitting antenna, and because these wavelengths (12 or 33 cm) can be focused toward the patient, loss between the antenna and patient rarely exceeds 10 percent, even though the antenna may be as far away as 15 cm. The microwave antenna is commonly referred to as a director because it beams energy toward the patient. Such focusing is possible because microwave wavelengths are short enough to have some of the properties of visible light. On the other hand, the shortest short wave diathermy wavelength in clinical use is 11 m. This and longer wavelengths cannot be adequately focused for efficient clinical use at a practical cost.

In order to meet the FCC regulation for frequency tolerance at microwave frequencies, approximately $\pm$ 2 percent, the insulation between the metallic conductors which transfer this extremely high frequency energy from generator to antenna must be far superior to the insulation needed for similar transfer of the lower frequency shortwave energy. Furthermore, because of the higher voltages needed to drive the microwave oscillating frequency circuit, 15,000 to 30,000 volts, the insulation between the outer conductor and any living tissue which could touch the lead cable must also be superior. The only practical way to meet these transmission requirements is to use a coaxial cable to deliver energy from the machine circuit to the patient. In order to deliver a significant quantity of energy, i.e. enough to cause a TTR, the insulation must be relatively rigid. The net result is that the lead cable from the machine to the antenna is far less flexible than that which is used for shortwave transmission. This can make ideal positioning of the director a problem. Figures 4-4 through 4-6 illustrate various aspects of director design.

a. Patient Surface

b. Side View

Figure 4-4. Typical microwave director for uniform output throughout the patient surface.

A. Bare metal antenna 5 to 10 cm in length, 3 to 4 mm in diameter.

B. Solid block of clear plastic completely enclosing the antenna.

C. Patient surface of the metal reflector. The two large dimensions make a nonadjustable 90° angle. Dimensions are approximately 1 mm thick × 10 cm wide × 15 cm long.

D. Coaxial cable lead from antenna to generator.

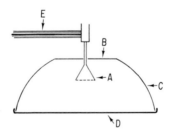

Figure 4-5. A typical microwave director for maximum focusing of energy midway between the center and the periphery.

A. Bare metal antenna 1 to 2 cm in diameter.

B. Flat surface of metal reflector (5 to 10 cm in diameter) Distance from B to D is 2 to 5 cm.

C. Curved surface of reflector (10 to 15 cm).

D. Detachable translucent plastic covering 1 mm thick.

E. Coaxial cable lead from antenna to generator.

Figure 4-6. Microwave coaxial cable.
A. Inner conductor wire.
B. Layer of insulation surrounding inner conductor.
C. Outer conductor wire (a slightly flexible hollow cylinder).
D. Outer insulation surrounding outer conductor.

In microwave treatment, the antenna is aimed at the surface of the body segment to be treated. The closer the antenna is to the skin, the greater the amount of energy available for absorption, but the smaller the area which can be treated at one time. Most clinical directors will have labeling clearly affixed indicating the approximate percent of power which can safely be used at any given distance from the typical patient. If this restriction is followed, the patient with normal sensation will perceive a comfortable *sensation* of warmth without risk of causing a dangerous deep tissue temperature rise. For directors in common clinical use, the closest distance is 2.5 cm and the greatest about 15 cm, with the director perpendicular to the skin surface. These distances permit safe use of 20 to 75 percent of available power if sensation and circulation in the tissues being exposed are within normal limits and there are no contraindications for utilization of diathermy.

Only one surface and one area can be treated at one time. A number of director sizes and shapes have been developed and used over the years. Perhaps the most widely used antenna at this time is one which is enclosed in a rectangular metallic reflector which focuses the energy over an effective area of about 215 cm². If placed 2 to 3 cm from the skin, one should anticipate that approximately the same skin area will absorb a significant amount of the radiated energy at an approximately uniform level if the contour of the skin is flat. If the director is farther away, a slightly larger area can be treated. To produce an equal temperature rise in skin or in subcutaneous tissues, the power used must be increased as distance from antenna to skin is increased.

Other directors have effective areas as small as 54 cm² or as large as 470 cm². Some are designed for low energy transfer at the center and periphery as compared to the area in between. Such directors are usually hemispherical in shape, in contrast with the square or rectangular appearance of those designed for uniform energy transfer. The hemispherical directors are intended to be centered over a bony prominence. Because of its density, bone will absorb more of any diathermy wavelength energy as compared to any soft tissue. This design of the reflector is intended for use when a rise in soft tissue temperature is needed without causing a dangerous rise in the temperature of bone that is close to the surface.

Energy of clinical microwave wavelengths (12 or 33 cm) causes a TTR in living tissue largely through stimulation of polar molecules. The more asymmetric a molecule, the more polar. Water is the most polar molecule present in the body in large quantity. Polar molecules attempt to spin or oscillate in response to the alternate buildup and collapse of high frequency electric and magnetic fields.[3,10] In microwave diathermy application, the buildup and collapse occurs hundreds of millions of times per second. Molecular oscillation cannot occur under such conditions, but intraatomic vibration can. The increase in intraatomic vibration has a net effect of tissue temperature rise. The same response takes place upon absorption of short wave diathermy wavelengths of energy, but since the frequency is so much lower, the polar molecule vibration is not the dominant factor in producing a rise in absorbing tissue temperature.

Blood has the highest water content of all normally occurring tissues. Tissues with a good blood supply will exhibit a useful TTR upon absorption of microwave energy. However, if the subcutaneous fat layer is more than 1 cm thick, the fat temperature will rise to dangerous levels (above 45°C) before there can be adequate underlying soft tissue temperature rise. If the fat layer is 2 or more cm thick, there can be no deep temperature rise at intensities at which a patient can safely tolerate.

Because of its low specific heat and because of its resistance to penetration of electric field energy, subcutaneous fat is a very real obstacle to practical utilization of *any* form of diathermy. This is especially true for microwave energy at the originally assigned frequency of 2,450 MHz.[3] It is somewhat less of an obstacle with the newer allowed frequency of 900 MHz.[3,5,6] However, very few microwave diathermies of this lower frequency are in clinical use, since this lower frequency was not approved for clinical practice until 1972.

INDICATIONS FOR APPLICATION OF THE DIATHERMIES

Utilization of diathermy is indicated for treatment when chronic pain is a problem and when causing a transient local relaxation of skeletal muscle or a local increase in circulation is likely to relieve that pain. SWD and MWD will relieve pain significantly only if a rise in temperature in tissues 1 to 3 cm deep to the skin will be effective in interrupting or arresting muscle spasm or in causing vasodilation for brief periods of time. The TTR induced in muscle by diathermy will rarely last more than one-half hour after treatment and will rarely exceed 2° to 3°C.[7,8] The interrelationships between pain, muscle spasm, vascular insufficiency, and chronic edema are discussed in Chapter 1.

SWD or MWD may be preferred to other means of causing a TTR in the following situations:

1. When a concomitant dermatological lesion is exacerbated by skin hydration
2. When tissues cannot tolerate a significant increase in weight or pressure applied externally
3. When a patient cannot or will not stay in a position necessary for application of other forms of energy
4. When a mild rise in temperature within a volume of tissue deep to subcutaneous fat is desirable
5. When the muscular or vascular malfunction lies sufficiently

deep to the skin so that conductive heating cannot bring about the desired change

6. When the patient's psychological response to his medical problem(s) is intolerant of simple treatment—when only a complicated-appearing treatment is adequate for his emotional needs

In regard to skin hydration, although the patient who receives any diathermy treatment will usually perspire in the area being treated, it is quite rare that the perspiration will be present in sufficient quantity to cause hydration of the skin. Exposure to whirlpool, Hubbard tank, paraffin bath, or to hot packs would be more likely to raise skin temperature to the point where the skin would become transiently edematous.

Patients with subacute or chronic orthopedic lesions may become less comfortable during or after treatment with hot packs or immersion in large volumes of water because of the weight and pressure of the direct contact with the energy source. Diathermy electrodes or directors are never in direct contact with the skin and hence do not cause discomfort through weight or pressure. Although the patient needs to be willing and able to stay reasonably immobile during treatment with diathermy, minor movement of the part would require less readjustment or correction than could be the case with hot packs or paraffin. Utilization of either air-spaced plate electrodes or the induction field cable make it possible to raise tissue temperatures over a larger area and volume than is practical with hot packs, infrared lamps, paraffin, or ultrasound, within the same time period. The whirlpool or Hubbard tank can be used for areas as large or larger than can be done with diathermy, but their effects do not penetrate as deeply. None of the conductive heat sources available to the physical therapist can be as effective in causing a deep TTR.

Lastly, there are some patients who cannot accept the fact that treatment with anything so common and obvious as hot packs or whirlpool can be significant in relieving their pain. However, if exposed to what is so visibly a complicated and mysterious device as a diathermy, the patient may perceive considerable pain relief.

CONTRAINDICATIONS FOR APPLICATION
OF THE DIATHERMIES

There are several major contraindications for use of the diathermies. They should never be used in the presence of any metal in the area to be treated, regardless of whether the metal is internal or external to the patient. The diathermy generator transmits high frequency, high voltage electric and magnetic field energy into the patient, which is absorbed by various tissues and hardware within its depth of penetration. The transmitted energy is converted into heat by the absorbing tissues. Any metal within the field will concentrate this energy at points (screws) or edges (plates). This will cause adjacent tissues to get very hot. Consequently, the patient should *never* be treated with diathermy while sitting on a metal stool, lying on an innerspring mattress, or touching a zipper on a pillow, nor should there be any jewelry in or near the treatment area.

It is essential if there is any scar in or near the treatment area that the therapist check with the patient and with the patient's chart to determine if there is metal deep to the scar. With the current widespread use of internal fixation of fractures, joint replacements, and so forth, the presence of metal screws, wires, and plates deep to a scar is common. War veterans may have shrapnel buried in their soft tissues. It is the therapist's responsibility to avoid the use of any form of diathermy if it is suspected or known that metal is within the area to be treated.

Watches should not be worn by the patient or therapist while a treatment is being given. In addition to the possibility of a burn, the watch can become magnetized and will not keep accurate time until it has been demagnetized. This can happen even with watches that are labeled "antimagnetic."

The most important contraindication for treatment with any diathermy unit anywhere on the body is when the patient's cardiac status is such that any kind of a cardiac pacemaker is used. The high frequency, high voltage electric field can cause the pacemaker to become erratic or to stop. It is the therapist's responsibility to know if the patient utilizes a pacemaker. The presence of a pacemaker anywhere in the treatment area, i.e. on another patient, is an absolute contraindication for the use of any form of diathermy.

SHORT WAVE DIATHERMY TECHNIQUES

Electrode Terminals

Some models of short wave diathermy (SWD) generators are designed to use any of the common electrodes: air-spaced plates, the drum, or the cable. Others are designed for use with only one or two types of electrode. The machine terminals are commonly designed so that leads from one type of electrode cannot be inserted into an oscillating circuit designed for another type of electrode. There will always be at least two machine circuit terminals to which the two electrode leads must be attached unless the apparatus is designed for only one kind of electrode, in which case there will be a permanent connection between the machine and patient circuit. Lead cables from one manufacturer will not fit the terminals of another make of generator, although usually the electrode leads are interchangeable among the various models provided by one manufacturer. The therapist must then know which electrodes belong to which diathermy generator.

Support Arms

Most models of SWD are designed for use with several types of electrodes. Air-spaced plates and the drum electrode must be supported away from the generator and close to but not in contact with the patient surface. Since there must be two air-spaced plates to complete the circuit, there must be two support arms. Each is manually adjustable as to height, angulation, and rotation at several joints. The drum electrode requires only one support arm. The cable electrode does not utilize a support arm. The electrodes are detachable from their support arms, and their respective leads from the machine terminals, by snap-fit or by spring-loaded locking mechanisms. Electrodes should never be removed from their support arms or from the machine circuit terminals while the patient circuit is energized. The patient circuit should never be energized unless electrodes have been properly positioned over a patient. If the patient circuit is energized without a subject in the circuit, the life expectancy of the machine and patient circuits will be shortened, since both circuits are designed to work within a certain impedance range.[4] Any diathermy apparatus and its accessories are expensive. With reasonable care and with daily use, such a unit should last for at least ten years.

Treatment Time

The generally accepted treatment time for exposure of one body area to SWD is twenty to thirty minutes.[7,8,10,11] There is ample documentation that significant vasodilation will have reached its peak within this length of time if the patient's circulatory system is capable of normal function. If treatment is continued for a longer period, i.e. forty-five to sixty minutes, the risk of rebound increases. Rebound is a phenomenon which may occur within the vascular tree when living tissues are exposed to energy addition or withdrawal which causes a marked rise or fall in tissue temperature. The known mechanisms are discussed in Chapter 5. The rebound phenomenon is not a desirable effect of treatment. Its occurrence is unusual in a person whose nervous and circulatory systems are capable of normal function unless treatment time exceeds thirty minutes. Before and after treatment, digital temperature measurements will provide objective evidence as to whether rebound occurred. If digital skin temperature drops after treatment, a significant amount of vasoconstriction has taken place.[7,8]

Tuning the Oscillating Circuit

Most models of SWD designed after the 1940s have automatic control of the oscillating circuit such that it permits variation in machine circuit frequency as the patient impedance changes. Change in impedance is to be expected as skin temperature rises. Several mechanisms which are used for the automatic tuning, or resonance, of the machine circuit to the patient circuit are discussed in Chapter 8. Suffice here to say that manual or automatic tuning permits more efficient energy transfer from the oscillating machine circuit to the patient. Many SWD units which have to be manually tuned are still in clinical use.

When manual tuning is necessary, after the patient and the electrodes are in position for treatment, the intensity is turned up to 30 to 40 percent of available power. Next, the control labeled "Tuning" (or "Resonance") is rotated until a maximum swing to the right occurs by the *power indicator needle*. The patient will almost always indicate he feels a sudden surge of warmth when the machine circuit is in tune. In any diathermy treatment, the patient with normal sensation should have only a mild sensation of warmth. Therefore, if after tuning the patient states the area being treated feels hot, the intensity *(not the resonance)* control should be turned down. If the patient reports only a vague sensation of warmth after the power indicator needle indicates that tuning has been accomplished, the intensity *(not the resonance)* control should be turned up. If more than 50 to 60 percent of available power is needed to produce a comfortable sensation of warmth, something is wrong with the patient circuit setup—too much or too little dielectric is a common error—or something has deteriorated within the machine circuitry or the electrodes or their leads are malfunctioning. If the therapist is satisfied that electrode positioning is proper and that the machine circuit has been tuned, and the patient is still not perceiving energy input, then professional servicing of the apparatus is indicated.

When using manually tuned apparatus it is important to remember to check the tuning again after treatment has proceeded for about five minutes. Most of the skin temperature rise that is going to occur will have taken place within a five-minute period. As skin temperature increases, impedance decreases, and the machine circuit may have to be readjusted as to frequency. If the machine circuit is not tuned and retuned, no significant amount of energy will penetrate the skin and no appreciable deep TTR will occur.

Skin Inspection

No clothing should be permitted to remain in the area to be treated. The skin should be inspected for scars or other blemishes before treatment. Any and all blemishes should be described in writing at the time of initial treatment. If there is traumatic or surgical scar tissue in the area, it is the therapist's responsibility to find out if there is any metal in or deep to the skin. If so, diathermy should not be used. Any change in appearance of any blemish after a treatment should be recorded. If this is done, the patient cannot return a week or a month later and claim the treatment caused damage. Since vasodilation is likely to occur during and after treatment, and is desirable, constricting clothing proximal to the treatment area should be loosened or removed. Likewise, the treated part should be horizontal or elevated rather than dependent, to permit the effects of gravity to aid venous return. If the treated part is dependent, edema present may be increased rather than diminished.

After skin inspection, the area to be treated should be covered with a single layer of bath toweling. This is to prevent accumulation of perspiration. If skin folds in or near the area are touching, the part should be positioned so that the folds are completely separated or additional toweling inserted so that perspiration cannot pool or accumulate.

Air-Spaced Plate Electrodes

Two plates must be used, with a segment of the patient between them, if the patient circuit is to be complete. Each plate is attached to a support arm. Each plate has its own lead cord for connection to an apparatus terminal. The lead cords should never touch each other when the patient circuit is energized. The area to be treated should be covered with a single layer of bath toweling and the plate guard placed in contact with it. Either the plate can be manually adjusted within the fixed plate guard or the plate guard can be adjusted around a fixed plate. For deepest *penetration*, the further the plate from the skin the better. For strongest *sensation* of heat, the closer the plate to the skin the better. Reasons for this fact were discussed earlier in this chapter. The plates may be equidistant or at different distances from the skin, depending upon treatment and patient needs. The plate itself should never be touched when energized. A severe electrical burn can result, especially if the contracting skin is moist.

Air-spaced plate electrodes are especially useful if one wishes to cause a TTR in both upper or both lower extremities simultaneously. Because the *circumference* of most forearms is not much larger than the *diameter* of most plates, it is usually better to position the plates on the upper arms. With a standard twenty-minute treatment, such positioning will induce transient muscle relaxation and vasodilation throughout both upper extremities and the upper trunk. Axillary skin folds must not be permitted to touch. This treatment is contraindicated in the presence of significant cardiac pathology.

Placement of one electrode on each calf or thigh will produce similar results in the lower extremities and pelvis. Care must be taken that the thighs do not touch, by positioning or by use of additional toweling. This treatment should not be used during or immediately preceding the menstrual period since there may be a pelvic temperature rise.

Very occasionally, there is need for use of air-spaced plate electrodes to encourage liquifaction of a consolidated area of lung tissue which has not been resorbed with the use of antibiotics. In this case, one plate would be applied over the anterior thorax and the other over the posterior thorax, in the area of consolidation. This treatment would be contraindicated in the presence of cardiac pathology or a history of pulmonary hemorrhage or infarct.

Most other areas of the body can be better treated with other electrodes or with other physical agents. Therefore, unless air-spaced plate electrodes are the only ones available, they are not as widely used as they were twenty years ago. If they are used, the best deep TTR will usually be obtained when the plates are as far away from the face of the plate guard as possible.

The Drum Electrode

This is probably the most commonly used of all diathermy electrodes. It is by far the easiest to apply and can be used to treat most areas of the body so long as the area to be treated is not large. Most drums can adequately treat an area from 10 to 15 by 30 to 35 cm in size.

For reasons presented earlier, a single layer of bath toweling should always be placed between the skin and the patient surface of the drum. The drum should be adjusted to follow contour as much as possible and should be as close to the toweling as possible without touching the toweling. This positioning will allow the most nearly uniform TTR and will minimize the risk of "hot-spot" formation.

The drum electrode is frequently used in treatment of chronic low back pain. The setup most often used calls for the patient to be lying prone, with the lumbar area flattened as much as possible. In the thin individual, this flattening can be accomplished by the addition of one or more pillows underneath the abdomen (*not* underneath the hips). After the toweling is in place, the hinged drum is placed so that its long dimension is at right angles to the vertical axis of the trunk. Care should be taken that the edges of the drum do not touch the pelvic brim, sacrum, or inferior ribs. Because bone is more dense than soft tissue, it will absorb more electromagnetic energy than surrounding soft tissue if the bone is within the limits of depth of penetration of the energy (2 to 3 cm deep to the skin). The spinous processes of vertebrae are rarely a hazard because only a small volume and surface of the process will be close to the patient surface of the electrode. If bone is too close, it is likely the patient will report a stronger sensation of warmth there than elsewhere. This is because both skin and periosteum are more richly supplied with thermal receptors than are other body tissues. The visible warning sign of a "hot-spot" is a discrete area of marked hyperemia. If electrode placement is not altered when this occurs, the "hot-spot" will usually evolve into a burn. Diathermy burns usually have an iceberg effect, i.e. much less shows on the surface as compared to major damage deep to the skin.

It is then apparent that the therapist must orient the patient prior to treatment that the sensation of warmth that should evolve within a treatment should be uniform rather than spotty, and that the patient should inform the therapist of any irregularity of sensation rather than try to tolerate it. Such uneven sensation is more apt to occur with either the drum or cable electrode as compared to air-spaced plates. This is because the plates are more often positioned so as to cause a TTR in a larger volume of tissue than may be the case with the drum or cable electrode.

The drum is frequently used to treat a segment of an extremity. Most often, the drum is positioned so that any three contiguous surfaces of the extremity are close to the patient surface of the drum. Thus, if a thigh were to be treated with the patient supine, the center of the drum would be facing the anterior aspect while one wing would be close to the lateral and the other wing close to the medial thigh. When any part of a lower extremity is treated with a drum, care must be taken that the non-patient surface of the electrode does not touch nearby tissue. The drum radiates energy in all directions.

Since extremity circumferences tend to be conical as well as cylindrical, it may be difficult to follow contour evenly. Because joints have bony masses near the surface, as well as numerous protuberances, it can be very difficult to avoid "hot-spots" with the drum electrode. Either air-spaced plates or the cable electrode can be utilized for a greater uniformity of TTR in an area which includes a major joint. An equal or better TTR can be produced in distal joints, i.e. ankle or wrist, with conductive heating, as discussed in Chapter 5.

Treatment of the hip area by short wave diathermy is of doubtful benefit. The hip joint is deep—above 10 to 12 cm in the average adult. This is well beyond the depth of penetration of SWD under optimal conditions. Additionally, the posterior aspect is covered by 3 cm or more of subcutaneous fat, even in a slender adult. Hence, little hip muscle or joint temperature rise can be achieved with SWD. Fortunately, there are more deeply penetrating physical agents, i.e. ultrasound, which can achieve a significant TTR at the desired depth.

The Cable Electrode

When using a cable electrode, it may be wound in either a two-dimensional or three-dimensional form. The two-dimensional form most often used is the pancake coil. The pancake consists of three or four circular turns in one plane, with a uniform spacing of 1 to 3 cm between each turn. Symmetry of the turns will minimize "hot-spot" formation as well as assure long life of a cable electrode. Symmetry is readily achieved by use of spacers at several points throughout the pancake. Spacers are usually not interchangeable among cables for different brands of SWD units, since manufacturers will differ in the thickness of the insulation covering the woven copper wire by as much as 5 mm. The lead end of that segment of the cable which makes the innermost turn must cross over other turns en route to its machine terminal. Utilization of additional insulating material at least 5 mm thick is mandatory at the point of crossover. If not used, when the high voltage current flows through the cable, a short circuit will develop. This will damage the cable beyond repair and can cause a burn in nearby living tissue. A hollow rubber sleeve is furnished, as are spacers, with each cable. The sleeve is slit lengthwise for ease of application. Any insulating material, i.e. bath toweling, may be substituted. It follows that the cable leads going from the wound cable to the machine terminals should never be allowed to touch because of the risk of causing a short circuit.

For the pancake coil to function most effectively, the innermost turn should have a diameter not to exceed 15 cm (6 inches). Apparatus not designed for use with cables may not have adequate provision for tuning, automatic or manual, if the innermost turn is larger in diameter. For the same reasons, the leads from the two ends of the turns should be approximately equal in length. A difference in lead length of up to 15 cm will usually present no problem. With practice in using the cable electrode, attention to these points will become habitual.

The pancake coil is frequently used in treatment of chronic lumbar and/or thoracic back pain. Application of a drum electrode would be less time consuming. However, the pancake coil can be applied with the patient in the hook-lying position, whereas the drum cannot. In the hook-lying position, the patient lays on his back with hips and knees sufficiently flexed so that his feet are flat on the plinth. This position minimizes lumbar lordosis. Supine or prone positioning will tend to increase lordosis, especially in the thin individual. Patients with low back pain almost always benefit from a decrease in lordosis. The drum electrode cannot be used for treatment of the back if the patient is supine or in the hook-lying position. The pancake cable is well tolerated.

The other commonly used cable winding is three dimensional. It is used in the technique with the clinical designation of "wrap-around" application. This is useful in the treatment of a segment of an extremity. Since the cable is literally wrapped around the extremity with three to five turns, good uniformity of TTR can be achieved up to a depth of about 3 cm. The turns should be at least 3 cm apart. When used with apparatus specifically designed for cable (or drum) electrodes (operating frequency = 13.56 MHz), the turns can be as much as 10 cm apart. When applied in this manner, very large areas and volumes of tissues can be treated with excellent uniformity of tissue temperature rise. Bony protuberances are no problem since additional dielectric material can be easily added between cable and skin where the cable must be positioned close to bone. Spacers should be used to insure uniform distance between turns if they are only 3 to 5 cm apart.

A major problem with use of the cable electrode, with both the pancake coil and the wrap-around technic, is the amount of linen which must be used to provide an adequate dielectric between the cable and the skin. For best depth of penetration of energy from the cable, the dielectric thickness should be at least 1 cm (cable on body) to 1.5 to 2 cm if body weight is compressing the dielectric on the cable. Bath toweling should always be placed next to the skin, just as for any SWD treatment. The rest of the necessary space can be filled with any dry linen. Only the innermost layer needs to be changed with each treatment. Purchase and maintenance of the requisite linen can be a major cost if use of the cable electrode is high. Also, it takes time and patience on the part of the therapist to properly position the linen and to effectively wind the cable to fit the area to be treated. Many therapists will not take the time to do a good job, especially if they do not realize that at times the cable electrode can be more effective than any other means of causing a deep TTR in a large cylindrical volume of tissue.

Since the core of the cable consists of many small-diameter

strands of copper wire, and since it is wound in many different shapes for treatment of various areas, it is wise to check the cable regularly for deterioration. One easy way to do this is to plug in both ends of the cable to the appropriate apparatus terminals and lay the cable on a plinth in the form of an elongated **U**. The distance between the arms of the **U** should not exceed their distance apart at the terminals. Place appropriate dielectric material on the cable so that a subject can sit or lie on a small segment of both arms of the cable at about the midpoint of the **U**. The subject should feel a mild sensation of warmth at 30 to 50 percent of available power when the apparatus is tuned to the subject's impedance (either manually or automatically, as the case may be). If more than 50 percent of available power is needed to produce the sensation, the cable is defective and should be replaced. Another and simpler way to check for early signs of deterioration is to touch the cable, with no intervening dielectric, immediately *after* a full twenty-minute treatment. If it is hot to touch anywhere throughout its length, either the cable is becoming defective or the setup was less than optimal. If the cable tips are hot, they are no longer fitting properly into the machine terminals. Reasons for the overheating of the cable tips should be explored by the institution's electrician.

Thus, all three types of electrodes in common use with SWD have advantages and disadvantages. If diathermy is used daily, it is probably wise to have all three kinds of electrodes available, along with generators of each operating frequency (13.56 and 27.12 MHz).

MICROWAVE DIATHERMY TECHNIQUES

Microwave energy in medical use has a much higher frequency and shorter wavelength as compared to short wave diathermy. On the basis of physical laws discussed in Chapter 2, one might expect the depth of penetration would be less for microwave energy. This is *not* so for at least two reasons. First, the difference in wavelength (SWD at 22 and 11 m, MWD at 33 and 12 cm) is not great when one considers the wavelength range of the electromagnetic spectrum as a whole, from millions of kilometers to tenths of

Angstrom units. Secondly, subcutaneous fat is as much or more of an obstacle for penetration of microwave as it is for shortwave energy. It is true, however, that because microwave energy can be beamed or focused toward the part to be treated, if the subcutaneous fat layer is 0.5 cm or less, MWD can cause a significant TTR up to a depth of 5 cm in soft tissue.[5,6] The focusing allows more of the energy to strike the skin perpendicularly. This minimizes scatter and enhances absorption. Short wave energy cannot be focused with any practical clinical technic.

Areas to be Treated

Microwave energy can be beamed to only one surface at a time. For uniformity of TTR, the contour of that surface must be flat. Otherwise, that area closest to the director will exhibit a substantially greater rise in temperature as compared to those as little as 1 cm more distant. Bath toweling on the skin is not necesssary because the energy transmitted to the patient is absorbed by a larger volume of tissue than is the case with SWD of equal intensity per unit area, provided the layer of subcutaneous fat is less than 5 mm in thickness. The deeper penetration of MWD under these conditions results in a smaller surface temperature rise and hence less perspiration production. Under optimal conditions, SWD will cause a significant TTR to a depth of 3 cm, whereas MWD will cause a rise to a depth of 5 cm.[3,5,6]

Machine Circuit Warmup

It takes considerably more time for an MWD generator to modify house current into useful quantities of microwave energy than it does for an SWD generator to convert line current into short wave energy. All commercially available microwave units require a minimum warmup time of at least two minutes. As the unit continues to be used, the warmup time gradually increases, up to five minutes. The control panel will usually have some sort of indicator light to let the operator know when the machine circuit is ready to deliver a significant amount of microwave energy. Only then should the patient circuit be energized. Most therapists will spend the 2- to 5-minute warmup time positioning the director and the patient for safe and effective treatment.

Intensity

Intensity needed should be governed by the patient sensation of warmth. This should be mild, *never hot.* No tuning, automatic or manual, is possible because of the physical characteristics of the multiple cavity anode, which is the heart of the oscillating circuit in microwave generators.

Positioning of the Director

Depending upon the volume of soft tissue which is to absorb microwave energy, the patient surface of the antenna will be placed 2 to 15 cm from the skin. Each director should be clearly labeled by the manufacturer as to the average percent of power which is safe to use (no risk of overheating any soft tissue) at any given distance within the recommended range. The metallic reflector should be visually aligned so as to be as nearly perpendicular to the skin surface as is practical. In general, rectangularly shaped reflectors are designed for nearly uniform energy output throughout the reflector area, being only slightly less at the periphery as compared to the center.[3] The hemispherically shaped reflectors are designed for minimal energy output in the center 2 to 3 cm, with a band of high energy output several centimeters wide circumscribing the center area and diminishing again toward the periphery.

Neither the antenna nor the reflector should ever be touched by any living tissue when the antenna is transmitting this very high voltage, very high frequency energy. A severe electrical burn can result, especially if the contacting skin is moist.

Indications and contraindications for application of microwave energy are the same as for short wave energy and were given earlier in this chapter.

SUMMARY

Short wave and microwave diathermy energy can cause a deeper tissue temperature rise than any form of infrared energy. Consequently, in the management of clinical problems where a deep temperature rise is more likely to give pain relief, diathermy may be the treatment of choice. Reasons for penetration of this kind of energy under optimal conditions to a depth of 3 to 5 cm are discussed.

Each type of electrode and each frequency available has advantages and disadvantages over the others, so that the most effective treatment for the individual problem may require thoughtful selection of the best treatment parameters.

There are more *contraindications* for the use of either short wave or microwave energy than for any form of infrared application. Operation of diathermy generators safely and efficiently is complex. The risk of causing a burn is greater because there is less of a skin temperature rise and more of a deep tissue temperature rise. There are more thermal receptors in the skin than in underlying tissue. Hence, neither the patient nor the therapist may be aware of a dangerous subcutaneous temperature rise until pathological heating has occurred.

Diathermy in any form should never be used when there is a cardiac pacemaker anywhere in the clinical area, nor should it be used when there is any external or internal metal within or close to the field of this penetrating high voltage energy.

DEMONSTRATIONS FOR STUDENTS
I. To Demonstrate Differences in Temperature Rise of Oil and Water Depending Upon Type of Short Wave Diathermy Electrode Used

    A. Procure one two-liter and one three-liter glass or other non-conducting beaker. *Do not use metal beakers.* Fill the smaller beaker with tap water. Insert it into the larger beaker, letting the bottom of the small beaker rest on a folded dry washcloth or other insulating material so that the two beakers cannot touch. Fill the larger beaker with either paraffin or mineral oil, allowing a centimeter or so margin between the top of the small beaker and the oil level in the large beaker.

    B. The beakers and their contents should be allowed to sit at room temperature for at least one hour. Then, measure and record the temperature of each liquid.

    C. Wrap a cable electrode snugly around the outside of the

large beaker, using at least three turns with at least a 3 cm distance between each turn, holding this position with cable spacers.

D. Energize the cable at 50 percent available power. Tune the cable circuit if the generator requires manual tuning. Let the current flow for twenty minutes. After turning the power off, remeasure the temperature of the oil and of the water. *Do not* attempt to measure temperature while the power is on. The reading will be erroneous because of the magnetic field, and if an electronic thermometer was used, the probe and measuring circuits could be damaged beyond repair. Record the "posttreatment" temperatures.

E. The next day, repeat steps A through D, using a drum electrode designed for the same generator. Note the differences in temperature change. The change in water temperature will be smaller because the beakers were not exposed circumferentially. Likewise, the change in oil temperature will be smaller, for the same reason, but the difference will be greater for the water.

F. The next day, repeat steps A through D, using air-spaced plate electrodes designed for the same generator. It will be observed that the increase in oil temperature will be much greater and the increase in water temperature will be much less than was the case for either the drum or cable electrodes. This should help one to remember that where the energy coming from the electrode is primarily electric field, essentially no energy is transferred to the inner beaker as a primary process, whereas when the energy coming from the electrode is roughly 50-50 electric and magnetic, a significantly greater amount penetrates to the contents of the inner beaker and hence produces a greater deep tissue temperature rise.

G. Hence, one can conclude that when properly applied, the drum or cable electrode is more apt to give a greater deep tissue temperature rise as compared to air-spaced plates. The latter are more apt to heat subcutaneous fat layers to dangerous levels with a minimal rise in underlying muscle temperature.

II. To Demonstrate Significant Differences in Deep Tissue Temperature Rise Depending Upon Whether the Frequency Used Is 27.12 MHz or 13.56 MHz

A. The phantom setup should be as described in Demonstration I, steps A through D.

B. Use only cable electrodes, one for a generator of each of the above-assigned operating frequencies.

C. It will be noted that the temperature rise in the two beakers will vary on the basis of operating frequency. The generator operating at the higher frequency and shorter wavelength will produce a greater oil temperature and a lower water temperature rise as compared to the results when the lower frequency, longer wavelength unit is used, *if the energy added per unit volume* is equal in the two cases.

D. To insure that energy added is equal in both cases, first apply a cable electrode to a human subject. The coil can be wrapped around an upper arm or thigh, utilizing the standard treatment technics detailed within the chapter. Turn up the intensity until the subject reports a mild sensation of warmth. Note the percent of available power needed to achieve that sensation. Repeat, using the other generator on the contralateral area approximately one hour later. Note the percent of power needed to achieve equivalent sensation. Use these two power settings to achieve the most reliable results when measuring temperature change within the phantom.

E. A major reason for the difference in results observed when comparing the two frequencies is that the relationships among capacitance, inductance, and reactance vary with the SWD frequencies. The lower frequency achieves a more nearly 50-50 relationship between electric and magnetic field production. It is the magnetic field that is the major factor in water temperature rise and the electric field that is the major factor in oil temperature rise.

F. One can then conclude that if one wishes to achieve the best possible deep TTR with the cable (or drum) electrode, one should use the lower frequency.

III. To Demonstrate That with Both SWD and MWD Electrical Energy Is Transmitted to the Patient and That MWD Frequencies Can be Focused Whereas SWD Frequencies Cannot

A. Position a subject for treatment of any area.

B. Use any SWD generator in the standard fashion outlined within the chapter. Turn up intensity until the subject reports a mild sensation of warmth.

C. Another individual should then hold a 20 to 40 watt incandescent bulb or fluorescent light tube close to but not touching the energized electrode. *Do not* touch any metal on the bulb or tube. The bulb will light up.

D. This should indicate that a strong electric and/or magnetic field is present in the air around the electrode. If intensity is varied, the amount of light will vary in direct proportion. Intensity should be controlled by a third individual.

E. Move the light source along the electrode leads and around the generator. The bulb will stay lit, indicating the SWD generator emits significant energy in all directions.

F. Repeat steps A through D with any MWD generator. Note that the bulb will light up only when the bulb is between the director and the subject. As soon as the light source is moved to the surface of the director that is away from the subject, the light goes out. If moved along the antenna lead toward the generator, the bulb will not light up.

G. One can then conclude that MWD energy can be focused whereas SWD energy cannot, and that the transmission lead from generator to antenna is superior in insulation quality as compared to SWD.

REFERENCES

1. *Dorland's Illustrated Medical Dictionary,* 24th ed. Philadelphia, Saunders, 1965.
2. *Webster's Seventh New Collegiate Dictionary.* Springfield, Mass., Merriam, 1971.
3. Licht, S.: *Therapeutic Heat and Cold,* 2nd ed. New Haven, Licht, 1965.

4. Hall, E.L.: Diathermy generators. *Arch Phys Med Rehabil, 33*:28-36, 1952.

5. Lehmann, J.F. et al.: Modification of heating patterns with 2456 and 900 Mc energy. *Arch Phys Med Rehabil, 45*:555-63, 1964.

6. Lehmann, J.F. et al.: Muscle heating with 915 Mc microwave diathermy. *Arch Phys Med Rehabil, 51*:147-51, 1970.

7. Abramson, D.I. et al.: Change in blood flow, oxygen uptake and tissue temperature with shortwave diathermy. *Am J Phys Med, 39*:87-95, 1960.

8. Downey, J.A. et al.: Vascular response in the forearm to heating by shortwave diathermy. *Arch Phys Med Rehabil, 51*:354-7, 1970.

9. Pringsheim, P.: *Fluorescence and Phosphorescence.* New York, Interscience, 1949.

10. Glasser, O. (Ed.): *Medical Physics,* Volume I. Chicago, Year Bk Med, 1945, pp. 1091-2.

11. Scott, P.: *Clayton's Electrotherapy and Actinotherapy,* 5th ed. London, Balliere, Tyndall and Cassell, 1965.

Chapter 5

THE INFRARED ENERGIES

INTRODUCTION

THEORETICALLY, ANY OBJECT whose temperature is greater than 0° Kelvin (−273°C) is radiating energy of wavelengths classified as infrared. Practical clinical sources include cold and hot packs, the whirlpool (and Hubbard tank), paraffin baths, steam cabinets, and infrared lamps. The physiological effects are similar for all these forms of energy if the temperature of the energy reaching the patient is higher than that of the skin or subcutaneous tissue which absorbs the energy. If the temperature of the source is lower than that of nearby skin, a different pattern of reaction will take place because thermal energy always flows from a source of relatively high to relatively low temperature. Therefore, when the patient is exposed to an object whose temperature is lower than that of his skin, energy in the form of heat will flow from the patient toward that object. The local and whole-body response to loss of heat is different from the response to addition of heat.

NORMAL TISSUE TEMPERATURES

Normal human core (whole-body) temperature is 37 ± 1°C.[1] Skin and other tissue temperatures in the head, neck, and trunk are usually quite close to those values except in extreme environments. However, more distally in the extremities, normal skin and subcutaneous temperatures steadily decline, to a greater extent in the lower as compared to the upper limbs. The normal difference in arm and leg temperature is largely the result of the greater effects of gravity on circulation in the lower extremities resulting in greater circulatory stagnation.

In the normal individual in a temperate environment, subcutaneous temperature will be 1° to 2°C higher than that of overlying skin. Tissue closer to bone has a higher temperature than that close to skin. Under baseline conditions (no clothing, horizontally at rest for at least thirty minutes in a room whose temperature is constant at 21° to 22°C with humidity stable at 50 percent) a fingertip temperature of 32° and a toetip temperature of 28° would be the lower limits of normal skin temperature.[2]

During a twenty-four-hour period, the normal individual experiences fluctuation in distal extremity temperature, especially in the skin, in response to ambient temperature, caloric intake, and degree of skeletal muscle activity. Fluctuation on the order of ± 5°C is common in the fingers. They are usually exposed and normally play a major role in release or conservation of heat in maintaining core temperature. Fluctuation on the order of ± 2°C is more common in toes. They are usually encased in shoes.

If *local* tissue temperature reaches 45°C for an appreciable length of time, necrosis occurs from thermal damage. If local tissue temperature reaches 13°, necrosis occurs from intracellular ice crystal formation. These limits can be reached with brief exposure to a great temperature differential or with prolonged exposure to a lesser differential. *Core* temperatures above 42° or below 25°C are likely to be fatal, even if that temperature is maintained for only a short period of time.[1] The normal human has many mechanisms of local, nervous system, and humoral control to avoid such drastic changes in both local and core temperatures.[3,4]

Alteration in blood volume and flow rate are the major mechanisms by which the normal body strives to maintain core and peripheral temperatures within tolerable limits. The local reactions, nervous system, and humoral controls all have roles in variation of vasomotor tension. In general, when energy absorption causes a *local* tissue temperature rise (TTR), as would be the case with application of the diathermies, the infrareds, and ultrasound, vasodilation will occur transiently. If energy is withdrawn (cold application), vasoconstriction will occur transiently. A significant TTR occurs when the circulating blood does not dissipate energy as fast as it is being added. If the local temperature rises

and then levels off, the blood flow is then adequate to disseminate the added energy as fast as it is absorbed. If the local temperature drops (cold application), thermal energy is being withdrawn from the area faster than warmer blood can flow in from
other body areas.

CLINICAL SKIN TEMPERATURE PATTERNS

In the normal adult, when energy is absorbed at a comfortable
rate, maximum dilation will be achieved with a twenty- to thirty-
minute exposure to any form of infrared or the diathermies. The
anticipated skin temperature curve is a rather rapid rise for the
first ten minutes, followed by a plateau for another ten to fifteen
minutes, and either a rise or a drop if treatment continues beyond
thirty minutes.[7] The initial rise is due to energy being absorbed
at a faster rate than the gradually dilating arteriolar vessels can
bring cooler blood into the area. The plateau occurs when there
has been enough dilation so that a sufficient amount of cooler
blood is coming into the area being treated for energy to be carried away as fast as it is being added. If the arterial vessels continue to dilate further, they may reach the point at which absorbed
energy is carried away faster than it is added, at which time local
temperature will start to drop toward the resting level. More
often, the local arteries will have reached their maximum capacity
for dilation at some point between a ten- and 20-minute exposure
to thermal energy and will then undergo a rebound vasoconstriction. Because energy is no longer disseminated as efficiently as
before, the tissue temperature will rapidly increase.

If an infrared source is applied to cause a TTR, another anticipated reaction is uniform cutaneous vasodilation due to local
histamine release. This leads to a gradual change in skin color—
hyperemia—which is readily apparent in Caucasian or Mongolian
skin. If any form of diathermy is used to cause the TTR, one
would not expect to see as striking an amount of hyperemia because a considerable amount of this energy should be absorbed
deep to the skin. Because diathermy wavelengths are longer than
those for infrared, less energy is absorbed per unit *volume* of tis-

sue. Therefore, the visible reaction will not be as great *(see Chapters 2 and 4 for details)*.

MOTTLING

If exposure to and absorption of energy which causes a TTR continues appreciably beyond thirty minutes, a rebound vasomotor reaction usually occurs. If it does, and if it is ignored, an injurious TTR is likely to take place. This is more likely to take place with any form of infrared than with any form of diathermy because more energy is absorbed by superficial tissues when infrared is applied.[7]

The first warning that such a harmful reaction may take place is the appearance of mottling. In this situation, the skin will become abnormally white in patches, interlaced with angry red blotches. If this reaction appears, energy addition should be discontinued for that treatment period, or the rate at which energy is being added should be diminished. If no adjustment is made after mottling appears, a burn is likely to result. Once mottling has occurred, the skin is apt to retain its unique appearance for one-half to several hours after removal from the energy source. The angry red and pallescent patches gradually return to normal color as skin temperature reaches normal limits.

When energy is added with the intent of causing a TTR, one of the first tissue reactions to that change in environment is local release of histamine or histaminelike substances. Histamine is a potent vasodilator. Its release is seen clinically as hyperemia—a reddening of the skin. If the temperature change is fast and drastic, histamine is released in large quantities. Its massive release can cause a transient paralysis of the nerve supply to arteriole-sized vessels, forcing them to stay in maximum vasodilation until the histamine has been partially resorbed or metabolized. Recovery from the vessel paralysis may take several hours. Cells in the temperature-threatened area do not release histamine at a uniform rate. When arterial muscle is paralyzed in dilation, the associated capillaries are patent and engorged, yielding an angry red color. If the energy absorbing cells do not release enough histamine to cause paralysis but the cutaneous blood supply has been maximally dilated for a prolonged period, the muscle in vessel walls can go into spasm. This leads to local vasoconstriction. with subsequent closing of associated capillaries. When the vasoconstriction is extreme, patches of pallor are plainly visible. These reactions result in the mottled appearance of the skin.

CIRCULATORY IMPAIRMENT AND INFRARED

If the patient to whom energy is being added has a circulatory impairment, a TTR to safe limits may occur much more rapidly than would be the case if his circulation was normal. This is largely due to the fact that when flow is impaired and energy is added, the heated blood is not replaced with cooler blood as quickly as with normal circulation. Thus, when adding energy in the presence of known circulatory problem, the intensity should be lower than otherwise. A commonly used technic in the known presence of a circulatory problem is "reflex-heating." In this technic, energy is added in an area remote to the site where a TTR is desired. Since most chronic circulatory impairments are more severe in the distal portions of the extremities and more severe in the lower extremities, the low back is frequently the site of choice for "reflex-heating." The degree of TTR in the distal lower extremities is considerably less than if energy were added directly to the involved problem area. The distal arterial vessels are more likely to be able to achieve enough dilation under these conditions of remote heating to safely dissipate the energy being added. Conversely, if the local TTR is too great, the local arterial vessels could go into spasm, vasoconstriction would occur and serious tissue damage (burn) could be the result. Since any form of infrared will be less penetrating than any form of diathermy, the risk of skin damage with the application of infrared can be greater than with diathermy. However, cutaneous sensation is much more sensitive than that of underlying fat or muscle, because of the greater number of sensory receptors of all kinds, so the patient is more apt to be aware of a dangerous TTR if it affects the skin.

HOT PACKS

Hot packs are a very widely used form of infrared, with transfer of energy from source to patient primarily by conduction.

They are inexpensive, easy to apply, and highly effective in relieving pain caused by superficial muscle spasm.

Hot packs in their present form came into use in the 1940s, with development of suitable thermostatically controlled water heaters and development of the pack itself. Some kinds of silicon dioxide (SiO_2) are very hygroscopic. Each molecule of the "sand" used in these packs has the capacity to absorb approximately seventeen molecules of water. This sand is contained in a woven fabric which is tight enough to hold the sand, but loose enough to admit water. When immersed in water, the pack swells to several times its dry size. The affinity of this special sand for water is so great that, when removed from water, it takes from three days to a week for the pack to dry. The individual pack is divided into pouches of about $15 \times 5 \times 3$ cm when dry. They are supplied in various sizes, having as few as five and as many as thirty pouches in one pack, for application to any and all neck, trunk, and extremity segments. The division into pouches gives a reasonable degree of flexibility so that the wet pack can approximate body contour. The pack will not leak sand unless the fabric is ruptured. With reasonable care in handling, the pack should last for five years or more.

The Water Heating Unit

The standard stainless steel container for heating the water comes in many sizes, from that needed to hold three standard size packs (twelve pouches, divided into two rows of six each) up to containers large enough to hold twenty-five packs, each with thirty-six pouches. Depending upon container size, there will be one or more heating units in the bottom of the container. The packs are stored in racks which hold the packs vertically and are completely covered with water. When properly placed in the container, the pack never touches the heating unit. If it does, the fabric will scorch or burn and result in a sand leak. If this happens, the water becomes turbid, and the pack should be discarded.

The heating unit can be adjusted to maintain water temperature set for anywhere between 65° and 90°C. It is recommended that a good waterproof and relatively unbreakable thermometer be kept in the pack console. The heating unit can malfunction and cause the water temperature to go up or down beyond the practical temperature range. The thermometer should be read at least twice daily.

Precautions When Using Hot Packs

No one can tolerate direct contact with water at 65°C without tissue damage. Consequently, insulating bath toweling is standardly used between skin and pack. Toweling on the side of the pack away from the patient will also help to minimize heat loss from pack to room air. If initial pack temperature is lower than 65°C, by the end of the standard twenty-minute treatment the patient is likely to have a cold, clammy sensation, which will not encourage muscle relaxation. A reasonable rule of thumb for a first exposure to hot packs, if stored at that temperature, is three layers of bath toweling between packs and skin. If initial storage was at 90°C, there should be at least six layers of insulating toweling. The above suggestions are for when the pack is lying on the patient. If the patient is lying on the pack, the amount of toweling needed may need to be more than doubled, in compensation for body weight compressing the toweling.

Direct contact with water at these temperatures can also burn the pack handler. Therefore, the pack should be removed from the container with tongs, grasping the pack tabs designed for this purpose. The pack should be held out of water until the excess has dripped off (about thirty seconds) to avoid soaking the insulating toweling. The layer of towel next to skin must be dry. Otherwise, a burn can result. If the patient complains at any time during the treatment that the sensation is more than comfortably warm, more toweling should be added. If the patient reports no sensation of warmth within two or three minutes after the pack has been applied, one or more layers of toweling should be removed.

In any case, it is the therapist's responsibility to inspect the skin in the area to be treated, before, during, and after treatment, regardless of patient statement of sensation. Any blemish on the skin before treatment should be described and recorded. The anticipated skin reaction from the standard treatment is that within five minutes the patient's skin will be warm to touch, with or without the appearance of hyperemia. If the hyperemia is an angry red, or if mottling has occurred, more toweling *must* be added, or the pack removed, to prevent a burn. Ideally, the first time the patient receives a hot pack treatment, the skin should be reinspected every five minutes throughout the treatment period. Once that patient's reaction to the treatment is established, on subsequent treatment, skin inspection prior to treatment and five minutes later may be adequate.

If the patient is emotionally disturbed, has a neurological deficit, or is on medication which could impair sensation, regular skin inspection during each treatment is mandatory. Any lesion resulting from the treatment is the therapist's responsibility, regardless of patient behavior during treatment.

Because of the large volume of bath towels and other linen needed if the clinic has much demand for use of hot packs, many departments have installed automatic washers and dryers. Over a period of several years, this cost will be more than returned by the savings in commercial laundry bills and lower investment in the actual numbers of towels needed by the department.

THE PARAFFIN BATH

The paraffin bath has been in clinical use longer than the hot pack. It is especially useful for pain relief in *chronic* orthopedic lesions, such as in rheumatoid, osteo-, or mixed arthritis, involving joints distal to the elbow or knee.

The contents of the paraffin bath are actually a mixture of paraffin and paraffin oil, mineral oil, or petroleum jelly. Perhaps the most widely used mixture for a standard-sized upper extremity bath is 25 Kg of solid paraffin to 1 liter of paraffin oil. The paraffin is a solid at room temperature and is supplied in slabs weighing 4 to 5 Kg. This paraffin liquifies when stored at temperatures above 40°C. Hence, it is placed in a thermostatically controlled stainless steel container of suitable dimensions to immerse an arm (up to and covering the elbow) or a leg (up to the knee). The other ingredient is added to the bath to make it easier to remove solidified paraffin from hairy skin. If the bath is intended for upper extremity use, most clinics set the temperature within the range of 52° to 58°C. If primarily for lower extremity use, the temperature is usually within the 45 to 52 degree range.

Physical Differences Between Paraffin and Water

On might immediately wonder how a patient can tolerate immersion of a body segment into paraffin at these temperatures when it was previously stated that heating of normal tissue to 45°C is likely to cause irreversible damage. There are several physical reasons why paraffin, but not water, can safely come into contact with skin at these higher temperatures. One difference is in the quantity of thermal energy released per degree drop in temperature by water as compared to paraffin. The amount of energy needed to raise the temperature of water one degree is nearly double that needed to raise the temperature of paraffin. The specific heat (S.H.) of water is arbitrarily set at 1.0. The S.H. of clinically used paraffin is approximately 0.65. The S.H. of paraffin oil, mineral oil, and petroleum jelly is about 0.45. When cooling, therefore, less energy is released by these liquids.

Secondly, when living tissue is immersed in the bath, the paraffin in contact with the skin cools to a solid almost instantaneously because of the low skin temperature. This one or two millimeter layer of solidified paraffin now acts as a thermal insulator so that the surrounding liquid paraffin, which is of higher temperature, can no longer transmit as much thermal energy to the skin. A small volume of air also frequently becomes trapped between the skin and the solidified paraffin, especially upon repeated movement of the segment into and out of the paraffin. The trapped air acts as additional insulation.

For both of the above reasons, and possibly more, the starting temperature of the liquid paraffin mixture can be higher than if the applied liquid were water.

Physiological Differences Between the Paraffin Bath and Water

The next question might well be, why not substitute use of water at a lower temperature. This is done with both the whirlpool and Hubbard tank. Why bother to have both whirlpool and paraffin available? It is the clinical experience of many therapists and physicians that the patient with a *chronic* orthopedic lesion will usually perceive a greater and longer-lasting pain relief when the paraffin bath can be used as the source for adding thermal energy, as compared to water.

The reasons for this are not known. There is a useful working hypothesis. The paraffin close to the skin is a solid and a very effective insulator, especially if the solid layer is built up by repeated immersion to a thickness of more than 5 mm. The net result is that the cutaneous receptors are cut off from all extrinsic stimuli except the thermal stimulus. This enables the local cutaneous sensory system to be maximally flooded with thermal input. If one accepts the gate control theory of pain and pain relief (Chapter 1), optimal conditions are set up for pain relief. Furthermore, the insulating capability of paraffin diminishes heat loss by evaporation (in the area where the paraffin is applied). The end result is a greater local TTR, a more pronounced hyperemia, and pain relief which lasts for an hour or more.

It is not practical, however, to apply paraffin to the more proximal body segments, nor is it recommended for use when local circulation is impaired. The whirlpool (or Hubbard tank) then becomes more practical and safer.[7]

Technics of Application of Paraffin

Two technics are in common use when applying paraffin. One is usually called the "dip and wrap" technic. The distal extremity is slowly dipped into the hot liquid and withdrawn. This is repeated until a glove of solidified paraffin of 5 to 10 mm has been built up. The number of dips required will depend largely on the temperature differential between the skin and the liquid paraffin. The hotter the paraffin, the more dips needed to make an effective glove. When the glove is adequate, the segment enclosed by the glove is inserted into a loosely fitting plastic bag and then into an insulating fabric several layers thick. Paper toweling may be substituted for the plastic bag and bath toweling for the fabric bag. Any cloth which must be laundered should not come into contact with paraffin. It is difficult to separate one from the other. After the part is adequately insulated, the patient is allowed to rest comfortably for about twenty minutes. The paraffin glove is then removed and saved for reuse after reheating; whatever additional treatment is needed is then done. The skin will invariably be moist, supple, and hyperemic.

If mottling is present to a significant extent, the number of dips used at the next treatment should be diminished. Mottling is more apt to appear with treatment by paraffin than with treatment by any other form of infrared. This is due to the initial liquid temperature and to the extreme insulating capacity of paraffin, even at room temperature.

The other widely used technic of paraffin application is called "dip and leave in." The dipping procedure is as was described for the "dip and wrap" technic. After a thick glove of solidified paraffin has been built up, the distal segment and its glove are re-immersed in the constant temperature bath for a fifteen-to twenty-minute period. The patient should be seated comfortably during the "leave in" period. With this technic, the anticipated skin and subcutaneous TTR will be higher during and for a longer period of time after treatment. Therefore, it is recommended that bath temperature not exceed 52°C (hand) or 45°C (foot).

Precautions

The risk of burn is greater with paraffin application as compared to hot pack use, especially with the "dip and leave in" procedure. Therefore it is recommended that an easily readable thermometer be immersed in the liquid paraffin before each treatment. Until the thermometer stem warms up to a higher temperature than that at which paraffin solidifies, a coating will form on the stem and give a false low reading, by as much as 5°C. It is also recommended that the thermometer stem be placed deep in the bath and kept moving until the reading is stable. The heating units are in the bottom and the paraffin is frequently hotter toward the bottom of the bath.

The thermostats on paraffin baths are usually reliable, but they can fail. There is an additional danger with paraffin, that of a flash fire if a malfunctioning thermostat raises the paraffin temperature above 85°C. The paraffin and other ingredients all have flash points below the temperature at which water boils. Therefore, a working fire extinguisher should always be near but not too close to the paraffin unit. It should be of the CO_2 type rather than one of those in which water is a major constituent.

Because of the strain placed on cutaneous and subcutaneous circulation by application of paraffin, many therapists are reluctant to use it on lower extremities. Circulation is always less efficient in the lower as compared to the upper limb, and a majority of arthritic patients are of an age where they will have an appreciable circulatory impairment affecting the blood flow in the calf and foot. Hence, it is recommended that a separate bath, set at a lower temperature (48° to 52°C), be used.

Cleaning the Paraffin Bath

In normal usage, perspiration, dirt, and other skin debris will accumulate because of the immersion in the liquid paraffin. Water and most of the debris will settle to the bottom, since paraffin is of low density. Most baths will have some kind of perforated cover between the tank bottom and the immersion area. The heating elements are never open, so they cannot be touched, but the liquid near the bottom is always hotter, and the bottom itself is very hot to touch. Since the top several millimeters of the paraffin is usually solid, because of prolonged exposure to room air, the debris and water at the bottom are not usually visible to the therapist or patient.

If the bath is in repeated daily use, it must be taken out of service and cleaned about every six months. This is a two- or three-day procedure. The liquid paraffin does not drain out easily because of instant solidification at exposure to room temperatures. If an attempt is to be made to salvage some of the paraffin, it is common to add several tablespoons of powdered boric acid to the liquid. This will tend to pool the accumulated water. If the draining paraffin is run through a cheesecloth seive, most of the debris can be collected and discarded. The last several centimeters of sludge at the bottom should always be discarded. Mechanical scraping of the sides and bottom, followed by scrubbing with a fat solvent, will complete the cleaning. Alcohol, tolune, benzene, carbon tetrachloride, and ether are all useful for the scrubbing. All except alcohol are also highly volatile and toxic to humans. Hence, the room where this is done must be well ventilated, and smoking should be prohibited.

Debris accumulation can be kept to a minimum by thorough washing of the part to be treated, including rinsing and drying, before immersion.

Treatment by means of the paraffin bath is inevitably messy, even with careful technic. Some scraps of solidified paraffin will always reach the floor. This can be a major hazard because solidified paraffin is very slippery to walk on. The floor around the bath should be scraped at least at the end of each day and lightly scrubbed with alcohol or other fat solvent.

HOT MOIST AIR

Although not in widespread use because of equipment cost for safe and efficient utilization, if water is heated to form steam and the cooling vapor is transmitted to the trunk, hot moist air is a very effective way of inducing "reflex heating" to the extremities. The water temperature is thermostatically controlled so that the vapor reaching the patient's skin is readily adjusted within the range of 70° to 90°C. This will produce a strong hyperemia in all exposed skin and induce a distal extremity skin temperature rise of 5° to 10°C. Skin temperature does not return to pretreatment levels for up to six hours if ambient temperature is reasonably constant. Rise in body temperature is rare and not desirable. If it occurs, the patient's thermoregulatory mechanisms are not functioning adequately and treatment should be discontinued.

Practical and commercially available equipment consists of a stainless steel plinth of usual dimensions to which is attached a foldable platform extension large enough to hold the water heating unit. This hood-shaped unit is designed to roll freely into position over the supine or prone patient.

Technic of Application

The patient is placed on the padded plinth with all but essential clothing removed. The heating unit is then rolled into position over the trunk area. Plastic curtains attached to the inverted U-shaped hood are then tucked around the neck and shoulders, trunk, and hips. The heating unit is turned on. Within five minutes, an adequate quantity of hot water vapor fills the enclosed space. The heating unit is left running at the desired temperature for twenty to forty minutes. Pain due to orthopedic trauma (such as muscle spasm) is usually reduced with the shorter treatment time. Chronic arterial vasospasm usually responds better to a lower temperature and longer treatment time. If the room temperature is over 28°C, administration of salt tablets during or after treatment may be indicated since sweating will be profuse. Most patients go to sleep during the treatment. After treatment, the patient must be thoroughly dried and kept in a draft-free area for at least one-half hour. As a precautionary measure, it is recommended that for the first several treatments the patient's oral temperature, blood pressure, and toetip skin temperature be recorded before and after treatment.

The authors are unaware of any definitive study comparing attempts at pain relief by hot moist air and with any other form of infrared energy. If there is a significant difference, it may be due to the fact that a greater number of cutaneous thermal receptors are receiving maximum stimulation, resulting in thorough muscle relaxation and reduction in vasomotor tone, with exposure of a large part of the trunk to hot moist air.

INFRARED LAMPS AND BAKERS

As with the application of hot packs or a paraffin bath, when one uses an infrared lamp (IRL), a 5° to 10°C skin temperature rise is anticipated in the area of application. Infrared lamps and bakers have the advantage of being able to cause a superficial TTR in an area where the patient cannot tolerate the weight of a hot pack or where a skin lesion precludes significant temporary skin hydration. Furthermore, it is easier to control intensity of energy absorption with an IRL or baker as compared to the paraffin bath. Finally, the quantity of linen necessary when radiant heat is used, as compared to conductive heating, is negligible.

Despite the above advantages, radiant heat is not in common use at this time. It does not give as effective pain relief as either hot packs or paraffin. The reasons for this have not been explored in detail.[7] However, speculation, on the basis of the gate control theory of pain relief (Chapter 1), could indicate that because the patient is not in direct contact with the source of thermal energy, the cutaneous receptors are not as isolated from other external stimuli, such as air currents. Numerous studies in the 1940s and 1950s have shown that the depth of tissue temperature rise within a standard twenty minute treatment is essentially equal for any clinical source used to add thermal energy. These data have been well presented in earlier literature.[5-7]

Bakers are rarely used today. Presumably, this is because they are relatively heavy, bulky, and hard to move on and off the patient. Also, they fall easily if jarred by the patient or therapist. The standard baker consists of four to eight incandescent bulbs with a wattage rating of 25 to 60 per bulb. These are evenly spaced within an inverted U-shaped reflector. They are wired so that four, six, or eight bulbs are radiating infrared energy simultaneously, thus giving easy control of intensity. It is practical to use a baker to induce a superficial TTR on the posterior trunk, hips, or on segments of the lower extremities. It is rarely possible to use a baker to supply heat to the upper extremities because of awkwardness of patient positioning.

The authors are not aware of any company which manufactures a nonluminous infrared lamp at this time. Several manufacturers do continue to make luminous lamps. It was shown late in the 1920s that, because of certain unique characteristics of human skin, infrared at a wavelength of about 12,000 Å will penetrate slightly more deeply than either longer (nonluminous and carbon filament incandescent bulbs) or shorter wavelengths. Tungsten filament bulbs and special "quartz" rod sources produce significant amounts of infrared at the 12,000 Å wavelength. Both types of luminous sources present a major problem with glare from the source or its reflector. When a luminous lamp is used at an angle or in an area in which glare can irritate the patient's eyes, the lamp should be shielded. This is done usually by fastening a sheet around the reflector. When this is done, care must be taken to avoid covering the reflector's ventilating holes. Otherwise, the draping material may catch fire, as the source reflector becomes quite hot.

When an infrared lamp is indicated, the authors prefer a luminous source with a ruby-red colored glass envelope. Essentially, no radiation as short as 12,000 Å are passed by the colored envelope. The standard 250 watt incandescent bulb generates adequate thermal energy for treatment of surfaces in one plane up to 50 cm diameter at a distance of 50 cm from the skin. The colored envelope filters all the glare-producing visible radiation. This eliminates the need for draping the source. Most patients find the resulting visible red radiation very soothing psychologically, while receiving the same benefits as from any other source of infrared energy.

Technique of Application

Most infrared lamps are mounted on casters so that with reasonable care the lamp is easily moved. The lamp is adjustable in height through a wide range and can be tilted vertically and/or horizontally. Frequently, there is provision for moving the reflector and its bulb laterally with respect to the upright. When this adjustment is provided, the base should be weighted.

There are two physical laws which the therapist should keep in mind when applying either an infrared or an ultraviolet lamp (Chapter 6) to a patient.

THE COSINE LAW. The cosine law states,

The energy per square centimeter is proportional to a constant multiplied by the cosine of the angle made by a line connecting the source and the patient, and a line perpendicular to the patient's body. That constant is the light per square centimeter when the patient is perpendicular to the line joining the light and the patient.[8]

Clinically, this means that if energy is to be absorbed rather than reflected from the skin, the source should be approximately perpendicular to the surface being treated. In practice, deviation of 10° from the perpendicular is acceptable. Such an approximation of a right angle is easy to achieve without a measuring device.

THE INVERSE SQUARE LAW. The inverse square law states

The intensity of radiation from any source of light varies inversely with the square of the distance from the source.[8]

One might assume that when a light source is 40 cm from the surface to be treated, the amount of energy absorbed would be twice as great as compared to when the source is 80 cm away. This is incorrect. If the lamp is twice the distance away, the radiation intensity is only one fourth as great, if all other factors are equal. For example, if one squares 40 ($40\times 40 = 1600$), squares 80 (6400), and then divides 6400 by 1600, it is seen that the square of 80 is four times greater than the square of 40.

Clinically, if a patient reports that a source of radiant heat is uncomfortable, or if mottling becomes visible during treatment, two things could be done. One could either increase the distance between the source and the patient or cover the patient surface with a towel. In either case, energy reaching the patient will be decreased. If the distance is increased, the inverse square law should be kept in mind, thus realizing that an increase of a few centimeters can result in a significant decrease in energy reaching the patient.

The distance between source and patient will necessarily be different if the IR source is 250 as compared to 1250 watts (w). A 250 w lamp with an 18 to 40 cm diameter reflector would usually be placed 40 to 50 cm distant. A 1250 w source would commonly be positioned 75 to 90 cm away from the skin. The larger source will usually have a larger reflector. Because less energy per unit area may reach the patient when a larger reflector is used, the therapist must select the appropriate distance with both wattage and reflector size in mind.

Adequate provision for locking the source in place at the desired distance is critical for patient safety. It is the therapist's responsibility to see to it that the reflector cannot drop onto the patient during a treatment period. A serious burn could occur. The lowest temperature nonluminous source of infrared will have an operating temperature of about 400°C, and the common luminous source, a tungsten filament incandescent bulb, a temperature of about 3000°. In both cases, the reflector becomes too hot to touch.

Skin Inspection

Whenever treatment is given with the objective of causing a TTR, it is the therapist's responsibility to inspect the skin in the area to be treated *before* treatment and to descriptively record any skin lesion. Furthermore, the skin should be inspected after treatment to make sure no damage (burn) has occurred. Damage with application of any form of infrared is rare, *unless* the patient is emotionally disturbed or has diminished or absent cutaneous sensation. If either of the above circumstances are known to be a factor with an individual patient, the therapist should visually inspect the skin *at least* every five minutes during treatment and adjust intensity as necessary.

Movement of a Lamp or Baker After Treatment

For safety, as soon as the treatment is over, the lamp or baker should be removed from its position over the patient. Then the lamp should be lowered to its lowest adjustment in height and then moved out of the treatment area. When the lamp is at its lowest height, its center of gravity is as low as possible and it is less apt to tip over on lateral movement. The baker reflector will be too hot to touch except at its handles. Care should be taken to lift it *up* and then off away from the patient; it should then be placed on the floor until it is cool.

WHIRLPOOLS AND HUBBARD TANKS

The whirlpool (WP) and Hubbard tank (HT) are convenient sources of infrared energy which can be used to cause either a mild tissue temperature rise (TTR) or a slight drop in superficial tissue temperature. If the water temperature is at or above the skin temperature of the area being treated, a superficial TTR will occur. If the water temperature is more than $1°C$ less than the skin temperature, the net effect produced within the standard ten- to twenty-minute treatment will be a drop in temperature of the exposed skin and superficial subcutaneous tissues. The WP is used to treat adult-size body segments, most commonly the distal segments of the upper or lower extremity. The HT is used when one or both lower extremities plus the trunk and upper extremities need a change in superficial temperature for relief of pain and/or increase in range of motion. The areas treated with WP or HT are usually larger than can be conveniently treated with other forms of infrared.

Water Temperatures for Causing a Tissue Temperature Rise

The surface and volume of tissues treated by hydrotherapy is larger than is the case with hot packs or other forms of infrared. Consequently, if the skin temperature of these large body segments is raised as high as it is with other forms of infrared, a rise in core temperature would be likely. This is rarely desirable. Hence, with rare exception, the water temperature should not exceed 40°C. When an HT is used, its water temperature should not exceed 38°. Also, when a larger body segment is exposed to heat, there is a greater demand on regional circulation. If the patient has a chronic arterial insufficiency in the segment being treated, the larger the area exposed, the less the capability of adequate dilation to supply the demand and the greater the chance of causing an increase rather than decrease of pain because of the vasospasm induced by rebound.

Water Temperatures for Causing a Tissue Temperature Drop

If the objective of the WP or HT treatment is to cause a drop in local tissue temperature, for both physiological and psychological reasons it is recommended that immersion should be started at or near a neutral temperature (33° to 36°C), followed by a gradual decrease in water temperature over the usual ten-minute treatment period. The extent of the gradual temperature drop should vary in proportion to the size of the body segment exposed to the cool water. Thus, if exposing one lower extremity, distal to the knee, the drop in temperature could be greater than if both extremities were simultaneously exposed. If both lower extremities plus the trunk are to be exposed, the temperature decrease should be smaller still.

The major indications for use of a cold WP are for *acute* orthopedic trauma, *acute* edema, and *acute* muscle spasm. The HT is more likely to be needed when dealing with moderate to severe *chronic* spasticity due to a central nervous system lesion. However, when using cold (or heat) with such patients, it must be predetermined whether their vasomotor regulatory controls are intact. If they were damaged by the lesion, the patient can undergo a critical *core temperature* crisis when large body segments are exposed to either heat or cold. A reasonable rule of thumb for water temperature drop in a Hubbard tank would indicate *no more than* a 5°C drop from the neutral starting temperature during the first treatment while never exceeding a 10°C drop in water temperature on any subsequent treatment. Knowledgeable personnel should be on hand at all times whenever a patient who has damage to his thermoregulatory controls is in a Hubbard tank.

Operation of Whirlpools and Hubbard Tanks

The smallest whirlpool in clinical use will have the capacity to hold about 120 liters (30 gallons) of water. It is designed for immersion of an upper extremity from the elbow distally. Whirlpools of 200 to 300 liter capacity are used for immersion of one or both lower extremities distal to the knee. The largest size permits an adult to sit in it and are used for immersion of the body distal to the navel. All such units require an additional 10 to 20 percent of the initial volume of water to clean the WP after each treatment. A standard Hubbard tank requires 3200 to 4000 liters for each filling. All hydrotherapy units require a large volume fast-recovery source of hot water as well as provision for mixing hot and cold water to obtain the desired temperature.

Each unit will have one or more electrically driven water pumps (turbine), with a manually adjustable flow rate for varying the degree of water aeration and provision for adjusting the height of the turbine impeller in the water. The pump shaft bearings are water lubricated. Hence, the turbine should never be switched on unless the impeller is immersed in water. Since warm water plus the turbulence created by the pump are excellent for loosening adhesive dressings and cleaning debris from the skin, the therapist must be alert to dressings floating loose and being sucked into the impeller. If this occurs, the turbine should be shut off immediately to prevent clogging, with subsequent damage to the impeller, its drive shaft, or its bearings. Since the pumps are electrically driven, care must be taken to avoid splashing water onto the motor housing or its electrical connections.

Patient Safety and Comfort

It is the therapist's responsibility to see that the patient is positioned safely and comfortably. When an upper extremity is treated, the patient sits in an armless chair, resting his lateral trunk against the outside of the whirlpool. If the patient is short, the top edge of the whirlpool may press into his axilla. If this is the case, some kind of padding should be added to the tank edge to minimize the pressure, or the chair seat should be raised. The chair should have a back rest, and the patient's feet should be supported by the floor or a footstool so that he can be safe and relaxed while receiving treatment.

If one or both distal lower extremities are treated, the patient often is placed in a special swivel chair whose seat is several centimeters above the brim of the WP. The patient climbs into the chair when it is facing away from the WP and then swings around, with or without assistance, until he can immerse the lower extremities. If only one leg is treated, the other foot should be supported outside the tank by another chair or stool. If there is any question that the patient could fall from his high seat, he should be strapped in. Care must be taken that the seat is high enough so there is no pressure from the edge of the tank on the posterior thigh.

When the patient is to be seated in the whirlpool, he would first climb onto the high seat, immerse his legs, and then slowly slide into the water and onto the seat in the whirlpool. Normally, his arms would rest on the padded edges of the tank. Care must be taken that the water level in the WP is not so high that when the turbine is turned on water is splashed out of the whirlpool.

If the patient has any past history of suicidal tendencies, or of fainting, knowledgeable personnel should be in constant attendance and should keep the patient in sight at all times.

For entrance into a Hubbard tank, the patient is manually transferred from a wheelchair or stretcher onto an immersible litter. The litter is then connected to a motor-driven, ceiling mounted hoist, manually transferred over the tank, and then lowered into the water. The head end of the litter is fastened to the head supports in the tank while the foot end of the litter continues its descent to the bottom of the tank. After the litter is in its final position, the connections to the hoist are removed from the litter and away from the tank area. If the patient's behavior is not under voluntary control, for either physical or psychological reasons, he may need to be strapped onto the litter for transfer and treatment.

It is recommended that anyone responsible for patient transfer into a Hubbard tank experience such a transfer as a patient, in order to fully appreciate the apprehension which the patient may feel.

Care must be taken to keep the patient's head out of water at all times. Adequate provision for rapid drying of the patient after removal from the tank is necessary to prevent chilling. Since HT (and WP) rooms will invariably be quite humid, provision should be made for good air circulation. Likewise, the floor of such rooms will be wet during treatment periods. Good nonskid floor surfaces and adequate floor drains will minimize the obvious hazards.

Physiological Advantages of Hydrotherapy

Whirlpools and Hubbard tanks are excellent for cleaning debris from skin and/or open wounds, for promoting muscle relaxation (heat) or reduction of muscle spasm or spasticity (cold), and for permitting a transient increase in passive or active range of motion.

Although the authors know of no comparative study, they prefer, as soon as the patient has some control over his joint motion, to let the patient rest and relax as completely as possible while in the WP or HT and then to guide the patient in performing any indicated exercise after transfer of the patient out of the water. Other therapists routinely supervise the indicated exercise while the patient is in the water, during the time the patient has the best chance to relax. The buoyancy effect of the water is not likely to be critical for the exercise, except in a few peripheral nerve lesion problems. The buoyancy makes it harder for the therapist to adequately stabilize the patient and to observe substitution of motion due to muscle imbalance. The buoyancy effect is important when a patient is relearning how to walk in a walking tank or therapeutic pool, but very few physical therapy departments have such expensive hydrotherapy sources available.

The Cleaning of Hydrotherapy Units

Bacteristatic or bacteriocidal agents are commonly added to the water when open lesions are to be immersed. Acute burn patients and all persons with open lesions will inevitably discharge pathogenic microorganisms into the WP or HT. Careful cleaning of the unit can be critical in preventing cross contamination. Most departments which treat open lesions with hydrotherapy rely on regular culture testing to prove or disprove the efficiency and thoroughness of their cleaning procedures. Discharge of urine or fecal material into the water can be as much or more of a problem than open lesions. Tank seams, water inlets and outlets, and the insides of turbine shafts are especially difficult to keep clean. Each department should establish its own cleaning procedures, usually on recommendation and monitoring from the institution's pathology or microbiology departments.

Costs of Hydrotherapy

The initial cost of whirlpools and Hubbard tanks are high. They are custom-made of heavy gauge stainless steel. If the area where they are placed was not designed for hydrotherapy, addition of floor drains can be a major item. The ceiling to hold the Hubbard tank hoist requires special design. Floors may have to be reinforced.

A department with, for example, five whirlpools and two Hubbard tanks in regular use may consume water at a rate in excess of 400,000 liters (100,000 gallons) per day. Much of that water has to be heated. For these reasons, more and more large hydrotherapy departments are installing water purification and recirculation systems. Initial costs are high, but a properly installed system will recover its cost in about five years.

The point to remember is that hydrotherapy is one of the most expensive physical agents, especially in the form of the Hubbard tank, in initial cost plus installation plus water consumption. Hydrotherapy is also high in personnel and linen costs.

COLD PACKS

Cold packs are similar in construction to hot packs. However, they are supplied in sealed, waterproof plastic bags so that if stored at temperatures below the freezing point of water they are not unusably stiff. It is possible to store the water-soaked pouch below freezing because the sand-water slurry has a lower freezing point than that of water alone. If the plastic cover is torn or removed, in time the ratio of water to sand will change (through evaporation). Then the pack will become stiff when frozen. The commercially available storage unit is thermostatically equipped to maintain pack temperature at any desired temperature between 20° below and 20° above 0°C. Many clinics store their packs at 0° to 10°C.

The storage cabinet should not be filled with water. The thoroughly soaked pack should be placed in its plastic bag and the bag sealed and placed into the dry storage cabinet. When first used, the pack needs to have been stored at the desired temperature for about twenty-four hours. After initial use, replacement in the storage cabinet for one-half to one hour should return the pack to an effective temperature.

Treatment Procedures

The pack (in its plastic bag) should never be placed next to the skin. At least one layer of bath toweling should be used. Clinics will vary in election as to whether the toweling toward the patient should be wet or dry. Wet toweling will speed the process of withdrawal of thermal energy from the patient. Water plus moist air are better thermal conductors than dry toweling and dry air. Several layers of dry toweling are standardly placed on the side of the pack away from the skin, so that not as much of the cold effect is lost to room air.

The usual treatment time is ten to fifteen minutes. Depending upon the differential in temperature between the pack and the skin, after five minutes of application, one may expect to see hyperemia, or a marked pallor of the skin. If hyperemia is present, it indicates that the normal vasomotor regulatory system has been able to bring in enough warm blood so that even though the skin temperature may have dropped 5° to 10°C, the cutaneous blood supply is adequate to prevent tissue damage. Damage will occur if the temperature of the skin approaches 13°C.[9,10]

Pallor indicates that arterial dilation has been inadequate to maintain skin temperature within physiological limits, and so cutaneous vasoconstriction has occurred to conserve heat loss from underlying tissues. If the pack was applied to a distal extremity, by the time ten minutes has elasped, few patients will have hyperemia, and pallor should be anticipated. Since cutaneous temperature and circulation is normally better in the trunk areas, pallor rarely appears here. If the temperature differential between the pack and skin was initially great and was maintained by replacement with a fresh pack after five minutes, by ten minutes pallor is very likely to appear. If the skin becomes cyanotic in appearance, severe vasoconstriction has occurred and the treatment should be discontinued.

Physiological Effects of Cold Pack Application

The cold pack is widely used in *acute* orthopedic lesions in an attempt to control traumatically induced edema. It is better to use cold for ten to fifteen minutes out of each half hour rather than a single longer application. Injured tissues must receive some nutrition even in the presence of massive swelling. It should also be realized that the pack will come to equilibrium with skin temperature within ten to fifteen minutes after application. If an intense cold application is indicated, the pack should be changed every five minutes. The temperature change in the patient will be confined to the skin and adjacent subcutaneous tissue rather than penetrating to muscle unless the pack is changed frequently and the cold differential is maintained for at least one-half hour.[9,10]

A decrease in axon temperature will slow condition velocity. If the temperature drop is great enough, no conduction will take place. The critical axon temperature has not yet been established, but in most patients a decrease in skin temperature of 5°C will be adequate to cause a reduction in *motor nerve* activity, with subsequent reduction of muscle spasm. It has been shown that in the presence of a CNS lesion, spasticity is dramatically reduced within one minute after exposure of the skin to cold.[11] The mechanisms involved are not understood.[12,13] It cannot be due to decrease in motor nerve or muscle temperature within such a short time period. However, if pain is due to acute muscle spasm or to spasticity, local application of cold can be very effective in temporarily decreasing muscle hyperactivity and hence reducing pain.[14]

Many patients with a CNS lesion will have diminished or absent sensation. This is especially true for patients with a spinal cord lesion. If this is the case, the spasticity will not be accompanied by pain, but even so the spasticity can be transiently reduced with appropriate application of cold. If the volume of muscle in spasticity is small, this can be done with cold packs. If the area to be treated is large, a cold whirlpool or Hubbard tank (as described earlier in the section on hydrotherapy) may be indicated.

Precautions for Cold Application

It is probably wise prior to first exposure to cold on any patient to check blood pressure before and after treatment. There have been occasional clinical notes of a sharp transient rise in systolic pressure. This could be hazardous if the patient has a history of high blood pressure. Presumably, the pressure change is due to a massive reflex vasoconstriction.

SUMMARY

Infrared sources of various kinds have been in use over the centuries to transmit thermal energy to or from a patient. In the last several decades, increasing use of various types of cold applications has evolved.

Both moist and dry heat, as well as moist and dry cold, are part of the electromagnetic spectrum. Their wavelengths are short, and hence their effect is chiefly on cutaneous circulation, cutaneous axons, and the skin itself. Pain relief is achieved through application of heat or cold of infrared wavelengths which act directly on the skin and structures in the skin and, through these structures, cause certain reactions in deeper lying tissues.

Rationale and technics for judicious use of the many forms of the infrared energies through conduction, convection, and radiation are discussed, with emphasis on technics in widespread use at this time. The relative safety and ease of use of infrared as compared to the hazards associated with conversive heating (Chapter 4) are discussed.

REFERENCES

1. Sodeman, W.A. and Sodeman, W.A., Jr.: *Pathological Physiology*, 4th ed. Philadelphia, Saunders, 1967, p. 202.
2. Eddy, H.C. and Taylor, H.P.: Experiences with the Dermatherm in relation to peripheral vascular disease. I. Normal studies. *Am Heart J, 6*:683-9, 1931.
3. Shepard, J.T.: *Physiology of the Circulation in Human Limbs in Health and Disease.* Philadelphia, Saunders, 1963.
4. Davson, H.: *A Textbook of General Physiology*, 4th ed. Baltimore, Williams & Wilkins, 1970, Chapter II.
5. Glasser, O. (Ed.): *Medical Physics,* Volume I. Chicago, Year Bk Med, 1945, p. 1158.
6. Hollaender, A. (Ed.): *Radiation Biology*, Volume I. New York, McGraw, 1954, p. 20.
7. Licht, S. (Ed.): *Therapeutic Heat and Cold,* 2nd ed. New Haven, Licht, 1965.
8. Krusen, Frank H.: *Physical Medicine.* Philadelphia, Saunders, 1942, p. 235.
9. Wolf, S.L. and Basmajian, J.V.: Intramuscular temperatures deep to localized cold stimulation. *Phys Ther, 53:*1284-8, Dec., 1973.
10. Beirman, W.: Therapeutic use of cold. *JAMA, 157:*189-92, 1955.
11. Miglietta, O.: Electromyographic changes with application of cold. *Arch Phys Med Rehabil, 45:*508-12, 1964.
12. Newton, M. and Lemkuhl, D.: Muscle spindle response to heating and cooling. *Phys Ther, 45:*91-105, 1965.
13. Negrin, R.: Hypothermia to the spinal cord for relief of spasticity and rigidity. *Arch Phys Med Rehabil, 47:*169-73, 1966.
14. Mecomber, S. and Herman, R.: Effects of local hypothermia on reflex and voluntary activity. *Phys Ther, 51:*271-81, 1971.

Chapter 6

ULTRAVIOLET LIGHT

INTRODUCTION

U NLIKE the diathermy and infrared portions of the electromagnetic spectrum which are used to induce a tissue temperature rise in absorbing tissue, ultraviolet wavelengths are used to stimulate a variety of chemical reactions in microorganisms, epidermis, and dermis. The desired effect on microorganisms is to kill them. Taylor[1] has published a useful clinical study on the value of ultraviolet light (UV) in infectious dermatoses. Epstein[2] has presented a useful discussion of the use of UV in various dermatological problems.

When the healing of an open wound such as a bedsore is delayed by the inevitable infection which results from the loss of the body's first barrier against microorganisms (the skin), regular exposure of the wound to UV is superior to either local or systemic administration of antibiotics, provided that regular debridement precedes the exposure. Bailey[3] states that antibiotics are useful in the management of pressure sores only if a streptococcal cellulitis is present. The general lack of usefulness of antibiotics in control of infection in this type of wound is due to the poor blood supply. Formation of granulation tissue is essential for the repair of any open wound. Formation of this tissue is stimulated by exposure of the wound to UV.

Normal skin is dehydrated and thickened by even a single exposure to UV. Repeated exposure increases stratum corneum thickness (hyperplasia) by as much as fifty times.[4] The dehydration and thickening are effective in treatment of acne and related diseases. When an intense skin reaction is desired, photosensitizing chemicals may be administered systemically or topically prior to exposure to UV.[4,5] This is standard practice in the treatment of vitiligo and psoriasis. More often, the therapist needs to be aware that if the patient is on medication which enhances the effects of UV, the combination can exacerbate rather than alleviate the skin pathology. Appendix A at the end of this chapter lists generically those drugs which are presently known to increase the hazard of exposure to UV.[5]

Photochemical conversion of provitamin D (7-dehydrocholesterol) into the active compound (cholecalciferol, or possibly 25-hydroxycholecalciferol) is a well-established reaction.[6,7] Provitamin D is a normal constituent of human epidermis. Vitamin D deficiency is a major factor in the bone disease, rickets (osteomalacia). It is still a sufficiently common problem that three major articles appeared in the Journal of Bone and Joint Surgery between 1968 and 1972. When children have an adequate supply of vitamin D, *and are able to metabolize it normally,* calcium absorption becomes normal and the disease disappears.[6] Control of diet and oral administration of vitamin D are standardly adequate procedures in the management of rickets. Whole-body irradiation with small doses of UV are indicated if the patient does not respond to routine care. The mechanism by which UV absorption stimulates conversion of provitamin D into the active compound is not known. It is known that the interaction of vitamin D and calcium is markedly increased by the use of UV. Exposure of skin to UV is effective in initiating the mechanism. Sources which produce UV of the 297 nm wavelength are superior to those which produce more of either shorter or longer wavelengths.[5,6,7]

CLINICAL SOURCES OF ULTRAVIOLET LIGHT

There are two major types of ultraviolet sources in clinical use in this country. They are classically designated as "Hot Quartz" (HQ) and "Cold Quartz" (CQ) mercury vapor arc lamps. It is easy to tell whether a given lamp is HQ or CQ (Figs. 6-1 and 6-2). The transparent envelope which contains the arc will appear as a straight hollow cylinder or it will be seen at a flat coil (grid). HQ envelopes are straight, rarely exceeding 20 cm in length or 2 cm in diameter. CQ envelopes are coiled, usually in a circular fashion, with a uniform distance between turns of 0.5 to 1 cm. The number of turns will vary with the size of the lamp. Very large CQ sources may have rectangular coils more than a meter in length and be 10 to 15 cm in width. The envelope diameter in CQ sources rarely exceeds 1 cm.

All clinical UV sources contain small quantities of mercury, a semisolid at room temperature, and argon. Argon is an inert gas which is a very efficient conductor of electricity at ambient temperatures. When the metallic arc is energized, excitation of the argon, not the mercury, gives rise to the characteristic blue radiation. This visible radiation is *not* UV. UV is invisible to the

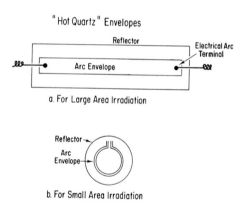

Figure 6-1. (A) *The HQ Envelope for Large Area Irradiation.* The envelope will range from 10 to 20 cm in length and 1 to 2 cm diameter, depending upon the size of the reflector and intensity of the arc. The envelope is usually made of quartz in order to withstand extreme temperature changes. Commonly, the envelope is positioned 50 to 75 cm from the surface to be treated.

(B) *The HQ Envelope for Small Area Irradiation.* The envelope may be coiled into a single ring, as shown, or may be a single straight tube. In either case, the reflector diameter will be 3 to 5 cm. Modern lamps for high intensity area clinical use are air cooled by high speed fans. This permits their use as close as 10 cm from the surface to be treated with negligible risk of thermal tissue damage so long as the exposure does not last more than sixty seconds.

"Cold Quartz" Envelopes

a. Rectangular Coil

b. Grid Coil

Figure 6-2. (A) *The CQ Envelope for Large Area Irradiation.* The long
dimension of the rectangularly coiled envelope may be as
much as 90 cm, with a 5 to 10 cm distance between the sides
of the rectangle. The reflector may be as much as 150 cm
long and 30 cm wide. The diameter of the envelope is usually 0.5 to 1 cm. Distance from source to surface to be treated
is usually 20 to 40 cm.
(B) *The CQ Envelope for Small Area Irradiation.* The reflector
is usually circular in shape, with an envelope coiled into several turns wound in a grid fashion closely adjacent to the
reflector. The diameter of the reflector often ranges from
10 to 20 cm. Diameter of the envelope is usually 0.5 to 1
cm. This type of lamp is commonly used at a distance of 1 to
2 cm from the surface to be treated.

human eye. As the temperature of the gas within the envelope
begins to rise, the mercury starts to vaporize (at about 357°C).
When the average temperature of the mercury atoms reaches more
than 8,000°C, an appreciable amount of UV, along with infrared
and visible light, is emitted. The more intense the arc, the greater
the thermal energy production, the more visible light production,
and most importantly, the broader the UV spectrum.[8] No mercury vapor source will have more than 25 to 30 percent of its total
radiation as UV.[8,9] Those designed for use without medical
supervision will radiate less than 5 percent as UV. The stronger
the arc (wattage), the more intense the radiation. Clinical HQ
sources require 5 to 20 amperes and a step-up transformer.
Clinical CQ sources rarely require over 2 amperes. They do not

need transformers. Ballast similar to that in residential fluorescent lights provides the short-duration high voltage needed to excite the CQ arc. Appendix B summarizes the physical differences between clinical HQ and CQ sources.

The arcs may be conveniently classified as high, medium, or low pressure. These designations are relative to atmospheric pressure at sea level (760 mm Hg). High and medium pressure arcs are always HQ and always have a broad UV spectrum with strong peaks at 2537, 2800, and 2967 Å. The only high pressure arc in clinical use is the Kromayer type, which is used for application of intense radiation to a small area of diseased skin or infected subcutaneous tissue, as in bedsores. The total arc output is so great that the arc must be cooled to avoid thermal damage to the patient. Models built prior to 1940 were usually water cooled. Since the waterlines must be flexible in order to position the arc, leaks are inevitable in time. If any water should leak onto the high voltage transformer, the noise, damage to the lamp, and the risk to the therapist are very real. Development of small, high speed fans now permit safer cooling of these high pressure arcs. However, the closest distance permitted between source and absorbing tissue is 10 cm because of the tremendous infrared output.

For research *(not clinical)* use, extremely high pressure xenon arcs have been developed. The internal envelope pressure may be as high as 100 atmospheres. In addition to UV radiation at the previously mentioned wavelengths, they also have large output between 3200 and 4000 Å,[8] which is not needed in clinical UV treatment.

Most clinical UV sources are medium pressure (approximately 0.5 atm.) or low pressure (about 0.2 atm.) for safety reasons and for ease of control of the UV output. If a high pressure envelope is shattered, the contents are diffused with explosive force. Pieces of the envelope and the mercury vapor could badly burn the patient and the therapist. When the pressure inside the envelope is less than atmospheric (partial vacuum), if the envelope loses its seal for any reason, the envelope pieces and the mercury would not be driven towards the patient or therapist, but the laws of gravity would still be in effect. As manufacturing

techniques and quality control have improved, explosion or im-
plosion of envelopes has become rare, but if the lamp, and
especially the envelope, receives a sharp blow, it will still shatter.

Even more important, as manufacturers have learned to
achieve better vacuums while sealing the essential electrodes inside the envelope, they have been able to reduce arc intensity and
the quantity of mercury needed to produce an adequate UV output. It has been known for many years that absorption of radiation at 2650 Å is the most lethal for all kinds of microorganisms.[8]
To have a mercury arc produce adequate quantities of this wavelength and little other UV, the arc intensity must be low.[8] The
clinical CQ sources have better than 90 percent of their UV output at a wavelength of 2537 Å, which is quite close to the 2650 Å
wavelength insofar as its bactericidal effects are concerned. The
total pressure within the envelope is low, the quantity of mercury
is low, and the arc wattage is low. The net result is a CQ source
whose envelope temperature rarely exceeds 60°C, even though the
average mercury vapor temperature is more than 8000°C. In any
gas, the interatomic and intermolecular distances are vast in comparison with the same distances for a solid. The higher the
temperature of the gas, the more this is true. Hence, the confining solid which makes up the arc envelope will get hot but will
not even remotely approach the temperature of the contained
vapor because of the vastly greater number of molecules per unit
area to absorb the thermal energy. The greater the vacuum (and
therefore the fewer the number of gas molecules to transmit
energy), the less the rise in envelope temperature. Hence, the
low pressure (high vacuum) CQ sources are ideal for use close
to any tissue. Because CQ arc intensities are low, these lamps are
rarely used at distances greater than 25 cm from the area to be
treated. However, one must bear in mind that they have no
significant output at 2800 or 2967 Å.

Modern clinical HQ sources are in the medium pressure category. The quantity of mercury is larger than in the CQ envelope,
the arc intensity is greater, and there is far more thermal energy
radiated, along with a broad spectrum UV output. The envelope
temperature will be higher, usually reaching a temperature of

500° to 1000°C. Therefore, unless the HQ source is air cooled, it is rarely used at a distance closer than 50 cm. With an efficient HQ source of a size intended to cover one surface of the trunk or one surface of an extremity with one exposure, a distance of 75 cm from source to tissue is usual.

The envelope confining the mercury must be able to transmit UV, to stand repeated, severe temperature changes, and be sufficiently rigid to contain low or high pressure. HQ source envelopes are usually quartz cylinders. The melting point of the quartz used is about 1500°C. Quartz is expensive and hard to work with. Hence, it is rare to see an HQ source large enough to give whole-body irradiation in less than four exposures (two anterior, two posterior). CQ source envelopes usually use a UV transmitting glass such as *Vycor*®* which readily withstands the temperature of low pressure arcs. Both quartz and UV transmitting glasses block all radiation shorter than 1850 Å. Since most investigators agree that wavelengths longer than 3200 Å produce effects similar to visible light, clinical UV should be regarded as having a wavelength range of 1850 to 3200 Å.[7,8,9]

Hot quartz lamps require warmup time of at least two minutes before their UV output is stable. Where precise dosage is important, it is probably better to allow at least five minutes, especially after the first 100 hours of operation. Once shut off, HQ sources require at least a two-minute cooling period before they can be restarted. When mercury has been vaporized and is cooling toward room temperature, as long as its temperature is above approximately 100°C, the random motion of the cooling molecules is still so great that they will not conduct enough electrical energy to restart the arc. For both of the above reasons, if one is to give several HQ-UV treatments in a morning or an afternoon, once the lamp is started for the first patient it is wise to leave it running until all treatments are finished for that day. However, it is important that care be taken that the radiation be confined by shutters or a fiberglass hood when a lamp is left running in a treatment area. Most HQ sources have adjustable shutters for this

---

*Vycor® is the trade name for the 96% silica content UV transmitting glass manufactured by Corning.

purpose. The shutters are manually opened only during actual intended patient exposure. If the lamp does not have shutters, the therapist must *not* use a pillow case or other linen for this purpose. If the HQ source is of any appreciable size, the concomitant heat production may scorch or set fire to any linen attached to the reflector. A fiberglass hood will easily withstand these temperatures; it is easy to make and easy to put on or remove. Small HQ sources (Kromayer) will usually have a snap-on, clear plastic cover which blocks all UV radiation. More than a few times, the therapist has forgotten to remove the cover for treatment and has wondered why there was no apparent response to the exposure.

Because of the higher starting voltage, the smaller quantity of mercury, and the greater vacuum, CQ lamps do not need a warm-up period. Within a matter of a few seconds, their UV output is at maximum. Because of the smaller quantity of mercury and lower envelope temperature, the CQ lamp cools much more rapidly when shut off. Hence, a CQ lamp can be started and shut off many times a day with no worry about uniformity of output.

TECHNIQUES OF ULTRAVIOLET TREATMENT
Cleaning the Lamp

Any dust or oil or water film on the envelope or reflector will diminish the UV energy reaching the patient. If not removed before starting the lamp, the contaminants can become baked onto the envelope or reflector. Output will be permanently impaired and nonuniform. Therefore, wiping off the envelope and reflector daily, if used daily, or before each treatment if usage is sporadic, is advised. Ether, toluene, carbon tetrachloride, or 95% ethyl alcohol are all good. Most other readily available and inexpensive alcohols contain a high percentage of water. Repeated use of water can cause rusting of areas of the reflector. All of these cleaning agents are volatile and flammable. Hence, they should be used in a well ventilated room when the envelope and reflector are at or near room temperature. Nap– or lint-free toweling are preferred to cotton balls or terrycloth because of the likelihood of leaving fibers behind with the latter materials.

Output of the Lamp

All clinical sources of UV deteriorate with use. This is more of a problem with HQ lamps as compared to CQ sources and less of a problem with lamps built within the last several decades. When the electrical arc is energized and the mercury is vaporized, some of the mercury is inevitably baked onto the inside of the envelope. Therefore, there is always a decrease in intensity of output by about 20 percent during the first 100 running hours and by about 5 percent per year thereafter if the lamp is in daily use. Also, even with the best sealing techniques, over a period of years, the vacuum will decrease so that there will be more air molecules within the envelope to absorb more energy from the arc, causing more nonuseful collision of mercury and argon molecules with the increased air molecules. For these reasons, it is wise to regularly check on lamp intensity. The accepted clinical test is to do a sleeve test on the most lightly complected staff member, recording the number of seconds required to produce a standard visible response at a standard distance. In lamps used once daily, such a test should be done at least every six months. When the time required to produce an equivalent response has approximately doubled, it is time to consider repair or replacement of the lamp. This should be done for each UV source in the department, as each lamp will deteriorate at a different rate. The standard response time should be plainly visible and permanently attached to the lamp. There are a lot of variables to such a clinical test, especially medication the subject may be on and whether the test area is more or less pigmented than at the time of previous tests. Currently available UV meters are expensive and must be recalibrated at least twice a year. Since no one meter is valid for both HQ and CQ sources, few departments can justify this expense.

Eye Protection

The eyeball and adjacent structures are extremely sensitive to UV of any wavelength because of their relative avascularity. Since blood supply is poor, absorbed energy is not diffused rapidly. In addition, UV penetration is poor, leading to concentration of the energy in a small volume of tissue. Exposure to small quantities can lead to a painful conjunctivitis lasting several days. Exposure to larger quantities can lead to temporary blindness. Hence, eye protection is mandatory for patient and therapist alike. Glass commonly used in eyeglasses is effective as a UV filter, as are *Uvinyl®** and *Mylar®*.† Unless tinted, they do not diminish the quantity of glare (from the reflector) or visible light which can reach the eyeball. Because it is possible for UV to be reflected from skin to eyeglass lens and be redirected toward the eyeball, the glasses should fit snugly. Since the therapist should be able to see during treatment in order to time the treatment, he cannot wear heavily tinted glasses and may prefer a clear or lightly tinted full face shield. These are inexpensive and lightweight. Many therapists recommend the patient keep his eyes closed even when wearing goggles as a further precaution.

The Sleeve Test

Because each lamp will have its own output characteristics, and since human skin is very sensitive to UV, it is always wise to perform a sleeve test on an individual who is to receive clinical UV if skin is to be the absorbing tissue. This can be done in a number of ways. It is probably wise to select an area of skin which has not been appreciably exposed to sunlight for at least six months. Such areas are becoming increasingly difficult to find, especially in the younger population, but the skin of the abdomen inferior to the navel or the skin on the inside of the upper arms is usually less exposed. A series of holes at least 2 cm in diameter are cut into UV filtering cloth or paper. As few as four and as many as fifteen holes have been recommended by various authors. This author prefers five or six holes unless the dosage must be extremely precise. The paper is attached snugly to the skin, with all holes exposed for a period of time (usually seconds) which, on the basis of past experience, should produce no visible re-

---

*Uvinyl® is the trade name for benzophenone compounds manufactured by the Antara Chemical Co., a division of General Aniline and Film.

†Mylar® is the trade name for polyester plastics manufactured by DuPont. Both are excellent filters for all UV wavelengths shorter than 4200 Å.

sponse. Then, one hole at a time is covered at specified intervals until all holes are covered. The times used should be marked adjacent to each exposed area. The therapist should observe the exposed skin approximately twenty-four hours after the test exposures. Although there is a difference in opinion, a majority of therapists regard that exposure time needed to produce a faintly visible reddening of the skin present twenty-four hours after exposure as the minimal erythemal dose (MED). Test skin which has no erythema present twenty-four hours after exposure has received a suberythemal dose (SED). Test skin which retains reddish coloration for up to forty-eight hours after exposure will have been exposed to UV approximately two and one half times as long as the skin which showed an MED. The visible reaction lasting up to forty-eight hours is usually called a first degree erythemal response (1st D). If the response lasts from forty-eight to seventy-two hours, it is usually considered a second degree erythemal dose (2nd D). The 2nd D response skin will have been exposed approximately five times as long as the MED skin. Thus if the MED was established with a thirty-second exposure, a 2nd D response would result upon exposure to 5×30 (150) seconds. With exposures causing erythema to last more than seventy-two hours, blistering will usually occur in less than one hour after exposure, indicating destruction of epidermis and sometimes the dermis (3rd D). This is clearly a pathological dose and has no place in modern use of ultraviolet in treatment of diseased skin. However, one should remember that mucous membrane and subcutaneous tissues are far less responsive to UV than is skin. Therefore, in treatment of urine scalds, Vincent's angina ("trench mouth"), and other mucosal infections, such a dose may be used beneficially. These pathologies usually respond routinely to antibiotic therapy, and UV is needed only in stubborn cases. When 2nd or 3rd degree doses are used intentionally, care must be taken to prevent exposure of adjacent skin. Otherwise, a painful burn is likely to follow. When UV is used to control infection in a pressure sore, 2nd or 3rd degree doses are routine. Protection of surrounding skin with adequate draping is necessary.

The use of a sleeve test on a patient prior to treatment is becoming more important as medical therapy is becoming more complex. The dose that may yield an MED on a person not under medication may yield a 3rd D response when they are taking any photosensitive drug. Therefore, it is prudent to perform a sleeve test on each patient, especially if the skin is lightly pigmented.

The visible reddening of the skin (erythema) is brought about by a series of events to be discussed later. Erythema due to exposure to UV is always a delayed reaction, rarely appearing before two hours after exposure. Exposure at intensities which can later be classified as MED usually are visible by seven to eight hours after exposure and reach maximum intensity at eleven to twelve hours.[9] Stronger intensities may cause earlier appearance. It is well to remember that erythema from a CQ source will usually appear earlier and disappear sooner than will erythema from an HQ source.[7,8,9]

Doses of MED or greater intensity are followed by epidermal exfoliation, hyperplasia, and pigmentation. The hyperplasia and pigmentation appear to make the skin more resistant to UV. Hence, if it is desired to maintain a given level of reaction over a period of several weeks, repeated exposures must be of slightly greater intensity. For example, if the MED was established as thirty seconds at 75 cm and the treatment is to be given daily, progression of exposure might well be thirty, thirty-five, forty, forty-five, and fifty seconds. UV is not commonly given more than five days in a row. For each day of "rest," using the above scale, one should cut back five seconds. If on a Friday a fifty-second exposure was used, on Monday, the treatment would be resumed at forty seconds. If treatment is scheduled three times weekly, a more nearly constant dose would be used to maintain equivalent reaction.

The Inverse Square Law

This law states that as distance between source of radiant energy and absorbing tissue is altered, intensity is decreased (or increased) geometrically rather than arithmetically. Formal statement and significance are discussed in Chapter 5. At one time, therapists had to be able to calculate alteration in intensity with change in distance to maintain the prescribed dose level. With modern equipment this is rarely necessary, since it is unusual that a single exposure will require over sixty seconds. It is essential, however, when the sleeve test is done and when treatment is given that the distance used is accurately recorded, to minimize the possibility for error in dosage. Equally important is accurate timing and recording of each actual exposure in seconds. This used to require a stopwatch, but wristwatches with sweep second hands are entirely adequate, readily available, and usually more convenient. If the department has more than one UV source, it is wise to record which lamp was used on which patient.

The Cosine Law

This law states that for maximum absorption of radiant energy, the source should be perpendicular to the absorbing surface. Deviation of ± 10° from the right angle does not create a major energy loss problem. For this reason, visual positioning of the source is usually adequate, although when large areas, i.e. posterior trunk, are subject to a single exposure, the erythema production will be noticeably less where surface contour is curved rather than flat.

Reflection of UV

It is the therapist's responsibility to drape areas of the patient which should not be exposed to UV. A single layer of an ordinary sheet, bath or linen towel, or a pillowcase is adequate to block UV unless the linen is threadbare or torn. It is equally important that the therapist realize that white cloth is a very good reflector of UV. Many a therapist has received an inadvertent exposure to his arms and face by standing near the patient draping while the patient is being treated. Such reflection from cubicle curtains is a good reason for remembering to tell the patient to keep his eyes closed when being treated, even though his face is remote from the source and the area of exposure.

Therapists vary in opinion as to the merits of drape versus no drape. If a patient is to receive a series of treatments to a small area, it will be difficult to place the draping precisely the same way for each treatment. Yet if a first or second degree dose is indicated, and if nearby previously unexposed skin is exposed at a third or fourth treatment intensity, a serious burn can result. Some therapists advocate the use of fabric or paper templates, with cutouts to be placed over the lesion. If the lesion is becoming worse, or if it is responding to treatment, the cutout has to be revised on a regular basis. It would seem simpler to leave adjacent areas exposed at each treatment so that no margin receives a sudden intense exposure. Where draping might be called for on the grounds of modesty, it would seem simpler to have female therapists treat female patients rather than to drape for modesty alone. Nipples and external genitalia tolerate exposure to UV considerably better than less pigmented skin. Also, many a skin lesion has been inadequately treated because the therapist did not expose adipose or pendulous skin folds.

Patient Positioning

Thoughtful attention must be paid to patient positioning, especially if whole-body irradiation is to be used. One half of the face and either the anterior or posterior surfaces of the upper extremities and the lateral aspect of the lower extremities are very likely to receive a painfully uneven dosage. To illustrate, suppose the patient is prone. For comfort, his neck will be fully rotated to the right or left and his forearms will be in full pronation so that the volar surface is exposed. When he is turned over and lies supine for the next exposure, unless the neck is rotated so that the other half of the face is exposed, one side will have received a double exposure. When lying supine, the forearms are commonly pronated, which is fine because the dorsal surface of the forearm and the anterior surface of the upperarm will be exposed. But if the patient happens to lie supine with forearms in full supination, the volar surface will receive a double exposure. In both the prone and supine position, many patients lie with their lower extremities in moderate external rotation. This is more readily visible when the patient is supine. If the therapist instructs the patient to keep the extremities neutral while supine but does not do so when the patient is prone, the lateral surfaces can receive excessive exposure. It is the therapist's responsibility to see to it that no surface is under– or over-exposed.

Preparation of the Surface to be Treated

It is necessary to remember that ultraviolet light is not a penetrating form of energy. All investigators agree that more than 50 percent is absorbed within the first 0.1 mm (100 microns) and all is absorbed within the second 0.1 mm. Therefore, the treatment surface must be cleansed, rinsed, and dried before each exposure for best results. If a photosensitizing liquid or ointment has been applied to the diseased skin, only a very thin residue is needed or desirable upon exposure. This can be effectively achieved by gently rubbing the area with soft, dry toweling. If the medication stains fabric, use soft, disposable toweling. If an open wound is to be treated, it should be debrided before each exposure. Institutions will vary as to whether the task of debridement is assigned to physicians, nurses, or therapists. Hand-held electric dryers are very effective and efficient in temporary drying of both skin and open wounds.

PHYSIOLOGICAL EFFECTS OF CLINICAL ULTRAVIOLET LIGHT

Cold quartz (CQ) lamps produce more than 90 percent of their UV output at the 2537 Å wavelength. Hot quartz (HQ) lamps produce a substantial peak at that wavelength, as well as a strong peak at 2800 Å, and radiate very srtongly throughout the range of 2900 to 3200 with a peak at 2967 Å.[7,8,9] Early studies indicated that less than 1 percent of any UV penetrated to the dermis. The conclusion was that all response to absorption of UV started in the epidermis and diffused to the dermis. Recent data[7,9] indicate that 10 to 20 percent of UV reaches the dermis of lightly pigmented skin, especially when the epidermis is of normal thickness. Where the epidermis is thick (palms, soles of feet), none of the radiation penetrates to the dermis.

Human skin is classically described as having two major divisions — the epidermis (outermost) and the dermis. The epidermis has five layers. From the outside in, they are as follows: the stratum corneum (horny or keratinized layer) and stratum lucidium (clear layer), followed by the granular, prickle cell, and basal layers. Pigment cells (melanocytes) are within the basal (Malphigian) layer. No part of the epidermis has a direct nerve or blood supply.[4,5]

Extensive study by Kligman (1964) has indicated that in most areas of the body, the epidermis is much thinner than was previously thought.[10] Except in atypical areas (callous), the epidermis is 60 to 100 microns in depth. Normal stratum corneum has a maximum depth of 15 microns and an average of 11 microns, regardless of degree of pigmentation. Both the stratum corneum and the entire epidermis are much thicker on the sole of the foot and, to a lesser extent, on the palm of the hand. Observable reaction to UV by the epidermis of the sole or palm is rare, irrespective of degree of pigmentation prior to treatment or of the dose administered.

Production of Erythema

The best known and most studied reaction of human skin is production of erythema. UV-induced erythema is a *delayed reddening* of the skin. It first appears several hours after exposure and lasts in direct proportion to intensity of exposure. The intensity of the erythema also varies depending upon which region was exposed. The chest is usually the most sensitive, followed by the abdomen and then the posterior trunk. The skin of the extremities ordinarily requires a significantly higher dose to produce an equivalent erythema.

There are differences in erythema production which depend on whether the skin was exposed to CQ (2537 Å = 254 nm) or to a HQ source (2967 Å = 297 nm).[7-9] Both the intensity and duration of response are significantly less when exposed to CQ, but the onset of erythema is earlier, in normal skin.

In all cases where erythema appears, there is active vasodilation of the cutaneous capillaries. Arteriolar dilation occurs only with an intense exposure.[9,11,12] Neither the mechanism nor the site of the reaction causing either type of dilation is known. For many years, it was thought that absorption of UV caused a photo-chemical decarboxylation of histadine, which is the usual pre-cursor of histamine (Fig. 6-3). This reaction does occur when skin is exposed to a strong dose of infrared (Chapter 5). Such a reaction has yet to be demonstrated *in vitro* using UV sources with major output in the 290 to 320 nm range. However, one well-known deamination product of histadine is urocanic acid (Fig. 6-4). Urocanic acid is normally present in human skin and is a major factor in protection of the skin from damage due to ex-posure to either natural or artificial sources of UV.[7] When urocanic acid absorbs at 290 nm, it undergoes a *cis-trans* isomeriza-tion.

Histidine   Histamine

CONVERSION OF HISTIDINE TO HISTAMINE

Figure 6-3. *Conversion of Histidine into Histamine.* For many years it was *assumed* that this reaction took place in human skin upon absorption of UV and that this reaction was the basis for erythema production. To date this reaction has never been demonstrated *in vitro,* even at intensities far above those clinically feasible.[7]

If urocanic acid is applied to the skin prior to exposure to UV, erythema production is suppressed. There is some evidence that decarboxylation of 5-hydroxytryptophan to 5-hydroxytyptamine may be a factor in UV induced capillary dilation (Fig. 6-5). The present theory is that all mercury arc sources have a direct action on the dermis and that the longer wavelengths (290 to 310 nm) also act directly on the epidermis.[13,14] Apparently, some vasodila-

Histidine   Urocanic Acid

Figure 6-4. *Conversion of Histidine into Urocanic Acid.* Urocanic acid is a well-documented deamination product of histidine. This reaction is known to take place when human skin absorbs UV. Urocanic acid is a vasodilator.[7]

5 – Hydroxytryptophan   5 – Hydroxytryptamine

Figure 6-5. *Conversion of 5-Hydroxytryptophan into 5-Hydroxytryptamine.* This reaction is well established as taking place in human skin upon absorption of UV. It is a vasodilator. It *may be* a significant factor in erythema production.[7]

tor substance is produced or activated within the stratum corneum by any UV wavelength.

It has been known since 1950 that erythema production is *not necessary* for bactericidal or other effects of UV.[15] The major usefulness of erythema production is as a clinical dose scale.

Pigmentation Augmentation

Melanin is the pigment which protects skin against damage from overexposure to any source of UV. Although human skin, irrespective of racial genetics, contains the same number of

melanocytes, darker-complected individuals produce more melanin.[16]   Melanin is synthesized from the amino acid tyrosine,
through a series of reactions, and combines with a protein.[17] Figure 6-6 illustrates the known steps in the reaction.

Pigmentation occurs when these pigment granules are transferred from the melanocytes to the keratinocytes. Both types of
cells are found in the basal layer of the epidermis. The pigment
granule remains colorless until it is oxidized. Exposure of the
epidermis to either natural or man-made UV brings about the
oxidation. Smaller quantities of HQ radiation cause more pigmentation than occurs with CQ sources. This makes sense if one
recalls that natural sunlight at sea level has no wavelengths shorter than 290 nm. HQ sources have a large output between 290 and
320 nm. CQ sources have an insignificant output within that
range.

In lightly pigmented skin, the level of activity of *tyrosinase*
always increases when the skin is exposed to UV. Tyrosinase is the
enzyme which catalyzes oxidation of tyrosine into dihydroxy-
phenylalanine. If the level of tyrosinase is increased, more tyrosine will be metabolized. One of the results will be augmented
pigmentation. There is some evidence that genetically darker
skin contains more of a tyrosinase *inhibitor*.[7] The net effect of the
inhibitor is to prevent already pigmented skin from darkening
further upon exposure to wavelengths longer than 290 nm.

Certainly it can be shown in patients with vitiligo, a depig-
menting disease, that vitiliginous areas will sunburn far more
easily than the surrounding darker skin. A standard treatment
for this disease is oral administration of 8-methoxypsoralen (a
photosensitizing chemical) followed by suberythemal doses of
HQ-UV.[4,5]

Most redheads and blondes are far more apt to suffer from
overexposure to the sun. Few brunettes or blacks need fear the
sun. However, there are notable exceptions among both lightly
and heavily pigmented individuals. These exceptions, plus individual treatment source differences in output, plus differences
in recent over-the-counter or prescription medication make performance of a sleeve test almost mandatory if large areas of the

TYROSINE

   Tyrosinase

3, 4 DEHYDROXYPHENYLALANINE
(DOPA)

   Tyrosinase

DOPAQUINONE

INDOLE 5, 6 QUINONE

5, 6 DEHYDROXYINDOLE

5, 6 INDOLEQUINONE

   Polymerization

MELANIN

Figure 6-6. *Conversion of Tyrosine into Melanin.* One way in which melanin is formed is by absorption of UV by the amino acid tyrosine, which is

skin are to be treated with clinical UV. Details of this test procedure are given in the technique section of this chapter. It is the therapist's responsibility to see that the same lamp that was used for testing is used for treatment. The sleeve test is not as critical when mucous membranes (inside of the mouth) or open wounds (pressure sores) are treated. These tissues will tolerate and benefit from far heavier doses. Doses standardly used on open wounds would cause a 3rd degree burn if applied to healthy skin.

The Bactericidal Effect

It is now well established that when any microorganism absorbs UV of a wavelength at or near 254 nm, the pyrimidine base fraction of deoxyribonucleic acid (DNA) known as thymine is the most strongly affected part of the molecule.[7,9,17] When DNA absorbs UV in the 250 to 270 nm range, thymine dimerization occurs. Only 1 to 2 percent of the thymine in a given molecule needs to be affected to suppress the ability of the cell to synthesize new DNA. Normally, no thymine fraction of DNA is ever directly linked to another thymine fraction. With dimerization, two thymine fractions break their normal linkages and join together. Figure 6-7 schematically portrays the theoretical appearance of a thymine dimer.

A UV dose several times *weaker* than that needed to produce an MED is completely lethal to the absorbing microorganism. Appendix C gives in tabular form the known physiological mechanisms excited by various UV wavelengths and intensities needed.

When human epidermis absorbs wavelengths in the 250 to 270 nm range in sufficient quantity, DNA synthesis is suppressed for twenty-four to forty-eight hours. This is followed by a period of increased synthesis, and hyperplasia.

The CQ-UV lamp major output is at 254 nm. Because its infrared output is low, there is little risk of concomitant thermal damage when massive doses of UV are needed. There is some recent evidence (1973) that the presence of histidine in the skin at the time of exposure will tend to block absorption of longer wave-

---

normally present in human skin. The steps outlined in this series of reactions are known to take place in human skin.[22]

A Thymine
(as part of DNA)

B Thymine Dimer
(shaded area indicates
linkage between two
Thymine molecules)

Figure 6-7. *Conversion of Thymine into Thymine Dimers.* Thymine is a pyrimidine base fraction of human DNA and RNA. Absorption of UV by human DNA or RNA causes some of the thymine to dimerize. This prevents normal metabolism of the DNA. If enough thymine is converted, the cell dies.[7]

lengths of UV by the pyrimidine bases of DNA.[18] The molecular mechanism of this attenuation is unknown. Whether this has clinical significance is unknown. It is well known that HQ-UV, which produces significant quantities of UV in both the 250 to 270 nm and 290 to 320 nm ranges is also highly effective as a bactericidal agent.

Photosensitization and Photoreactivation

The term *photosensitization* refers to the process by which an object becomes abnormally sensitive to light. The furocoumarins (psoralens) constitute a class of compound which, when administered either orally or topically to humans, enhances the effects of UV.[4,5] It has been recently shown that the psoralens bind to the pyrimidine bases in both DNA and RNA, forming a new cyclobutane ring. This reaction is strongly enhanced when the skin is exposed to HQ-UV (290 to 310 nm) but is attenuated when exposed to CQ-UV (254 nm).[19] Thus, if one wishes to increase the effectiveness of UV by use of a psoralen, one should remember to use a hot quartz rather than a cold quartz lamp.

The authors are not aware of any similar study on the effects of crude coal tar preparations on DNA or RNA. Crude coal tar has been used for years as a topical ointment to enhance the effects of UV in the treatment of acute generalized psoriasis. It would be interesting to test the effectiveness of HQ versus CQ sources when the Goeckermann regimen, or some modification of it, is used in the management of psoriasis. There are many modifications of the Goeckermann regimen in use. Basically, it consists of topical application of some form of crude coal tar as a paste or ointment to the psoriatic skin several times daily, and especially within one hour before exposure to UV. The ointment is removed immediately before exposure to UV, using a dry towel (no solvent). This mechanical removal of the ointment leaves a *thin* residue, which is excited by the absorption of UV. The excitation markedly enhances the visible and other effects of the radiation upon the epidermis and dermis. Frequently, the UV exposure is immediately followed by a ten– to twenty-minute immersion in a dilute starch or bran bath, which, at least in some patients, seems to further intensify the effects of the UV.[20]

Photoreactivation is the name given to the process which decreases the effects of UV. The process was discovered by Kelner in 1949.[21] He observed that bacteria which had been exposed to 100 percent lethal doses of 254 nm UV would survive if later exposed to daylight which had reached the bacteria through window glass. In time, it was shown that wavelengths from 320 to 400 nm were essential for photoreactivation, with exposure to radiation at 340 nm being the most effective. In the mid 1970s, conclusive evidence was reported demonstrating that human epidermal re-action to UV is attenuated by later exposure to similar longer wavelengths.[22]

This becomes important clinically if a patient is inadvertently given a massive overdose of UV. When this is known to have happened, the overexposed skin should be treated with a lumin-ous infrared lamp (see Chapter 5) or to a residential type fluores-cent light within one hour after the overexposure to UV. The attenuating radiation should be applied for at least ten minutes. This will usually diminish the injurious effects of overexposure to UV.

INDICATIONS FOR ULTRAVIOLET THERAPY

There are three major categories of indication for the clinical use of UV. These are infections, noninfectuous skin diseases in which transient exfoliation and hyperplasia are adjunctive in the return of the epidermis to its normal state, and in excitation of calcium metabolism.[1-6]

The mechanism by which UV disrupts microbial infection is the dimerization of the thymine fraction of DNA.[7,9,21,22] DNA and/or RNA is present in the nucleus of all microorganisms as well as in all human cells. Theoretically, CQ-UV should be more effective for this disruption because absorption of the 250 to 270 nm wavelengths without the presence and absorption of addition-al longer wavelengths does not stimulate histidine inhibition of the thymine dimerization.[19] The presence of histidine in the intra– or extracellular fluid blocks or suppresses DNA disruption.

It has been the authors' clinical experience that HQ-UV is equally or more effective in combatting infection as compared to CQ-UV. The reasons for this are not known. It may be that the mixture of both long and short wave UV brings about additional chemical reactions which have not yet been isolated but which are synergistic to DNA alteration, or it may be simply that the total UV output per unit area is significantly greater with any clinical HQ-UV source.

With the evolution of antibiotic therapy since the 1940s, the need for UV to combat infection has markedly declined, except in the treatment of pressure sores. These open wounds do not respond well to antibiotics, presumably because of their poor blood supply.[3] It will be interesting to see whether development of new antibiotics will keep pace with the evolution of antibiotic-resistant strains of microorganisms.[24]

The use of UV in the management of infections has a major drawback — its lack of depth of penetration. The absorbing microorganisms must be within a few microns of the surface being exposed in order to absorb the radiation. This requires cleansing and drying of the skin or debridement of the open wound prior to each exposure in order to achieve maximum effect.

The skin lesions which respond to UV but which are not caused by contagious pathogens are acne, seborrheic dermatis, psoriasis, and pityriasis rosea.[2,4,5] The role of dehydration, hyperplasia, exfoliation, and pigment augmentation in the treatment of these lesions is not known. The mechanism of increasing UV effectiveness through the use of photosensitizing drugs may, at least in the case of the psoralens, be the disruption of DNA by 290 to 310 nm UV.[19] It is known that these pathologies respond better to HQ sources of UV and that the best approach is to start the series of treatments with an SED, working toward an MED.[2,4,5]

The authors would like to see the results of a carefully designed comparative study on patients whose clinical diagnosis indicates the likelihood of onset of pressure sores, with half the patients receiving regular suberythemal doses of UV to skin over bony prominences long before there is any sign of incipient breakdown and the other half not receiving UV until the ulceration is self-evident. It would be interesting to determine whether the difference in number and severity of the pressure sores would be statistically significant in a series of 100 patients.

Although it has been known for years that epidermal absorption of UV stimulates interaction between calcium and provitamin D, and that it stimulates calcium absorption, no clue to the mechanism has yet been published.[6,22] To the best of the authors' knowledge, there has been no definitive study published on the possible role of UV in arresting or reversing osteoporosis or in arresting or reversing soft tissue calcification. Since both the latter lesions are far more common than osteomalacia, at least in the nongeriatric population, this could be a useful investigation. It is probable that a significant number of cases could be assembled by a small number of cooperating institutions within a matter of one or two years.

CONTRAINDICATIONS FOR ULTRAVIOLET THERAPY

There are a few clear-cut contraindications for the clinical use of UV. These are mostly in rare metabolic disorders such as in the porphyrias and pellegra[6] or in the presence of either systemic or discoid lupus erythematosus, sarcoidosis, or xeroderma pigmentosum.[2,4,5] Because of extreme individual differences in skin reaction to exposure to UV, it is strongly recommended that a sleeve test be performed prior to treatment to enable the therapist to achieve the desired level of response. For this same reason, a detailed record should be kept of the source used, distance, and duration of each exposure. This should minimize the chances for error resulting in either over– or underdosage. Whenever skin absorbs UV, enough energy is absorbed per unit volume to bring about a massive stimulus-response reaction. Therefore, whole-body irradiation should also be avoided in patients who have severe cardiac, pulmonary, renal, or hepatic pathology.

SUMMARY

The physical and physiological differences between broad and narrow spectrum clinical ultraviolet sources are discussed, including advantages and disadvantages of each type of source. Differences in utilization on skin as compared to other tissue is stressed. Standard clinical treatment techniques, along with indications and contraindications, are reviewed. The importance of performing a sleeve test, especially when large areas of skin are to be exposed, is emphasized. Presently known mechanisms in erythema and pigmentation production, bactericidal effects, and excitation of calcium metabolism are discussed. The possible significance of photoreactivation in all of the above mechanisms is presented.

APPENDIX A

PHOTOSENSITIZING DRUGS*

I. Sulfonamides

II. Sulfonylurea Hypoglycemics
   Tolbutamide
   Chlorpromamide
   Acetohexamide

III. Antibiotics
   Demethyltetracycline
   Griseofulvin
   Tetracycline

IV. Chlorthyazide Diuretics
   Chlorothiazide
   Hydrochlorothiazide
   Cyclothiazide
   Methylchlorothiazide

V. Phenothiazines
   Chlorpromazine
   Promazine
   Perchlorperizine
   Promethazine
   Neprazine

VI. Psoralens (Furocoumarins)
   8-Methoxypsoralen

---

*From G. Sauer, *Manual of Skin Diseases,* 3rd Ed., 1973. Courtesy of J.B. Lippin-cott Company, Philadelphia.

APPENDIX B

PHYSICAL DIFFERENCES BETWEEN HOT AND COLD QUARTZ ULTRAVIOLET LAMPS

	Spectral Output (UV)	Electron Temp.	Average Mercury Temp.	Envelope Temp.	Starting Voltage	Running Voltage	Starting Amperes	Running Amperes	Arc Warmup	Restart Characteristics
COLD QUARTZ	Narrow – more than 90% at 2537 Å	Higher than for Hg vapor	7000° to 9000°C	60°C	High – 1800 to 2000	Low – 110 to 120	Low – Less than one	Low – Less than one	Instant	Instant
HOT QUARTZ	Broad – Strong at 2537, 2800 & 2967 Å	Equal to that for Hg vapor	7000° to 9000°C	500 to 1000°C	Moderate – 800 to 1000	Moderate – 400 to 500	High – 5 to 20	High – 5 to 10	2 to 5 minute *minimum*	2 minute minimum after lamp is shut off

APPENDIX C

ESTABLISHED *PHYSIOLOGICAL* EFFECT DIFFERENCES BETWEEN HOT AND COLD QUARTZ ULTRAVIOLET LAMPS

	Bactericidal Effects	Conversion of Provitamin D into the active compound	Excitation of Calcium and Phosphorous	Erythema Production	Pigmentation Augmentation
COLD QUARTZ	Excellent	None	None	Moderate — early onset, short duration	Usually poor, short duration
HOT QUARTZ	Good	Excellent	Excellent	Strong — delayed onset, long duration	Variable, usually strong

Under optimal circumstances, it requires about 20 microwatts/cm²/second for ionization of Ca and P.[6]
Under optimal circumstances, it requires about 100 microwatts/cm²/second for thymine dimerization when DNA is exposed to UV at 2537 Å.[18]
Under optimal circumstances, for lightly pigmented Caucasian skin, it requires about 700 to 800 microwatts/cm²/second for production of a minimal erythemal dose when skin is exposed to UV at 2967 Å.[4,24]

REFERENCES

1. Taylor, R.: Clinical study of ultraviolet in various skin conditions. *Phys Ther, 52*:279-82, 1972.
2. Epstein, J.: Ultraviolet light in office practice. *Postgrad Med, 37*:70-4, 1965.
3. Bailey, B.N.: *Bedsores.* Baltimore, Williams & Wilkins, 1967.
4. Sulzberger, W., Wolf, J., and Witten, V.: *Dermatology: Diagnosis and Treatment,* 2nd ed. Chicago, Year Bk Med, 1961, pp. 85-96, 558.
5. Sauer, G. (Ed.): *Manual of Skin Diseases,* 3rd ed. Philadelphia, Lippincott, 1973.
6. Thompson, R. and Wootton, I.: *Biochemical Disorders in Human Diseases,* 3rd ed. New York, Acad Pr, 1970, pp. 774-82.
7. Giese, A. (Ed.): *Photophysiology,* Volume IV. New York, Acad Pr, 1968, Chapter II.
8. Hollaender, A. (Ed.): *Radiation Biology,* Volume II. New York, McGraw, 1955.
9. Urbach, F. (Ed.): *Biological Effects of Ultraviolet Radiation.* New York, Pergamon, 1969.
10. Montagna, W. and Labitz, W. (Eds.): *The Epidermis.* New York, Acad Pr, 1964, p. 408.
11. Holti, G.: Measurements of the vascular responses in skin at various time intervals after damage with histamine and ultraviolet radiation. *Clin Sci, 14*:143-55, 1955.
12. Sams, W. and Winkleman, R.: The effect of ultraviolet light on isolated cutaneous blood vessels. *J Invest Dermatol, 53*:79-83, 1969.
13. Van der Leun, J.C.: Theory of ultraviolet erythema. *Photochem Photobiol, 4*:453-8, 1965.
14. Tronnier, H.: Zur Bedeutung der Hornschicht fur die Lichttreaktionen der menschlichen Haut. *Strahlentherapie, 132*:128-33, 1967.
15. Grynbaum, B. et al.: Prevention of ultraviolet induced erythema. *Arch Phys Med Rehabil, 31*:587-92, 1950.
16. Gordon, M. (Ed.): *Pigment Cell Biology.* New York, Acad Pr, 1959, pp. 107-9, 127-37.
17. Giese, A. (Ed.): *Photophysiology,* Volume V. New York, Acad Pr, 1970, Chapters VI and VII.
18. Giese, A. (Ed.): *Photophysiology,* Volume VI. New York, Acad Pr, 1971, Chapter III.
19. Peak, M. et al.: Inactivation of transforming DNA by ultraviolet light. II. Protection by histadine. *Mutat Res, 20*:137-41, 1973.
20. Krusen, F.H.: *Physical Medicine.* Philadelphia, Saunders, 1971, Chapter V.
21. Kelner, A.: Photoreactivation of ultraviolet irradiated eschericoli, with special reference to the dose reduction principle and to ultraviolet induced mutation. *J Bacteriol, 58*:511-22, 1949.

22. Giese, A. (Ed.): *Photophysiology,* Volume VII. New York, Acad Pr, 1972, Chapters V and IX.

23. Nicolaus, R.A.: *Melanins.* Paris, The Hermann Co., 1968, Chapters 3, 5, and 8.

24. Pringsheim, P.: *Fluorescence and Phosphorescence.* New York, Interscience, 1949.

25. Dulaney, E.L. and Laskin, A.I. (Eds.): The problems of drug resistant pathogenic bacteria. *Ann NY Acad Sci,* Vol. 182, June 11, 1971.

Chapter 7

ULTRASONIC ENERGY

INTRODUCTION

U TILIZATION of ultrasonic energy for relief of pain and/or soft tissue relaxation was introduced into this country in the early 1950s. Prior to that time, extensive basic research, with subsequent clinical application, had been carried out in Europe, especially in Germany. Basic and clinical research has continued there and has developed in this country. Clinical application of ultrasonic energy for pain relief is now widespread and is perhaps second only to the use of hot packs.

Ultrasonic energy is a component of the acoustic spectrum of energy rather than a segment of the electromagnetic spectrum. Acoustic energy production, transmission, and absorption differ in major ways from that of electromagnetic energy. Acoustic energy of any wavelength cannot penetrate a vacuum. It must be conducted by molecules or larger units of matter. Electromagnetic energy travels best through a vacuum and does so at the speed of light (approximately 300,000,000 meters per second). Acoustic energy travels very inefficiently through any gas or mixture of gases. Electromagnetic energy travels well through gases. At sea level, its velocity is about 296,700,000 m/s. At sea level pressures, acoustic energy travels at a rate of about 330 m/s. Acoustic energy is transmitted well through degassed or gas-free liquids and travels best through high density solids. Since velocity equals wavelength times frequency, and wavelength equals velocity divided by frequency, any acoustic frequency will have a far shorter wavelength than electromagnetic energy of the same frequency.

Ultrasonic energy by definition is any vibrational energy of a frequency too high for stimulation of the sensory receptors of the human ear. Obviously the cutoff point between audible and ultrasonic sound will vary, particularly with age, but in no case will audible sound have a frequency over 20,000 Hertz (Hz). Ultrasonic energy is almost entirely absorbed by the nitrogen, oxygen, and carbon dioxide in the atmosphere. Hence, in order to transmit ultrasonic energy to a patient, a liquid or a semisolid (ointment) must be used to insure significant transfer of energy from the source to the patient. Human skin is not a smooth surface, even when the transmitting applicator is applied with pressure. When the radiating surface is in contact with skin, air is always trapped within the pores of the skin. This leads to non-uniform energy transmission from the patient surface of the applicator into absorbing tissues. If the applicator (sound head or transducer) and the skin are immersed in a liquid or semisolid, the amount of interfering air is markedly reduced. Both the efficiency and uniformity of energy transmission is greatly enhanced. Use of a coupling agent is standard clinical procedure.

Since human soft tissues consist of 70 to 90 percent water, plus proteins and other solids, the velocity of sound in water is standardly considered to be equivalent to that of sonic and ultrasonic energy in soft tissues. At ambient temperatures, that velocity is about 1500 m/s. Ultrasonic velocity in cortical bone, the body's most dense solid, is approximately 3500 m/s. For various reasons, to be discussed later in this chapter, the standard clinical ultrasonic frequency is 1 megacycle (1 Mc = 1000 Kc = 1000 KHz), although there are commercially available clinical generators with an operating frequency as low as 750 Kc and as high as 2 Mc. The relationship of operating frequency to depth of penetration is well documented.[1] With a frequency of 1 Mc, approximately 50 percent of the ultrasonic energy will penetrate to a depth of 5 cm within soft tissue. At 90 Kc, 50 percent will reach a depth of 10 cm. At 4 Mc, 50 percent will penetrate to a depth of 1 cm. It is then obvious that clinical ultrasound is indicated when good depth of penetration is needed. Ultrasonic energy has another important clinical advantage over any electronmagnetic energy that physical therapists utilize, namely the more homogenous the tissue, the less the absorption. Subcutaneous fat is the most nearly homogenous human tissue and presents many problems when electro-magnetic energy is being added for the purpose of causing a deep tissue temperature rise (TTR). Excessive fat temperature rise is no problem when ultrasonic energy is used. This fact, coupled with the depth of penetration, makes ultrasound the most effective physical agent when a TTR is required in a deeply seated joint.

A further advantage is that ultrasound may be safely used even though metallic implants are well within the depth of penetration of 50 percent of the energy.[2] The metal does not absorb or concentrate the energy as would be the case if short wave or microwave energy were used, although there will be reflection, especially if the radiating surface of the application is not at a right angle to the implant's largest dimension. Hence, the presence of metallic implants does not give rise to tissue "hot-spots" with subsequent risk of damage to adjacent tissue. Actually, it has been shown that the metals used in the various wires, screws, plates, and joint replacements do not get as hot as surrounding tissues. Presumably, this is because the metal is more homogenous than living tissues and therefore transmits rather than absorbs the ultrasonic energy.

In the past, there has been major controversy as to whether the pain-relieving effects subsequent to exposure to ultrasonic energy are entirely due to the TTR, which always occur under clinical conditions, or to a combination of thermal and nonthermal (mechanical or chemical) effects, or to the nonthermal effects alone. Three of the leaders of ultrasonic research in this country, Schwann, Lehmann, and Gersten, now (1975) agree that there are significant nonthermal effects. Possibly Gersten and coworkers[3,4] were the first to demonstrate nonthermal effects of ultrasonic energy on peripheral nerve. In publications appearing as late as 1965, Schwann classified ultrasonic energy as a form of diathermy.[5] In 1969, he stated that he wished he could tear up that section of his chapter and give equal emphasis to the thermal and nonthermal effects of ultrasound.[6] Lehmann was well aware of the existence of nonthermal effects of ultrasound in the 1950s[7] but did not regard them as clinically significant until much later.[8]

The reluctance of many investigators to conclude that non-thermal effects of ultrasound on intact tissues might have clinical significance is understandable if one reviews the intensive efforts made in the 1930s and 1940s to demonstrate nonthermal effects from exposure to short wave and microwave diathermies. It is now well accepted that the only effects of these latter forms of energy are due solely to the TTR which results from absorption of these electromagnetic frequencies.

Thus, treatment with ultrasonic energy can lead to pain relief where the lesion is beyond the reach of an infrared– or diathermy-induced TTR because of its superior penetration. It can be used safely in the presence of metallic implants whereas the diathermies cannot (*see Chapter* 4), and it can give pain relief by mechanisms not related to tissue temperature rise.

GENERATION OF CLINICAL ULTRASONIC ENERGY

Any unit of matter exposed to a pulsating stimulus will be set into vibration by the absorption of energy. Vibration is standardly defined as periodic motion in alternately opposite directions from a position of equilibrium. The rate of vibration will be in direct proportion to the rate of alternate periods of stimulus — no stimulus — stimulus, etc. In the case of a solid of finite dimension, there will be a certain rate of stimulus which will produce the maximum excursion of vibration for a given quantity of energy absorbed. That particular rate is called the resonant frequency. What that rate will be depends largely on the dimensions of the solid and, of course, upon its composition. When the vibrating object is of homogenous composition, i.e. a crystalline material, its resonant frequency is controlled largely by the ratio of thickness to width or diameter. In general, the higher the ratio, the higher the resonant frequency.

One convenient way to set crystals into vibration is to attach two wires at some distance apart on the face of the crystal. If a direct current (DC) voltage of adequate amplitude is applied, the mass of the crystal will tend to deform as long as the voltage is applied, but in one direction only. This would not result in vibration in the usual sense, and if the energy applied were great enough, the crystal would eventually shatter. If an alternating current (AC) is applied, with each half cycle the crystal would bend first in one direction and then in the other, with maximum excursion if the AC frequency matched the ratio of thickness to diameter. If a liquid or solid is in contact with a face of the vibrating crystal, much of the energy applied to the crystal would be transferred to that other material in a periodic fashion.

When ultrasonic energy began to come into clinical use, most ultrasonic generators produced the mechanical energy by applying AC of appropriate frequency to natural quartz crystals. Quartz is expensive and hard to work with. Furthermore, quartz is a very poor conductor of electricity. Hence, high voltage is required to set quartz crystals into vibration. Fortunately, the technology for precise controlled growth of synthetic crystals developed rapidly immediately after World War II, and some synthetic crystals are admirably suited for being driven by low voltage, high frequency AC. At this point in time, almost all clinical ultrasonic generators utilize either barium titanate, lead zirconate, or a grown mixture of the two kinds of crystals to convert high frequency, low voltage AC into high frequency sound energy. For protection of the patient and of the crystal, the crystal is bonded to a metal plate (usually nickle-plated brass) or to a thin layer of glass. This surface is applied to the patient. The dimensions of the plate or glass are carefully selected so that their resonant frequency exactly matches that of the driven crystal. These synthetic crystals are cheaper to prepare for clinical use and require far less voltage to set into useful vibration as compared to quartz, so the cost of the necessary transformer for modifying house current is far less. The net result is that it is now possible to buy a clinically adequate ultrasonic generator for as little as 250 dollars, although extremely sophisticated models may cost nearly ten times that much.

A crystal which has an operating frequency of 1 Mc will have a thickness of 3 to 4 mm. Clinically useful crystals will have a diameter of anywhere from 0.5 to 10 cm. Most of the transducers in use have an effective patient surface of from 2 to 10 cm². Different manufacturers vary widely as to how much of the apparent patient surface is actually producing a significant quantity of ultrasonic vibration.[9] One should bear in mind that an operating frequency of 1 Mc means that the crystal is deforming one million times per second in each of two directions — toward and away from the patient. When the operating frequency is lower the crystal is thicker. When the frequency is higher, the crystal is thinner. For any given diameter or thickness, the synthetic crystals will have a more nearly uniform energy output from the entire radiating surface as compared to natural quartz crystals. The latter are very apt to have a high intensity output at the center of the radiating surface and much less toward the periphery. Thus, if the radiating surface had an area of 5 cm^2 the center square centimeter might be producing two to five times more ultrasonic energy than that surface as little as 0.5 cm distant. Such a "hot-spot" effect is much less evident with barium titanate or lead zirconate crystals. The synthetic crystals respond to an applied AC voltage with a more nearly true piston action rather than a deforming or bowing effect.

To drive either kind of crystal, house current (60 cycle 110 v AC) is converted into whatever is the resonant frequency of the crystal to be driven. This frequency conversion is done by some form of oscillating circuit (*see* Chapter 8). The high frequency current is then led into a step-up transformer to supply a high voltage (quartz crystal, 2000 to 3000 v) or an intermediate voltage (synthetic crystal, 200 to 300 v). The modified electromagnetic energy is then coupled to the crystal, usually through a coaxial or triaxial cable. Since clinical use of ultrasonic energy frequently necessitates immersion techniques, there must be a good seal between the lead cable and the crystal and between the crystal and its metal or glass patient surface.

Early ultrasonic generators had problems with bonding the metal or glass face to the crystal and to the metal covering housing the disc edge. One could tell that the bond was becoming defective when audible as well as ultrasonic energy was being produced. Apparatus manufactured since about 1965 rarely becomes defective in this manner.

The crystals are driven with either continuous or pulse modulation AC. The former is in more common use. In apparatus designed to deliver pulsing ultrasound (US), there frequently is a manually controlled variation in ratio of power on to power off. Some arrangements for this duty factor control are very precise. Others leave much to be desired insofar as accuracy in timing and uniformity of intensity is concerned, especially when a given piece of apparatus has been in regular use for more than six months.[9] With pulsed ultrasonic energy, it is possible to use higher peak intensities with less risk of tissue damage.

CLINICAL ULTRASONIC FREQUENCIES

Perhaps more than 90 percent of all the clinical ultrasonic generators in use in this country are intended for operation at a frequency of 1 Mc. This frequency was deliberately chosen as a compromise frequency between those which produce predominantly thermal effects (2 Mc and higher) and those which produce nonthermal (mechanical and/or chemical) as well as thermal effects (500 Kc or lower) in human soft tissues. Theoretically, if the ratio of crystal thickness to diameter is kept constant, frequencies below 300 Kc should *not* produce a significant TTR.[10] This is true for at least two reasons. At lower ultrasonic frequencies, the energy spreads laterally to a much greater extent than is true for frequencies at or above 1 Mc, so that there is less energy available for absorption per unit of volume of tissue. Also at low frequencies, the time between significant radiation pressure changes becomes great enough so that there is no net TTR. In practice, since it is not feasible to keep the ratio constant in a clinically useful transducer because of size of the patient surface, the lower frequencies also produce a strong TTR, in large part due to the thermal *(not acoustic)* energy production and transmission as well as US (ultrasonic) energy production.[11] A barium titanate crystal with a resonant frequency of 250 Kc will be about 2 cm thick. If its total patient surface area is 5 cm, its diameter will also be about 2 cm. Thus, the crystal would be very nearly symmetrical in its critical dimensions. Such a crystal will become quite hot when an AC voltage is applied with an intensity great enough to produce more than a few tenths of a watt per cm² of ultrasonic energy. Because of the liquid or semisolid coupling between the transducer and the patient, much of the thermal energy, along with the ultrasonic energy, is transmitted to the patient. The Acoustics Branch of the Bureau of Radiological Health is in the process of establishing regulations which will include requiring the manufacturer to state the expected crystal face temperature rise under standard operating conditions for any ultrasonic generator intended for clinical use.

PHYSIOLOGICAL EFFECTS OF CLINICAL ULTRASONIC ENERGY

This discussion will be limited to effects that have been demonstrated when the operating frequency is between 750 and 2000 Kc at intensities not exceeding 3 watts per cm²(w/cm²). Almost all ultrasonic generators in clinical use in this country have an operating frequency within that range and a maximum output of 3 w/cm²/or less.

Effects of Ultrasonic Energy on Peripheral Nerve

It has been known at least since 1950 that peripheral nerve *in situ* is more responsive to exposure to ultrasonic energy than is any other soft tissue.[12] It has been shown that there is more cortisol present in normal untreated peripheral nerve than in any human soft tissue except the adrenal cortex.[13] It has also been demonstrated that when the peripheral nerve (lumbosacral plexus) of swine is sonated *in situ* its cortisol content increases significantly.[14] Farmer established that there is significant change in conduction velocity when human subjects are exposed to ultrasound.[15] When ultrasonic intensity is between 0.5 and 1.5 w/cm², conduction velocity decreases. At intensities below 0.5 or above 2 w/cm², conduction velocity increases. When electromagnetic energy is absorbed in sufficient quantity to cause a TTR, conduction velocity invariably increases. Reasons why absorption of intermediate intensities of ultrasonic energy result in decrease of nerve conduction are not known at this time. It has been shown that the change in conduction velocity takes place when provision is made to prevent TTR as well as when a TTR is allowed to occur. The latter is the normal clinical circumstance.[4]

Molecular Effects

Piersol and coworkers established that about 80 percent of ultrasonic energy is absorbed by proteins, in comparison with carbohydrates and lipids, and that absorption is equal in protein in plasma and in membranes.[16] Lota and Darling demonstrated that clinical intensities alter the diffusion of potassium and sodium across the red blood cell membrane.[17] When ultrasonic energy is applied with an intensity of about 1 w/cm², radiation pressure changes on the order of $\pm$ 1.5 atmospheres take place within the absorbing tissues. This has been calculated to represent a change of about $\pm$ 4 milligrams per cell and is not regarded as destructive.[10] Both the pressure change and the normally occurring TTR could be factors in the well-established alteration of cell permeability. The pressure changes are usually considered to have a micromassage effect on the absorbing tissues.

Tissue Temperature Rise

Schwann,[18] Lota,[19] and Lehmann and others[20,23] have shown that with clinical intensities applied with a continuously moving sound head, muscle temperature rises on the order of 1° to 2°C are common. Subcutaneous fat temperatures are about half that of the underlying muscle. If cortical bone lies within the limit of penetration of 50 percent of the energy being added, the bone temperature rise will be 5° to 6°C. All temperature changes due to exposure to ultrasonic energy occur much more rapidly than is the case when electromagnetic energy is the cause of the TTR. With ultrasound, the temperature rise occurs within twenty to thirty seconds. Presumably, this difference in rate in rise is due to the fact that a large percentage of ultrasonic energy applied to the skin is transmitted through the skin and subcutaneous fat, which in turn permits primary absorption in underlying muscle and connective tissue much more efficiently than can occur when electromagnetic energy is added. Subcutaneous fat acts as an insulator against penetration of electromagnetic energy at frequencies in clinical use. Hence, deeper tissue temperature rise is predominantly due to reaction by cutaneous nerve and/or secondary conduction. Demonstrable increase in local blood flow may persist up to an hour after a five-minute exposure to ultrasound. When electromagnetic energy is used, a treatment time of nearly ten times as long is necessary to produce equivalent change in deep blood flow.[22,23]

One must remember there is considerable reflection of ultrasound at any tissue interface, i.e. skin-fat or tendon-bone. The reflection results in the more superficial tissue being exposed to greater intensities than would be the case if significant reflection did not occur. Reflection is greatest from tissues of high density. Theoretically, reflection from cortical bone should be on the order of 70 percent.[10] Actual *in vivo* measurements indicate it is more likely to be about half that amount.[20,24] The reflection of energy can give rise to sharply localized pathological temperature increases within the periosteum and to tendon at or near bone-tendon junctions. Both tendon and periosteum have a poor blood supply and a low water content. Hence, these tissues are poorly equipped to disseminate the reflected energy. The periosteum is richly supplied with sensory receptors, including thermal sensors. Therefore, if the patient has a normally functioning sensory nervous system, he will become aware of a characteristic noxious stimulus if the periosteal temperature approaches the critical level (45°C) and will move away from the source of energy before damage is done. The clinical response to periosteal overheating is commonly described as a deep, dull ache of very sudden onset. The sensation may occur at anytime within the treatment and may recur several times during a single treatment. Whenever this sensation is reported, the intensity of the ultrasonic energy being applied must be decreased rapidly or long-lasting thermal damage can occur.

Alteration of Connective Tissue

There are numerous clinical reports which indicate that exposure to ultrasonic energy is effective in permanently diminishing pain due to the presence of neuromas and adhesive scars.[25-27] Also, it has been the authors' clinical impression that when patients with Dupuytren's contracture receive appropriate local sonation, there is long-lasting relaxation of the tight palmar fascia. On the basis of *in vitro* study, where pain is due to excess proliferation of connective tissue, relief of pain may be due to relaxation of polypeptide bonds after the absorption of ultrasonic energy.[3,18] Joseph has reported that experimentally induced wounds heal faster upon exposure to ultrasonic energy. He presented evidence which indicates that improvement in tissue regeneration parallels systemic increase in the "male sex hormone" and that this increase occurs with local sonation at intensities which do not cause a significant TTR.[28]

Exposure to ultrasonic energy is also an effective way of increasing range of motion where limitation is due to massive hypertrophic scar tissue formation, as occurs in burns which have destroyed the dermis. Distinction must be made between hypertrophic and true keloid scars.[29-31] Exposure to ultrasound is not effective in regaining range of motion lost because of formation of a true keloid.[30] The histological distinction between hypertrophic and keloid connective tissue proliferation is that in the former, proliferation comes entirely from the epidermal margin. In keloid proliferation, collagen production is predominantly from dermal rather than epidermal tissue and there is massive hyalinization. Furthermore, hypertrophic scarring occurs with no predilection for race or age, whereas keloid scarring is considerably more common in Negroes, Malaysians, and Hindus and is more common at ages between ten and thirty than at any other time of life. Keloids occur most commonly after trauma which has lacerated the dermis. The biochemical error, if any, which results in the formation of a keloid is not yet known. Recurrence after surgical excision occurs in more than 50 percent of the true keloids as compared to 15 to 20 percent in the more common hypertrophic scar. There is no known surgical, physical, or chemical technique which is consistently reliable in permanently removing the true keloid. Careful radiation therapy is the most reliable treatment to date.[32]

Regeneration and repair of connective tissue after injury is characterized by (1) watery edema, followed by (2) mucinous edema, containing at first hyaluronate and later chondroitin sulfate, and then (3) collagen cicatrization, and in the skin still later by epithelialization.[29] Fibroblasts synthesize the collagen precursors. Mast cells synthesize the acid mucopolysaccharides, i.e. heparin and hyaluronic acid, as well as histamine and serotonin. Repair of damage seems directly proportional to the amount of histamine produced. *In vitro* exposure of hyaluronic and chondroitin sulfuric acids to ultrasonic energy of intensities and duration of exposure close to those used clinically results in a sharp decrease in their viscosities.[33] With prolonged exposure (20 to 30 minutes), their viscosity approaches that of water. It is presumed that the viscosity change is due in large part to disruption of glucoside bonds. It has also been established that there is significant increase in tendon extensibility[34] and relaxation of skeletal muscle[35] upon absorption of ultrasonic energy.   Hence, the therapist should anticipate being able to bring about the regaining of range of motion where the limitation is due to contracted fascia, muscle, tendon, and most scar tissue.

Mineral Deposition in Soft Tissues

A small percentage of patients with a clinical diagnosis of some form of periarticular pathology, i.e. tendonitis, bursitis, or fibrositis, have apparent calcium salt deposition upon or within the irritated tissue, as evidenced by x-ray visualization. Ultrasound has proven useful in relieving pain in many of these cases both with and without hard evidence that there has been mineral deposition within soft tissues.[36-39] Pain relief in such periarticular pathologies could be due to relaxation of skeletal muscle[35] and/or the apparent net result of resorption of abnormal calcium deposition on bone (spur formation), tendon (calcified tendonitis), or in muscle (myofibrositis). It is curious that with the widespread use of ultrasonic energy for relief of pain, no definitive study has been reported wherein pre– and post-treatment x-ray evaluation was used consistently. The author conducted an intensive search of American, British, and Canadian literature up through 1973 for clinical reports where abnormal calcium deposition was a likely cause of pain and was unable to find any study where x-ray evaluation of results was used through the reported series.

As of 1975, there was adequate documentation to state that absorption of ultrasonic energy as it is applied clinically will cause a physiological tissue temperature rise in underlying muscle, nerve, tendon, and bone. Furthermore, because it penetrates more deeply than any electromagnetic energy that physical therapists use, ultrasonic energy is more effective than other physical agents when stimulation of cutaneous nerve and vascular supply does not play a significant role in relief of pain. The significance, if any, of the fact that peripheral nerve is more sensitive to stimulation by ultrasonic energy than any other soft tissue is not yet understood. The fact that exposure to ultrasonic energy relaxes connective tissue in a more nearly lasting fashion than does any form of electromagnetic energy may be due to effects on plasticity, as opposed to elasticity, or to polypeptide bond disruption, or to reaction to radiation pressure changes. Much more laboratory study utilizing clinical parameters of ultrasonic energy needs to be done before the possible significance of nonthermal changes induced by absorption of this form of energy can be clearly stated.

TECHNIQUES OF APPLICATION OF ULTRASONIC ENERGY

Heating of the Skin Prior to the Application of Ultrasonic Energy

Some clinicians prefer to induce a rise in skin and subcutaneous tissue temperature prior to the use of ultrasonic energy (US). This is usually done with some form of infrared or diathermy. When it is done, the "preheat" treatment is usually given for about ten minutes. Clinicians who use this procedure feel that more of the US energy penetrates more deeply if immediately preceded by a local rise in superficial temperature. Other clinicians feel this procedure is unnecessary. The authors know of no published study which would support either school of thought. Until such time as a well-designed comparative study is reported, it would seem logical to try ultrasound alone for three or four treatments. If there is no lasting pain relief and/or gain in range of motion, preheating might then be tried for an equal number of treatments.

"Direct Contact"

This is the standard technique when the area to be treated is of reasonably regular contour. Some form of coupling material, liquid or semisolid (lotion, cream, or ointment) must be applied to the skin to minimize trapping of air in the skin pores when the transducer is applied to the skin and to minimize friction between the moving sound head and the skin. Degassed (boiled) water is the most efficient couplant for transfer of acoustic energy from the patient surface of the transducer into the patient because its acoustic impedance is reasonably close to that of the patient's soft tissues. However, its viscosity is too low to be practical when the direct contact technique is indicated. The sound head is likely to push all the water away so that the pores refill with air. Also, it is difficult for a clinic to maintain an adequate supply of degassed water since as the boiled water returns to room temperature, the nitrogen, oxygen, and carbon dioxide which had been removed by boiling rapidly reenter the water. Hence, many commercially available coupling agents intended for use with the direct contact technique will have water mixed with some kind of thixotropic gel. Since their viscosities are greater than that of water, they will have less of a tendency to be pushed away by the weight or the movement of the sound head. Reid and Cummings measured the transmission of US through several readily available coupling agents, using near field measurement technics.[40] They found that a thixotropic gel transmitted better than 70 percent of the radiated energy, glycerol about 68 percent, water about 60 percent, and mineral oil about 20 percent. Mineral oil is perhaps the most widely used couplant because it is cheap and gets the job done.

In a later study, Warren and colleagues measured transmissivity through various couplants, using far field measurement technics through a thin layer of couplant and then a large volume of degassed water. Using water as a reference standard for transmissivity, Warren found that glycerine was 75 to 100 percent as efficient as water and that mineral oil was as efficient or more efficient compared to water, under several experimental conditions.[41] It is then reasonable to conclude that when the direct contact technic is used, it does not matter which coupling agent is applied, insofar as transmissivity is concerned. There has been no study yet reported which has attempted to establish whether transmissivity is altered under the usual conditions for an immersion technic.

Various emulsions of water and animal or vegetable fats are also in clinical use. One must remember the transducer will always become warm during a direct contact treatment, so the gels and emulsions will tend to liquify during treatment. One should then compromise between couplants which will remain as a semisolid with a relatively high viscosity and hence require more effort on the part of the therapist to keep the sound head moving and the couplants which are liquids or become liquid during the treatment. A couplant which is adequate in body segments where the skin temperature is relatively low may be inadequate in segments that are more proximal. Furthermore, an agent which is adequate for use with a moving sound head may not be adequate with a stationary technic.

The coupling agent should be applied to the skin and the sound head should be in place on the skin before the transducer is energized. Otherwise, if the crystal is set into vibration and there is no provision for unloading the vibrational energy, the crystal will develop standing waves which can interfere with resonant vibration within the crystal. In extreme cases, the standing wave load can cause structural damage to the crystal. When this has occurred, the sound head must be replaced and the oscillating circuit must be recalibrated.

In the most common clinical usage, once energized, the sound head is kept in continuous motion on the skin over the area being treated. Since the patient surface of the applicator is hard and rigid, care should be taken to avoid running into a bony prominence such as a vertebral spinous process or a greater trochanter. Such contact can be painful if the subcutaneous fat layer is thin. The authors feel strongly that movement of the sound head should be slow and steady — on the order of 60 cm per minute — for best relaxation for the patient. Other clinicians feel that by moving the sound head faster, they can use a higher intensity without causing periosteal overheating. In either case, two types of motion are in general use — a slow circle within a circle with concomitant translatory motion, or a pure stroking movement. There is more risk of hot-spot development if the pure stroke is used, since inevitably there will be deceleration of motion as the direction of the stroke is reversed. Possibly, the circle-within-a-circle technic results in a slightly more uniform pattern of energy absorption within the area being treated, especially if the radiating surface of the sound head has an area of 5 cm² or less. If the effective radiating surface is 10 cm² or greater, it is simple to achieve adequate overlap with either technic and hence more nearly uniform application of energy.

Intensity to be used should vary depending upon whether the objective of treatment is to cause a maximum tolerable TTR or whether nonthermal effects are also desired. Connective tissue relaxation and relief of periarticular pain do not require intensities in excess of 2 watts/cm.[2,3,4,7,8,15,18,46] In general, the greater the volume of soft tissue, the higher the intensity. One needs to remember that the intensity indicated on the generator meter is not reliable, especially in apparatus which has not been calibrated within the last six months.[9] At least until such time as the federal government standardizes and enforces acoustic rather than the present electric power output measurement, it is better to use an intensity which produces a gentle sensation of warmth as the sound head is kept in slow motion rather than blindly picking a meter reading and adhering to it regardless of the patient sensation of warmth. Obviously, there can be dosage problems when ultrasonic energy is applied to patients who have a deficit in their sensory nervous system and/or an emotional disturbance. Significant damage to the patient is unlikely to occur if the intensity used on the trunk or proximal extremity does not exceed 1.5 w/cm² and on the distal extremity does not exceed 0.5 w/cm², assuming an area of about 150 cm² is being treated over a five-minute period with a steadily moving sound head.

Stationary Technique

There are occasions when a direct contact stationary technic is preferrable to a direct contact moving sound head technic. If there is a small, sharply localized area of pain and/or muscle spasm and/or organized hematoma, the stationary technic may be more effective. Specially designed transducers are more apt to be used for this procedure. Those in widespread use have a patient surface area of 50 to 100 cm². Very few pain-producing ortho-pedic lesions will be so sharply localized that the more common 5 to 10 cm² radiating surface will be adequate.

There are two important procedure differences when the stationary technic is used. The intensity must be far lower, and the coupling agent should have a greater viscosity as compared to when the moving technic is used. Although intensities up to 2 w/cm² are common with the moving direct contact technic, very few individuals can safely tolerate 0.2 w/cm² for more than two or three minutes with the stationary treatment, regardless of the volume of underlying soft tissue. Intensity on the order of 0.02 to 0.1 w/cm² is usually comfortable when the stationary sound head is in place for five minutes or more. The usual treatment time is ten to fifteen minutes, with the therapist always remaining close by to lower intensity as needed. Thus, if one is treating a small, sharply delineated organized hematoma within an adult-sized anterior thigh, the starting intensity might be 0.2 w/cm². Within three minutes, it is likely that the intensity will need to be reduced to 0.1 and by ten minutes to 0.01 w/cm² because of patient sensation of discomfort. Periosteal overheating (to 45°C or higher), with concomitant sudden onset of a deep, dull ache, is much more apt to occur with the stationary procedure. Also, since the transducer is not in motion, the *thermal* energy which is inevitably generated within the crystal is going to be trans-mitted to a much smaller area and volume of tissue for a longer period of time. Of course, the same holds true for the transmitted and absorbed acoustic energy. Both types of energy will cause a TTR, and since the sound head is not moving, there is less chance for the absorbing tissue to cool down during the treatment period in comparison with the moving technic. Hence, one should select a coupling agent whose viscosity will not decrease significantly until the couplant temperature is over 40°C. If the previously viscous couplant liquifies and drains off the area being treated, energy transmission to the patient can become very nonuniform.

Lotions, creams, or ointments with no more than a 50 percent water content and with a high glycerol content would seem very useful when the stationary technic is indicated.

Immersion Technique

Immersion of the part to be treated in a relatively large volume of coupling fluid is needed in treatment of elbows and distal upper extremity joints as well as for the ankle and more distal lower extremity joints. Since there is much bone close to the surface in these areas, it is difficult if not impossible to maintain uniform contact between the skin and the radiating surface of the sound head. The net result if direct contact is tried is that where there is a bony protuberance, the quantity of absorption may be painfully great, but immediately adjacent tissue may absorb an ineffective quantity of energy. There is also the factor of the rigid patient surface of the transducer being pushed against a protuberance and causing a painful pressure point. Both these problems are minimized if the part to be treated is immersed in a degassed liquid and the sound head is kept moving close to the skin (0.5 to 1 cm) over the area where the greatest absorption is desired.

Theoretically, water is the best couplant for the immersion technic because it transmits ultrasonic energy very effectively if it is degassed, and since the tissues exposed have a high water content, there is matching impedance. This means there is little change in frequency of the energy after it has left the sound head. However, water at or near ambient temperatures *always* has large quantities of the various gases which make up room air dissolved in it. When water at room temperature is exposed to ultrasonic energy, these gases collect together as visible bubbles and are attracted to the sound head in large quantity. The bubbles then proceed to absorb much of the energy emanating from the transducer so that very little actually reaches the patient. The only practical way to minimize such interference from the bubbles is to wipe off the radiating surface about once a minute throughout the treatment. Some therapists attempt to compensate for this bubble interference by increasing the intensity. This only serves

to increase the rate and volume of bubble formation. The problem of energy transfer from sound head to patient is immensely
compounded if a whirlpool is used and the volume of water is
unnecessarily large. The situation is still worse if the water is
further aerated by use of the turbine at the time of or shortly before the ultrasonic treatment. Under these very adverse circumstances, the quantity of energy available for absorption by the
patient must be very small.

It would seem simpler to avoid the use of water when an immersion treatment is indicated. Glycerol is more efficient than
distilled water in transmission of energy. It is substantially superior to mineral oil in the near field[40] and approximately equal to
it in the far field.[41] Glycerol does not contain significant quantities of room air gases at ambient temperatures. Hence, more
energy is likely to reach the tissues where the energy is needed.
Glycerol is more expensive than mineral oil, but it can be reused
with impunity if there are no open lesions in the area to be
treated and if the area has been washed with soap and water to
remove epidermal debris prior to treatment. Since the boiling
point of glycerol is well over 100°C, if there is ever any question
of cross contamination, glycerol can be heated to sterilizing temperatures with neglible risk of catching on fire. In the authors'
experience, good clinical results are obtained faster when mineral
or paraffin oil or glycerol are used as immersion coupling agents,
in contrast to water. There have been no reported differences
whether the immersion container is metal, ceramic, or plastic.

The Fluid-filled Bag

There are certain body areas where it is not practical to use
either direct contact or an immersion technic for sonation. If, for
example, it is desired to treat the anterior aspect of the knee,
including the patella, or the lateral hip, including tissues attached
to the greater trochanter, or the perianal area, via immersion, the
volume of couplant needed would be so great that little energy
would actually reach the target tissues. Most of the radiated
energy would be absorbed by the large volume of couplant. If
the direct contact procedure is used, because of irregular contour,

with or without bony protuberances in the examples given, it would be difficult to get uniform energy distribution from the transducer to the absorbing tissues, and since the radiating surface is rigid, it can cause pain when sliding into a protuberance.

Under such circumstances, it is feasible to fill a finger cot (condom) with degassed water or glycerol or mineral oil and attach the lateral margins of the transducer to the open end of the finger cot with heavy rubber bands or adhesive tape. Care *must* be taken that no air is trapped between the surface of the transducer and the coupling liquid, or essentially no energy will reach the patient. The same coupling fluid is also applied to the outside of the finger cot and to the skin over the target area. The fluid-filled bag is then applied to the skin, using either the moving sound head or stationary direct contact technic. The elasticity of the bag permits a more nearly uniform energy transmission to areas of irregular contour. If there is abrupt contact with a bony prominence, it will not be painful, as could be the case if the radiating surface was in direct contact with the skin. The same fluid-filled bag can be reused many times.

Phonophoresis

Phonophoresis is the movement of a substance away from the patient surface of the transducer by virtue of having been exposed to ultrasonic energy. The movement is due to radiation pressure changes caused by the transmission of the high frequency sound waves through the couplant and into tissues.[10] In clinical physical therapy, a liquid or an ointment containing the desired ingredient is applied to the skin over the area to be treated. Medication strengths on the order of 0.5 to 10% (5 to 100 milligrams per gram of vehicle) have been reported.[46,48] The vehicle functions as the coupling agent. The radiating surface of the transducer is placed into the couplant and energized in the usual manner, using either the moving or stationary technic. Laboratory data indicate that large, complex whole molecules such as hydrocortisone and lidocaine are easily driven through skin *in situ* and can be recovered from deeply underlying muscle and nerve using standard treatment parameters.[3,11,14,42] Significant amounts of the medication can be recovered 10 cm deep to the skin after a five-minute exposure with the stationary procedure. Early in the 1950s, Aldes and Jadeson[43] and Fellinger and Schmid[44] reported that chronic periarticular and osteoarthritic symptomatology responded better when intramuscular or intraarticular injection of hydrocortisone was immediately followed by exposure of the injected area to ultrasonic energy than do these pathologies when treated with either ultrasound or injected hydrocortisone alone. Presumably, the well-established ability of US energy to transiently increase membrane permeability is responsible for the improvement in pain relief, since diffusion of an analgesic, anesthetic, or antiinflammatory agent is increased by external application of ultrasound. The technic of phonophoresis minimizes the possibility of a pain increase immediately following intramuscular or intraarticular injection where the pain increase was caused by the quantity of liquid injected.

Phonophoresis seems to be superior to iontophoresis *(see* Chapter 3) as a method of driving topically applied medication deep into underlying soft tissue. There is no hazard of skin damage when ultrasound is used. There is a very real hazard of an electrical burn when DC with continuous modulation is used as a driving agent. Very few individuals can tolerate iontophoresis at an intensity of more than 30 milliwatts/cm².[45] Ultrasound is standardly used at intensities of 1 to 2 w/cm² with a moving sound head and at 0.1 to 0.2 w/cm² with a stationary transducer, with no risk of injury to the skin and only a remote possibility of periosteal overheating.[46] If the latter should occur, the patient is far more apt to become aware of it and report it than he is apt to be aware of warning signals for skin damage from absorption of too much continuous modulation DC.

With phonophoresis, there is no dissociation of the driven compound into ionized fragments. Hence, one does not need to know whether the ionized fragment which is physiologically active is driven in from the positive or negative pole. When iontophoresis is used, one must know this factor. Neither does one need to know about the ideal pH of the solution or ointment used when ultrasonic energy is the driving agent. At best, penetration of the driven compound will be to a depth of 1 cm with iontophoresis.[49] When US is the driving agent, there can be significant penetration to 5 cm with the standard clinical frequency (1 Mc) and to at least twice that depth in soft tissues when lower frequencies are used.[1,10,11] Lastly, if the area to be treated is no greater than 150 cm², a five-minute treatment appears adequate to drive in enough medication to provide substantial pain relief.[47] Iontophoresis requires at least a ten-minute treatment. Treatment for twenty to thirty minutes at a time is more common.[45]

INDICATIONS AND CONTRAINDICATIONS FOR ULTRASONIC THERAPY

Chronic Arthritis

Ultrasonic energy is in widespread use for relief of pain due to osteoarthritis, chronic rheumatoid arthritis, and the nonarticular pathologies which are usually grouped together as periarticular arthritis. Chronic bursitis, myositis, fibrositis, and tendonitis are classical examples of periarticular pathology which responds well to exposure to US. Assuming that pain relief is due to a rapid rise in muscle temperature, with subsequent vasodilation and reduction in skeletal muscle tension, ultrasonic energy is the treatment of choice if vasodilation and muscle relaxation is needed in tissues that are 2 cm or more deep to the skin. It is well documented that ultrasonic energy penetrates more deeply and that there is a faster deep temperature rise when tissues are exposed to US as compared to tissues exposed to hydrotherapy or other forms of infrared or to the short wave or microwave segments of the electromagnetic spectrum.[1,5,19,20,21,23,38]

In addition to being useful in pain relief in the more common arthritic and/or collagen disorders, ultrasonic therapy appears to be at least as effective as x-ray therapy for pain relief in ankylosing spondylitis (Marie-Strumpell arthritis) and does not present the hazards which are well-documented when x-ray therapy is used in the management of this problem.[50,51] Since the distance from skin to the bodies of the vertebrae in adults is more than 2 cm, the superior penetration of US over other forms of energy whose absorption causes a physiological tissue temperature rise, the transient increase in temperature could be a factor in pain relief. However, the authors have observed that patients suffering from the residual effects of gouty arthritis sustain excellent lasting pain relief and rapidly regain pain-free range of motion of the meta-tarsophalangeal joint upon one or two exposures to US, using the glycerol immersion technic. The patients were treated after their blood uric acid levels had returned to normal. The reasons for the apparent superiority of US in aiding return of damaged joints to normal function are not known. X-rays taken before and after treatment might provide part of the answer. Depth of penetration should not be a factor in treatment of such superficial joints.

Neuromas

Exposure of posttraumatic neuromas to ultrasound seems highly effective in relieving the pain. Such neuromas may be seen in patients who have had an amputation.[25,26] It is usually not difficult to pinpoint the location of neuroma, so the stationary technic can be used with good results. The pain relief could be due to a deep TTR or to relaxation or dissolution of the excessively proliferated connective tissue. Since most neuromas cause more pain when subjected to externally applied pressure, as occurs when a prosthesis is worn, it would seem more likely that absorption of ultrasonic energy has caused a permanent relaxation or dissolution of the neuroma rather than just intermittently warming it up.

Adhesive Scars

Adhesive scars resulting from natural repair of lacerated tissues or from surgical intervention also show excess connective tissue proliferation. The range-limiting effects of adhesion formation are effectively and permanently relieved by exposure to ultrasonic energy.[25,27] Exposure to US is also an effective means of increasing range of motion where limitation is due to massive hypertrophic scar tissue formation, as in the residual phase of a burn which has destroyed the dermis. Distinction must be made between the hypertrophic scar and the true keloid.[29,32] The histologic distinction is that, in the hypertrophic scar, the proliferation comes entirely from the epidermal margin. In the keloid, the collagen proliferation is predominantly dermal rather than epidermal in origin, and there is massive hyalinization. Ultrasound does not seem effective in releasing tissues bound by a true keloid scar.[30] The reasons for this difference are not known.

Plantar Warts

There is sharply divided clinical opinion as to the benefit of treating plantar warts with ultrasonic energy. Some have reported excellent results.[52,53] Others have indicated that ultrasound is of no benefit.[54] There has been wide variation in treatment parameters. There has also been debate as to what are the proper criteria for arrival at the clinical diagnosis of a plantar wart as compared to other causes of indurated skin. The most careful diagnosticians require demonstration of the virus verruca plantaris.

Laboratory investigation of deactivation of viruses by exposure to ultrasound indicate that far higher intensities are required for such deactivation *in vitro* than are feasible clinically.[33] Study of verruca plantaris was not included in that report. If exposure to ultrasonic energy is going to remove the wart, it would seem necessary that absorption of the energy would lead to the dissolution of the connective tissue binding between the normal and abnormal tissue or that the wart itself would have to be softened. Detailed pathology reports of removed tissue have yet to be published. When treatment has been reported as successful, both direct contact and immersion technics have been used. Direct contact with exposure at about fifteen minutes per treatment and for a series of ten to fifteen treatments seems most likely to obtain removal of the wart. There have been no reports of harm to adjacent normal tissue with the use of ultrasound; the treatment is less painful than when chemical technics are used, and the patient does not suffer through a postsurgical severe pain period. Hence, at this point in time, it would seem that ultrasound should be given a reasonable trial before more drastic methods are used.

Pressure Sores

Exposure of pressure sores to ultrasonic energy appears to significantly increase the rate of healing.[55] At each treatment, the cavity is filled with mineral oil. The sound head is then energized in the liquid. Obviously, eschar and other debris would be removed prior to each treatment, and there should be no evidence that a sinus runs from the wound to deeper lying tissue. If the wound is pale in color prior to treatment, a visible hyperemia is likely to appear within a five-minute treatment, and a better local blood supply will be maintained until external pressure again diminishes local blood flow. Sonation of adjacent intact tissues immediately before sonation of the ulcer itself would probably enhance duration of the improved circulation. To the authors' knowledge, no comparative study has been reported using infrared energy in any form as compared to ultrasonic energy for transient improvement of local circulation. Certainly infrared in the form of radiant energy, as well as hydrotherapy, had been used for this purpose long before US was available. Infrared is not often regarded as effective in helping to maintain the blood supply to a pressure sore area.

Chronic Systemic Peripheral Arterial Diseases

In the early and moderately far advanced stages of arteriosclerosis and atherosclerosis, arterial vessels react to the salt and lipid deposition with persistent vasospasm in varying degree. Vasospasm can be transiently relieved by local exposure of the affected vessels to ultrasonic energy and by paravertebral sonation of the sympathetic nervous system. It is not known at this time whether the local sonation has any effect on the rate of deposition or dissolution of the material which is decreasing lumen diameter. It would seem reasonable as part of the overall management of such chronic arterial insufficiency problems to try three or four treatments, using paravertebral sonation to the lumbar and sacral areas, followed immediately by local sonation as indicated. Skin temperature testing, before and after treatment, and/or oscillometric index testing would indicate whether that particular patient obtains enough transient reduction in vasospasm to make continued treatment worthwhile. If posttreatment temperatures show a rise on the order of 2° to 5°C at the toetips, and a lesser rise more proximally, lasting for an hour or more, ultrasonic therapy would seem beneficial for that particular patient. Lota has shown that in normal individuals, paravertebral sonation will increase distal remote skin temperature by 1° to 2°C.[19] This rise in skin temperature is assumed to be due to the effect of ultrasonic energy on the sympathetic nervous system, leading to a transient reduction in vasomotor tension. Local sonation would be contraindicated when there is clinical evidence of thrombophlebitis or phlebothrombosis because of the possibility of fragmenting an attached thrombus, thus converting it into an embolus, with the risk of causing a life-threatening intrathoracic infarct.

The Organized Hematoma

Anytime soft tissue is subject to trauma, small blood vessels are likely to be crushed and/or ruptured. Edema always occurs as a result of the marked increase in interstitial fluid. The outpouring of blood from the circulatory tree lasts only a few seconds if the injury is minor. It can last much longer, and can be fatal, in major trauma. In the case of small arteries, not more than a millimeter or two in outside diameter, instantaneous vasoconstriction takes place. This reduces the blood flow to the area, and escaping platelets start to adhere to the rupture margins. The damaged mural cells release chemicals, which, in conjunction with platelet activity, rapidly leads to clot formation in three major stages.[56] For the purposes of this volume, the important point is that ionizable calcium must be present in the extracellular fluid for each of the stages to take place. The reaction of serum and/or interstitial fluid calcium with the proteins released by the injured cells leads to the formation of a hard lump. The complete process leading to this lump formation may take several days to a week, depending upon extent of injury and whether the patient's clotting mechanisms are functioning normally. After natural or surgical repair of the leak (s) in the vascular tree, further intrinsic chemical activity dissolves the indurated mass.

If the clot is large, occupying many cubic centimeters, natural dissolution may take weeks to months for complete resorption. If a slowly dissolving clot is pressing upon nerve, muscle, or periosteum, it can be quite painful, restricting muscle contraction and/ or joint motion. When this occurs, exposure of the clot to ultrasonic energy is one way to speed resorption. If the clot is deep, this is the treatment of choice because of the penetrating power of ultrasound. The US-induced TTR causes local vasodilation and transiently increases cell permeability. There is no hard evidence to date that US also decreases the binding of calcium ions to fibrin or other proteins which are essential to clot formation. However, it has been established that when whole blood is exposed to US *in vitro* clotting time is significantly increased.[33] This is not known to happen with any form of electromagnetic energy in use by physical therapists.

It follows that once there is clinical evidence that continuing vascular leakage has stopped, exposure of the injury site to ultrasonic energy is an effective way of minimizing the pain and other problems that can result from a large and fully organized hematoma. In the situation where there is evidence of a mural thrombosis in venous circulation, there is a very real hazard that exposure to US could fragment the thrombosis and lead to an intrathoracic infarct. If there is any possibility of a venous thrombus in the area to be treated, the intensity of the ultrasound should be exceptionally low in order to minimize the possibility of embolus formation. To the best of the authors' knowledge, no report has appeared indicating that conversion of a thrombus into an embolus was due to exposure to ultrasound.

Contraindications

There are very few contraindications for the use of ultrasonic energy. It should be contraindicated whenever a TTR would hinder return to normal function. It should probably not be used in the thoracic area if the patient is using a cardiac pacemaker of any kind. Absorption of ultrasonic energy by the pacemaker or by adjacent tissues could lead to error in pacemaker response to instant cardiac status. Since US energy absorption is far more localized than is the case for most other forms of energy that physical therapists use, there is no reason why it cannot be used on other body areas in the presence of a pacemaker. This is not true for the application of nerve and muscle stimulating currents (Chapter 3) or the diathermies (Chapter 4).

The use of ultrasonic energy is contraindicated in an area of the body where a malignancy is known to be present. This is because of the established ability of ultrasonic energy to increase local arterial blood supply, which would tend to increase the rate of growth of the neoplasm. If the malignancy has reached the stage where it is untreatable by surgery or medication, and the patient is not obtaining satisfactory pain relief from narcotics, exposure of the local area to US is occasionally helpful in giving transient pain relief. This is probably due to transient relaxation of muscle spasm, where the cause of the muscle irritation is pressure from an expanding lesion.

Ultrasonic energy should not be used on a regular basis over or near growth centers of bone until bone growth is essentially complete. Absorption of this form of energy by cells making up the growth center tends to disrupt normal growth. Damage to growth centers has been clearly demonstrated in experimental animals when the exposure has been a long series at clinical intensities or a short series at high intensities.[57] However, since a big factor in selection of ultrasound for pain relief is its superior depth of penetration, it is rarely needed in treatment of children. If the ultrasonic energy is being used to promote lasting extensibility of tendon, the series of treatments would be small; hence the risk of damage to a child's epiphyseal centers would be small, but it could happen.

It should follow that a healing fracture should not be exposed to US since this might delay or prevent completion of callus formation. When the radiologist is satisfied that bone repair is complete, and there is need of exposure to US for pain relief, then there should be no harm in such treatment.

SUMMARY

Physical and physiological differences between electromagnetic and acoustic energy absorption are discussed. Critical factors in equipment choice are given in broad outline. Factors which need to be considered in application of ultrasonic energy to patients are presented. Physiological effects which are known to occur at clinical intensities and with clinical frequencies are documented. On the basis of these known effects, indications and contraindications for the use of ultrasonic energy are given.

Much of the value of ultrasonic energy in providing pain relief is due to its superior depth of penetration and to its ability to induce permanent relaxation of connective tissues, especially when there has been excess proliferation of such tissue as a result of trauma or where a neurological deficit has lead to muscle or tendon shortening.

REFERENCES

1. Goldman, D.E. and Heuter, T.F.: Tabular data on velocity and absorption of high frequency sound in mammalian tissues. *J Acoust Soc Am, 28*:35-37, 1956.
2. Brunner, G.D. et al.: Can ultrasound be used in the presence of surgical metal implants? *Phys Ther, 38*:823, 1958.
3. Gersten, J.W.: Thermal and non-thermal changes in isometric tension, contractile protein, and injury potential produced in frog muscle by ultrasonic energy. *Arch Phys Med Rehabil, 34*:675, 1953.
4. Madsen, P.W. and Gersten, J.W.: The effect of ulstrasound on conduction velocity of peripheral nerve. *Arch Phys Med Rehabil, 42*:645, 1961.
5. Licht, S.: *Therapeutic Heat and Cold,* 2nd ed. New Haven, Licht, 1965.
6. Schwan, H.P.: Personal communication, 1969.
7. Lehmann, J.F. and Bigler, R.: Changes in potentials and temperature gradients in membranes caused by ultrasound. *Arch Phys Med Rehabil, 35*:287, 1954.
8. Lehmann, J.F. and Guy, A.W.: Ultrasound therapy. *Proc. Workshop on Interaction of Ultrasound and Biological Tissues.* Washington, HEW (FDA 73:8008), Sept., 1972.
9. Stewart, H.F. et al.: Survey of use and performance of ultrasonic therapy equipment in Pinellas County, Florida. *Phys Ther, 54*:707, 1974.
10. Summer, W. and Patrick, M.: *Ultrasonic Therapy.* New York, Elsevier, 1964.
11. Griffin, J.E. and Touchstone, J.C.: Effects of ultrasonic frequency on phonophoresis of cortisol into swine tissues. *Am J Phys Med, 51*:62, 1972.
12. Rosenberger, H.: Uber den Wirkungsmechanismus der ultrashall Be-

handlung insbesondere bei Ischias und Neuralgien. *Chirurg, 21:*404, 1950.

13. Touchstone, J.C., Griffin, J.E., and Kasparow, M.: Cortisol in human nerve. *Science, 142:*1275, 1963.

14. Griffin, J.E., Touchstone, J.C., and Liu, A.C.: Ultrasonic movement of cortisol into pig tissues, II. Peripheral nerve. *Am J Phys Med, 41:* 20, 1965.

15. Farmer, W.C.: Effect of intensity of ultrasound on conduction velocity of motor axons. *Phys Ther, 48:*1233, 1968.

16. Piersol, G.M. et al.: Mechanism of absorption of ultrasonic energy in blood. *Arch Phys Med Rehabil, 33:*327, 1952.

17. Lota, M.J. and Darling, R.C.: Changes in permeability of the red blood cell membrane in a homogenous ultrasonic field. *Arch Phys Med Rehabil, 36:*282, 1955.

18. Schwan, H.P.: Absorption of ultrasonic energy by tissues and biological matter. *Proc IRE, 47:*1959, 1959.

19. Lota, M.J.: Electronic plethysmographic and tissue temperature studies of the effects of ultrasound on blood flow. *Arch Phys Med Rehabil, 46:*315, 1965.

20. Lehmann, J.F. et al.: Temperature distributions upon exposure to ultrasonic energy. *Arch Phys Med Rehabil, 48:*662, 1967.

21. Lehmann, J.F. et al.: Comparative study of the efficiency of shortwave, microwave, and ultrasonic diathermy in heating the hip joint. *Arch Phys Med Rehabil, 40:*510, 1959.

22. Abramson, D.I. et al.: Oxygen uptake and tissue temperatures produced by therapeutic physical agents. I. Effect of ultrasound. *Am J Phys Med, 39:*51, 1960.

23. Abramson, D.I. et al.: Oxygen uptake and tissue temperatures produced by therapeutic physical agents. II. Effects of shortwave diathermy. *Am J Phys Med, 39:*87, 1960.

24. Lehmann, J.F. et al.: Heating of joint structures by ultrasonic energy. *Arch Phys Med Rehabil, 49:*28, 1968.

25. Rubin, D. and Kuitert, J.: Use of ultrasound vibration energy in treatment of pain arising from phantom limbs, scars, and neuromas. *Arch Phys Med Rehabil, 36:*445, 1955.

26. Rubin, D., Magovern, G., and Kallenberg, R.: Application of ultrasound to experimentally induced neuromas in dogs. *Arch Phys Med Rehabil, 38:*377, 1957.

27. Bierman, W.: Ultrasound in the treatment of scars. *Arch Phys Med, 34:* 209, 1954.

28. Joseph, J.: Healing with ultrasound. *Medical Chronicle,* 18, May, 1970.

29. Asboe-Hansen, G.: Regeneration and repair of connective tissue, trans. In Valette, D.G. (Ed.): *La Cicatrization.* Paris, Editions du Centre National de la Recherche Scientifique #145, 1965.

30. Wright, E.T. and Haase, K.H.: Treatment of keloids with ultrasound. *Arch Phys Med Rehabil, 52:*280, 1971.
31. Lewis, J.R.: *The Surgery of Scars.* New York, McGraw, 1963.
32. Inalsingh, C.H.: An experience in treating five hundred and one patients with keloids. *Johns Hopkins Med J, 134:*284, 1974.
33. El 'Piner, I.E.: *Ultrasound: Its Physical, Chemical, and Biological Effects.* New York, Consultants Bureau, 1964, pp. 154-6.
34. Lehmann, J.F. et al.: Effects of therapeutic temperatures on tendon extensibility. *Arch Phys Med Rehabil, 51:*481, 1970.
35. Brust, M., Toback, S., and Benton, J.G.: Some effects of ultrasonic energy and temperature on the contraction of isolated mammalian skeletal muscle. *Arch Phys Med Rehabil, 50:*677, 1969.
36. Bearzy, H.: Clinical application of ultrasonic energy in treatment of acute and chronic sub-acromial bursitis. *Arch Phys Med Rehabil, 34:* 228, 1953.
37. Echternach, J.: Ultrasound: an adjunct treatment for shoulder disabilities. *Phys Ther, 45:*865, 1965.
38. Lehmann, J.F. et al: Comparison of ultrasonic and microwave diathermy in physical treatment of periarthritis of the shoulder. *Arch Phys Med Rehabil, 35:*627, 1954.
39. Goodman, C.: Ultrasonic therapy for chronic acromio-clavicular separation with calcific deposits. *NY State J Med, 72:*2884, 1972.
40. Reid, D.C. and Cummings, G.E.: Factors in selecting the dosage of ultrasound. *Physiotherapy Canada,* March, 1973.
41. Warren, C.G., Koblanski, J.N., and Sigelman, R.A.: Ultrasound coupling media: their relative transmissivity. *Arch Phys Med Rehabil, 57:* 218, 1976.
42. Nowak, E.J.: Experimental transmission of lidocaine through intact skin by ultrasound. *Arch Phys Med Rehabil, 45:*231, 1964.
43. Aldes, J.H. and Jadeson, W.J.: Ultrasonic therapy in treatment of hypertrophic arthritis in elderly patients. *Ann West Med Surg, 6:*545, 1952.
44. Fellinger, K. and Schmid, J.: *Klinik und Therapie des Chronischen Gelenrhuematismus.* Vienna, 1954, p. 549.
45. Abramowitch, D. and Neousskine, B.: *Treatment by Ion Transfer.* New York, Grune, 1946.
46. Griffin, J.E. and Touchstone, J.C.: Low intensity phonophoresis of cortisol in swine. *Phys Ther, 48:*1336, 1968.
47. Griffin, J.E. et al.: Patients treated with ultrasonic driven hydrocortisone and with ultrasound alone. *Phys Ther, 47:*595, 1967.
48. Kleinkort, J.A. and Wood, F.: Phonophoresis with one percent versus ten percent hydrocortisone. *Phys Ther, 55:*1320, 1975.
49. Murray, W., Lavine, L.S., and Seifter, E., The iontophoresis of C_{21} esterified glucocorticoids: preliminary report. *Phys Ther, 43:*579, 1963.

50. Tschannen, F.: Effects of ultrasonic therapy on rheumatic diseases and circulatory disorders, *Br J Phys Med, 15:*7, 1952.
51. Aldes, J.H.: Ultrasound in arthritis. *J Arkansas Med Soc, 54:*39, 1957.
52. Cherup, N., Urban, J., and Bender, L.F.: Treatment of plantar warts with ultrasound. *Arch Phys Med Rehabil, 44:*602, 1963.
53. Vaughn, D.T.: Direct method versus underwater method in treatment of plantar warts with ultrasound. *Phys Ther, 53:*396, 1973.
54. Braatz, J.H., McAlistar, B.R., and Broaddus, M.D.: Ultrasound and plantar warts: a double blind study. *Milit Med, 139:*199, 1974.
55. Paul, B.J. et al.: Use of ultrasound in the treatment of pressure sores in patients with spinal cord injury. *Arch Phys Med Rehabil, 41:*38, 1960.
56. Sodeman, W.A., and Sodeman, W.A., Jr.: *Pathologic Physiology,* 4th ed. Philadelphia, Saunders, 1967, pp. 875-87.
57. DeForest, R.E. et al.: Effects of ultrasound on growing bone; experimental study. *Arch Phys Med Rehabil, 34:*21, 1953.

Chapter 8

PRINCIPLES OF INSTRUMENTATION

BASIC ELECTRICITY AND ELECTRONICS

THE PROJECTED TOTAL MARKET for medical electronic equipment in 1974 was 673.9 million dollars, as compared to 524.6 million dollars in 1972. In the same two-year span of time, the market for just diathermy and ultrasonic therapeutic equipment went from 12.4 to 14.9 million; it is projected to reach 20 million by 1977. If these figures are any indication, today's physical therapists can expect to find themselves confronted with an increasing amount of therapeutic instrumentation in the near future. Not only will the number of devices increase but also the sophistication and complexity of those devices. In order to competently use such equipment, the therapist must have an understanding of the fundamental physical principles employed in its design.

It is the purpose of this section to provide the physical therapist with a working knowledge of electricity, electronics, and the basic theory of instrumentation as employed in physical therapy.

It is assumed that the reader has a background in physics and algebra. However, the material is presented in a descriptive manner in order to accommodate the widest reader population, including those therapists whose physics and math are a "few" years behind them.

Fundamental Circuit Theory

The basis upon which all electrical and electronic instrumentation is founded rests on three fundamental quantities and six types of electrical components. The conclusion to be drawn from this all-encompassing statement is that with a good grasp of these nine items, the reader should be able to understand any electrical or electronic device and how it functions, once given the appropriate instrument data.

The three fundamental quantities mentioned above are as follows:

1. Voltage
2. Current
3. Resistance

These quantities are related by the following equation, commonly referred to as Ohm's Law:

$$i = \frac{v}{r}$$

Simplified definitions of the above quantities will suffice to give the reader a working knowledge of electrical activity; therefore, no rigorous analysis will be attempted.

Voltage, Current, and Resistance

VOLTAGE. Voltage is defined as the difference in electron population between two points. This electrical "difference of potential" can be used to cause the orderly, directed movement of electrons through a conductor; hence, it is also termed *electromotive force* (e.m.f.).

CURRENT. Electrical current can be defined as the *directed* flow or movement of electrons through a conducting medium, as opposed to the *random* drift of electrons.

RESISTANCE. Resistance is a characteristic inherent in any substance. It is related to the number of "free" electrons in a substance and hence to the ease or difficulty with which a current can be passed through the substance. The greater the number of free electrons in a substance, i.e. metals, the easier it will pass a current; hence, its resistance is termed *low*. Materials with few free electrons, i.e. glass, mica have correspondingly higher resistances.

A useful analogy often used to facilitate an understanding of electrical circuits is the "fluid system analogy;" however, the reader is warned not to be caught holding too firmly to the analogy as it can become confusing.

Simply stated, the fluid system analogy compares voltage to pressure, current to fluid flow, and resistance to pipe diameter. Hence, where

$$\text{current} = \frac{\text{voltage}}{\text{resistance}}$$

this is equivalent to

$$\text{fluid flow} = \frac{\text{pressure}}{\text{pipe diameter}}$$

It is obvious that where an increase in pressure will cause more fluid to flow, also an increase in voltage will cause a greater current to flow. In turn, a decrease in pipe size will decrease the fluid flow at a given pressure, while an increase in resistance will decrease current flow.

This simple law holds true in all metallic conducting systems and electronic devices, and no matter how complex an electronic circuit is, it can, with the appropriate calculations, be simplified down to the fundamental relationship between voltage, current, and resistance given in Ohm's Law.

Components

As noted in the previous section, all electronic instrumentation is made up of various combinations of six types of electronic components. They are as follows:

1. Resistors
2. Capacitors (condensers)
3. Inductors (coils)
4. Vacuum tubes
5. Semiconductors
6. Integrated circuits (I.C.s)

These components may differ in size and appearance from each other; in fact, in some instances, there may be no resemblance whatever between two components of the same type. Nevertheless, each *type* of component can be described by way of a brief operational description as given below. A more detailed operational description is included in a later section.

Resistors. A resistor is a device used generally in one of three ways: (1) to limit current, (2) to provide current-to-voltage transformation, (3) to produce voltage division. Resistors may be fixed or variable; they may be made of carbon, wire, or metallic film. The specific form of a resistor is dictated by its application.

Capacitors (condensers). A capacitor is a device that (1) stores energy in an *electric field* and (2) tends to oppose *voltage* changes. Capacitors may be small or large, fixed or variable, with solid dielectric interiors, mica or even air filled. They are used most often to decrease or dampen power supply voltage variations as well as to filter out unwanted signals.

Capacitors are also found as the drum electrodes in diathermy units; each drum acts as a plate, and the patient is the dielectric.

Inductors (coils). An inductor is a device that (1) stores energy in an *electromagnetic field* and (2) tends to oppose changes in *current*. (The reader should note the general similarity to the action of a capacitor but also should beware not to confuse the two.) Inductors also play a role in controlling power supply output variations and in selective filters. In addition, specialized applications of the principles of electromagnetic induction are found in transformers, galvanometers, motors, meters, and generators not to mention diathermy applicator coils.

Vacuum Tubes. Vacuum tubes are principally monodirectional current devices; that is, they allow current to flow in only one direction. Depending upon the number of electrodes they have, they are used (1) to *rectify* alternating current into direct current and also (2) to *amplify* small signal voltages into larger ones.

Semiconductors. This general class of components includes the ubiquitous "transistor." Semiconductors are all miniature solid-state crystalline devices having the same general capabilities as vacuum tubes and providing the additional advantages of smaller size, longer life, and less power consumption.

Integrated Circuits. These microminature devices are today's state of the art in electronic technology. Where a single conventional semiconductor discrete component (for example, a transistor) is roughly the size of the head of a pin, an integrated circuit "chip" the same size may contain 200 transistors and numerous resistors—truly the ultimate in miniaturization. All electronic functions that are adaptable to vacuum tubes and transistors can be accomplished using I.C.s, with the additional ability of housing complete circuits, i.e. voltage regulators, multivibrators, etc., in a single I.C.

Current Sources

The majority of medical electronic instruments in use today contain circuitry that requires direct current voltages to operate. To obtain D.C. voltages, one has two choices: (1) to use battery supplies, or (2) to use a power supply that converts wall power (117 VAC, 60 Hz) to the required D.C. values. The former method is used primarily in portable devices, while the latter method is the form of power source found in most instrumentation.

CELLS AND BATTERIES. The word *battery* is often used incorrectly by the layman to refer to a cell, as in the "battery" used in a flashlight (really a "dry cell"). Hence, a battery is a combination of two or more cells. In all cases, the terminal voltage produced by a cell or battery is generated by chemical means and hence can eventually be depleted.

Batteries are of two types, based on whether or not their cells can be recharged. A *primary cell battery* is nonrechargeable; a *secondary cell battery* is rechargeable. The common everyday flashlight cell is a primary cell; the automobile battery is an example of a secondary cell battery.

The three most common types of primary cells are (1) zinc-carbon cell (Leclanche cell), (2) zinc-mercuric oxide cell (mercury cell), (3) zinc-manganese dioxide cell (alkaline cell). These cells are predominantly of the low voltage variety, ranging from the 1.5 volt flashlight cell to the 9 volt transistor radio battery. A recent introduction into the primary cell market is the *lithium cell*. This type of cell generates as much as thirty times the energy per unit volume as a more conventional cell—15 watt-hours as opposed to 0.5 watt-hours for a zinc-carbon cell. The cost of a lithium cell is also proportionally larger

($11.48 for a D cell).

POWER SUPPLIES. Most commercial electronic devices, in order to operate, are plugged into wall receptacles which deliver 117 VAC, 60 Hz. Consequently, there must be some circuit within the instrument which changes that AC into DC; such a circuit is called a power supply. Power supplies will be covered in more detail in a later section; however, a brief summary will be given here.

The essential components of a power supply are as follows: (from AC in to DC out)

1. *A transformer*—to step up or down the input voltage and to provide one or more secondary voltages.
2. *A rectifier*—to convert the high voltage AC into a pulsating DC.
3. *A filter network*—to remove the "pulsations" from the DC leaving "pure" DC.

Additional items that may or may not be included in a power supply are (1) *voltage dividers* to provide multiple DC voltages from a single high DC voltage and (2) *voltage regulators* to provide a constant voltage supply even though the current demands change. The complexity of a power supply is dependent upon its application. The requirement for a perfectly steady DC output over a wide current range will necessitate more complexity than a low voltage, low current, unregulated DC output.

DC Series and Parallel Circuits

An electrical circuit simplified down to its constituent parts is made up of (1) a power source, (2) a closed (or complete) conduction path, and (3) some form of driven element (or load) which constitutes the circuit resistance (or resistances). The manner in which the loads are connected to the power source requires an understanding of series and parallel circuits.

Figure 8-1 shows a simple series circuit. In such a circuit, total current (I_t) flows through each component so that its measurement at any point in the circuit will yield the same value. ($I_t = I_1 = I_2 = I_3$, etc.) In turn, the total resistance (R_t) that must be overcome by the current is seen as the sum of the individual resistances. ($R_t = R_1 + R_2 + R_3$, etc.). The total applied voltage of the power source (V_t) is "dropped" proportionally by the resistances in the circuit such that the sum of their voltage drops equals the applied voltage ($V_t = V_{R1} + V_{R2} + V_{R3}$, etc.)

$$R_T = R_1 + R_2 + R_3$$
$$V_T = V_{R_1} + V_{R_2} + V_{R_3}$$

Figure 8-1. A simple series circuit.

The difference in potential (voltage) measured at the terminals of a load or resistance represents the energy lost (or voltage "drop") necessary to sustain a current through the resistance. Such lost energy is designated "power dissipation" and most often is given off as heat. Power is measured in watts, and the amount of power dissipated by a given load is found by the following formulae:

$$P = I^2R \qquad P = IV \qquad P = V^2/R$$

It is important to note that in all series circuits there is only one path for current to get from one terminal of the power supply to the other.

When two or more paths exist for current to pass between two points, A and B, in an electrical circuit, it is a parallel circuit. As shown in Figure 8-2, two paths (R_1 and R_2) allow current to flow between points A and B, each path represented by a resistive element. From Ohm's Law it is known that the current through a given resistance is dictated by the quotient of voltage over resistance, and from this one can conclude that when a second resistance is placed in parallel with the existing resistance, circuit current increases as each resistance feels the same voltage at its terminals. This points out the sometimes confusing (to the layman) fact that when resistances are added to a parallel circuit, the *effec-*

tive total resistance decreases. Looking at the example from another point of view; suppose R_1 was the only resistance (and
hence conduction path) between A and B. Any addition of a parallel conduction path no matter how high its resistance can only
increase the ability of current to get from A to B. This effect can
be observed in the home when too many electrical appliances have
been plugged into a single outlet by use of a three-way plug, and a
fuse has blown. Ohm's Law shows why. Resistances in parallel
equals decreased effective R. Therefore,

$$I = \frac{V}{R}$$

decreasing R means an increasing I. When calculating effective
resistance, the following formula is used:

$$R_{eff} = \frac{1}{1/R_1 + 1/R_2 + 1/R_3, \text{etc.}}$$

As a general rule of thumb, it should be remembered that the *effective resistance* of parallel resistors *is equal to or less than the
smallest resistance.*

—————▷ INDICATES DIRECTION OF CURRENT

Figure 8-2. A series-parallel circuit. From Terence Karselis, *Descriptive Medical Electronics and Instrumentation,* 1973. Courtesy of Charles B. Slack, Inc.,
Thorofare, New Jersey.

From the previous example, one can also conclude that total
current (I_t) in a parallel circuit is found by adding the currents
in the individual legs ($I_t = I_{R1} + I_{R2} + I_{R3}$, etc.). In addition,

since the potential felt at the terminals of parallel connected resistances is the same, then $V_t = V_{R1} = V_{R2} = V_{R3}$, etc.

Comparing and at the same time summarizing series and parallel circuits, the following may be observed:

In a *series* circuit,
- current is the same at all points
- voltage is the sum of the individual voltages
- additional resistances in series increases total resistance

While in a *parallel* circuit,
- voltage is the same across all legs
- current is the sum of the individual leg currents
- additional resistances in parallel decreases effective total resistance

Electromagnetism and AC Generation

Although the predominant form of voltage used to drive instrument circuits is DC, the method of choice of transmitting electrical energy is by way of alternating current (AC) voltage. All electrical power generated in the United States is commonly produced by a hydroelectric generating plant delivering 6600 volts at 60 cycles per second (referred to as 60 Hertz). This voltage is stepped up by way of a transformer to 66,000 volts before being applied to the high power transmission lines one sees crisscrossing the countryside.

At distribution substations, the voltage is stepped down again (via transformers) to 2200 volts (commercial power) and finally stepped down again on the utility poles in individual neighborhoods to 240 volts, two phase (two phases of 120 VAC each). Hence, heavy appliances (washer and dryer) can be driven by 240 VAC while wall power is 120 VAC, 60 Hz.

A closer look at the basic principle of AC generation will yield some insight into its cyclic nature. When a current is passed through a conductor, a magnetic field is generated around the conductor; a steady current (DC) produces a steady magnetic field, a fluctuating current a fluctuating magnetic field. The process is called *electromagnetism*.

A magnetic field produced in this way can be used to operate electromagnetic devices such as relays, but it is the same process acting in the reverse direction that is used to generate electrical currents. If a conductor is passed perpendicularly through the flux of a magnetic field, a current will be induced into that conductor; this process is called *electromagnetic induction*. It should be noted that the process will occur whether the field *or* the conductor is the moving element, as long as there is relative motion between the two. The direction of the conductor's motion determines the direction of the induced current such that a conductor moving down through a given magnetic field would have an induced current in one direction, while if it were moved up through the same field, the current would flow in the opposite direction. It is this principle that provides the basis for electric *generators, transformers,* and even *tape recorder* heads.

An *electric generator* consists of a series of conductors, wound on a rotating element called an armature and caused, by mechanical effort, to rotate in a circular path through a magnetic field. Since the conductors cross the field in one direction for one half of a rotation and the opposite direction for the second half, the result is induction of an alternating current (Fig. 8-3). At two points in the circular path of the conductor, the motion is parallel to the magnetic flux; hence, no current is induced at these points, i.e. at 0° and 180° there is no voltage. If the conductor makes sixty rotations in a minute, sixty waves or cycles are generated.

A *transformer* (Fig. 8-4) consists of two coils wound on a common metallic core. When an alternating current is passed through one coil (called the primary), the magnetic field generated cuts the second coil (called the secondary), inducing a current into it. By manipulating the number of windings in the secondary, the induced voltage can be stepped up (more coils) or down (less coils). The metallic core is used only to concentrate the magnetic flux.

If a metal such as iron or aluminum is brought into the flux of an electromagnetic field, it will take on the property of a magnet, i.e. it becomes temporarily magnetized. This process, as mentioned earlier, is called *electromagnetism,* and it is the basis upon

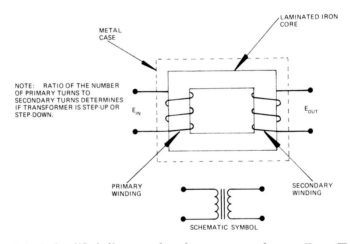

Figure 8-3. Electromagnetic induction. From Terence Karselis, *Descriptive Medical Electronics and Instrumentation,* 1973. Courtesy of Charles B. Slack, Inc., Thorofare, New Jersey.

Figure 8-4. A simplified diagram of an iron core transformer. From Terence Karselis, *Descriptive Medical Electronics and Instrumentation,* 1973. Courtesy of Charles B. Slack, Inc., Thorofare, New Jersey.

which such components as relays, solenoids, meters, and motors operate.

A *relay* is really nothing more than an electromagnetically activated switch. It consists of a coil with a fixed iron core and a movable arm with contacts. When current energizes the coil, the magnetized core attracts the movable arm, closing (or opening) the switch contacts.

A *solenoid* is similar to a relay except its core is movable, providing mechanical action that can open or close valves or engage gears (as the starter solenoid does in an automobile).

One should note that relays and solenoids function employing only *one* magnetic field, that of the energized coil. *Meters* and *motors* on the other hand employ the use of *two* magnetic fields, one stationary or fixed, the other capable of rotation.

A simple *meter* (Fig. 8-5) consists of a permanent magnet with a sensing or detecting coil suspended between the magnetic poles. A pointer is attached to the sensing coil. When a detected current passes through the sensing coil, it takes on the properties of a magnet and attempts to align its own field to the permanent field, thereby producing deflection of the pointer. Fine springs are used

Figure 8-5. A typical meter movement. From Terence Karselis, *Descriptive Medical Electronics and Instrumentation,* 1973. Courtesy of Charles B. Slack, Inc., Thorofare, New Jersey.

to return the movement back to its original (zero) position, and the whole sensing assembly is mounted in jeweled bearings providing minimal inertia.

The same "two magnetic field" principle applies also to electric motors, with some slight changes. The stationary field is not provided by a permanent magnet but by two electromagnetic field coils. The moving element is called the armature, and it consists of many coils whose terminals (called the commutators) are sequentially energized by current tapped from graphite brushes. As one coil is energized and its magnetic field provides motion, the armature turns, the first commutator segments leave the brushes, and another set comes in contact, thereby generating another magnetic field. This process is repeated, continually providing constant motion of the armature (Fig. 8-6).

Figure 8-6. Pictorial diagram of a simple motor. From Terence Karselis, *Descriptive Medical Electronics and Instrumentation,* 1973. Courtesy of Charles B. Slack, Inc., Thorofare, New Jersey.

Inductance, Capacitance, and Reactance

It was stated previously under the section on components that capacitors and inductors are capable of storing energy in electrostatic and electromagnetic fields, respectively. A slightly more detailed discussion will be helpful in showing *how* these devices function.

When a magnetic field is generated around a coil and then the current that produced the field is interrupted, the field will collapse; but in doing so, the conditions for electromagnetic induction, i.e. a moving magnetic field and a stationary coil, are present. Hence, a current is induced back into the coil. This action is called self induction, and it is property of all inductors. Since the field collapses in the opposite direction (inward) to which it was generated (outward), it is reasonable to expect that the current it induces will also be in the opposite direction to the current that caused its generation. Such is not the case. Self-induced currents are *always in a direction opposite* to the *change* that caused them. (If a current increases, the self-induced current *opposes the increase*. If a current decreases, the self-induced current tends to increase the net current—it *opposes* the decrease.) It should be noted that if the current originally passed through the coil is an alternating current, constantly increasing, decreasing, and changing direction, a continual self-induced current is generated in the coil. This property of an inductor to oppose a change in current is called *inductive reactance,* and it is a frequency-dependent property in that it increases with an increase in the frequency of the applied current. Inductive reactance (X_L; X $\times$ reactance, L = inductance) is measured in units of resistance—ohms—and is found by the following formula:

$$X_L = 2\pi FL$$

Where

F = frequency in Hertz
L = inductance inductance in Henries
X_L = inductive reactance in ohms
2π = a constant

The effects of inductive reactance are such that a *phase difference* between voltage and current is produced in inductive circuits. The result is that voltage changes appear to lead (or occur) before current changes.

The inductive components found in electronic devices are used in specific applications based on the exploitation of one of the above three effects. For example, relays and solenoids exploit the magnetic effects, filter inductors and chokes exploit the reactive effect, and oscillators use the phase shift effects.

Between any two charged objects there exists an electrostatic field; this is the basis for the operation of *capacitors*. All capacitors consist of two metallic plates separated by a material called the dielectric. By choosing an appropriate material to place between the charged plates, the amount of electrostatic energy capable of being applied (or stored) can be increased. Increasing the area of the plates will also increase the amount of charge that can be stored. When a voltage is placed across the capacitor's plates, electrons flow into one plate and away from the other plate until such a time as the plates are at the same potential as the applied voltage. The charge is "stored" by way of the applied field distorting the electric field of the atoms in the dielectric. A simple analogy is the energy stored when stretching a rubber band. When stretched and held that way, it represents potential energy; when released, it gives up its energy. In a capacitor, the dielectric atoms are "stretched" when a charge is applied, and if no discharge path is available, it will hold the charge. When the charge is allowed to bleed off, the atoms return to their normal condition. Capacitors can be damaged by too large a charge in much the same way as a rubber band can be broken by overstretching it. The overall effect of a capacitor's storage activity is a tendency to oppose changes in voltage. This effect leads to a primary application of capacitors as stabilizing devices in power supplies where they are used to smooth out fluctuations in DC voltages.

The charging and discharging currents of a capacitor are at a maximum as the charging process begins, gradually slowing down to eventual zero as the charging or discharging process is complete. For example, capacitor not charged—charging current maximum, and vice versa). This brings about a phase difference opposite to that found in inductive circuits; current changes appear to lead voltage changes. A simple memory aid for the phase relationships occurring in inductive and capacitive circuits is "ELI the ICE man," where I equals current, E equals voltage (or electromotive force), C equals capacitance and L equals inductance. E before I in inductive circuits, I before E in capacitive circuits.

The capacitor's action in opposing voltage changes gives rise to reactance in a similar manner in which inductive reactance arises from opposition to current changes. Capacitive reactance (X_c) is also measured in ohms and can be found by the following formula:

$$X_c = \frac{1}{2\pi FC}$$

Where

F = frequency in Hertz
C = capacitance in farads
X_c = capacitive reactance in ohms
2π = a constant

Note that for a given value of capacitance, capacitive reactance is proportional to $1/F$, indicating that it decreases exponentially as frequency increases. As with inductors, the reactive effects of a capacitor are employed in filter circuits. In addition, note that at zero frequency, i.e. DC, X_c is infinite, implying that capacitors can effectively block DC currents to which they exhibit an infinite opposition. This DC blocking effect is employed in filters as well as coupling circuits between amplifiers.

An important application of capacitors is in timing circuits. The time required for a capacitor to charge to 63.2 percent of the applied voltage is called a *time constant* (t) and can be found as follows t = R × C, where t is in seconds, R is in ohms, C is in farads. For any given capacitor, since the charging process is non-linear [it follows the equation $V_c = V_a (1 - e^{-t/RC})$], the time required to fully charge or discharge is five time constants. By altering the value of resistance through which the capacitor charges, the time constant is changed; hence, the frequency of the resulting signal is changed. For example, lowering R means a more rapid charge-discharge; therefore, more cycles per second equals higher frequency. This is a common method of making small changes in frequency. Also, if capacitance is changed, the frequency changes (since t = R × C). Switching in different values of capacitance is a method used to obtain large changes in frequency. This technique is used in some muscle stimulators as a method of varying pulse frequency.

Impedance, Selectivity and Loading

The combined current-opposing effect of resistance, capacitive reactance, and inductive reactance is termed *impedance* (Z) and is most often used in referring to the "AC resistance" of a circuit. The effects of capacitive reactance and inductive reactance are opposite in two ways: (1) (X_L) causes voltage to lead current, while capacitive reactance (X_C) causes current to lead voltage, and (2) as X_L increases in magnitude with an increase in frequency, X_C decreases with a similar change in frequency. Combining both effects into a single circuit means that at some frequency X_L equals X_C, and hence, reactance becomes zero (their effects cancel). This point is called *resonance,* and the frequency is termed the resonant frequency of the circuit. The circuit is then said to be "tuned." The property of circuit resonance is employed in (1) filter circuits, where the resonant frequency signals are allowed to pass but signals at frequencies other than the resonant frequency are attenuated, and (2) oscillator circuits, where at resonance any opposition to current in an oscillator is due to the tuned circuit's residual resistance alone, since X_L and X_C are equal and therefore cancel, and the absence of reactance enables the oscillating elements to charge-discharge and recharge, etc. with little energy loss.

An important item to be considered in discussing tuned RLC circuits is the *selectivity* of the circuit. Selectivity refers to a filter circuit's ability to discriminate between signals which are close in frequency or to an RLC tank circuit's ability to oscillate. The term used to describe selectivity is "Q" (or quality), which is circuit coil reactance divided by coil resistance. This is because the coil is the weak link in any tuned circuit. It should be obvious that the higher the Q of a circuit, the better its selectivity. It also appears that the higher the frequency involved, the better the Q, since ($X_L = 2\pi FL$) inductive reactance is directly proportional to frequency. This is only true, however, up to about 20 MHz; above that, tuned circuits become inefficient *(see* section on microwave oscillators) .

Impedance is also an important factor in considering circuit *loading.* When any two circuits are connected together in order to transfer a signal between them, each may draw current from the other; hence, each acts as a "load" for the other. In the case shown in Figure 8-7, all signal sources can be modeled as a voltage generator (V) and a series resistance (R_s; the impedance of the source). In the diagram shown, the objective is to measure accurately the source voltage. When a voltmeter with an internal impedance equal to the source impedance (20K or 2×10^4 ohms) is placed across the signal source, R_s and R_L are in series and the source voltage will be dropped across them according to Ohms Law; hence, the meter will actually measure only 5 volts, an error of 50 percent! If, on the other hand, R_L were 2 megohms (2×10^6 ohms), virtually all the source voltage would be felt across R_L. The conclusion to be drawn from this is that when the circuit objective is signal transfer (voltage transfer), the load impedance must exceed the source impedance by at least 100. On the other hand, if the circuit objective is power transfer (current transfer), source and load impedances should be equal. This concept is employed in some diathermy units where the patient is part of the output circuit and the output circuit must be "tuned" to obtain maximum efficiency.

Figure 8-7. An example of circuit loading and the solution.

Active Devices and Circuits

Basic Circuit Applications

Resistors, capacitors, and inductors are considered to be "passive" devices in that no excitation energy other than the signal voltage is required for them to perform their function. Vacuum tubes, semiconductors, and integrated circuits, on the other hand, are "active" devices in that they require excitation by a DC voltage in addition to the signal voltage.

All electronic instrument circuits, whether vacuum tube or semiconductor, are modifications of one or more of the following four basic circuits. These are as follows:

1. Rectifiers
2. Amplifiers
3. Wave generators
4. Logic circuits

RECTIFIERS. The purpose of rectifiers is to change AC voltages into DC voltages, primarily in power supplies. Rectifiers can be (1) metallic, (2) vacuum tubes, (3) gas filled, or (4) semiconductor in nature.

AMPLIFIERS. Basically, it is the function of an amplifier to take a small signal voltage and enlarge it to a useful magnitude. Amplifiers constitute the largest and most varied group of electronic circuits, and, as a consequence, special purpose amplifiers exist that will not only amplify but in addition will perform special functions such as integration, division, etc. Amplifiers can be of the (1) vacuum tube, (2) semiconductor, or (3) integrated circuit variety.

WAVE GENERATORS. Wave-generating circuits provide a wide variety of waveforms from simple sine waves to complex staircase-type square waves. The three most basic types of wave generators are (1) sine wave oscillators (2) square wave generators, and (3) sawtooth generators. Some wave generators, including all oscillators, require no trigger signal in order to operate; they are termed self excited in that they spontaneously jump into operation as power is applied. Other generators require some form of external excitation pulse to cause their operation. As with amplifiers, wave generators can be of the vacuum tube, semiconductor, or integrated circuit variety. As of 1974, one manufacturer has marketed a single I.C. chip that will provide sine, square, and sawtooth waveforms simultaneously.)

LOGIC CIRCUITS. Logic circuits constitute an area of electronics all their own—digital electronics. Although wave generators find wide application in digital electronics, the majority of digital circuits are of the "gate" variety, functioning in a go/no-go capacity. A typical example is the two-input *AND gate,* a circuit that will yield an output only when two input signals are present simultaneously. Although semiconductor logic circuits can be built from discrete compounds, today all digital circuitry is of the integrated circuit form.

Vacuum Tube and Semiconductor Theory

The overriding principle upon which all vacuum tubes and most semiconductors function is the principle of *monodirectional current flow* (current flow in one direction). This principle was first applied in the use of diodes as rectifiers.

DIODES. A vacuum tube diode consists of an electron-emitting cathode, an anode, and a filament which heats the cathode to facilitate electron emission. These components are encased in a "tube" of glass or metal from which the air has been removed, hence the name "vacuum tube." Since the cathode is the electron-emitting element, when a voltage is placed across the tube such that the anode is positive with respect to the cathode, electron current will flow from cathode to anode. If the polarity of the voltage is reversed, no current will flow, since the anode is not an electron emitter. Figure 8-8A shows how a diode is used as a rectifier. In the circuit shown, when an AC signal is applied, during the first half cycle the anode is positive, the tube conducts, and the signal is reproduced across R. During the next half cycle the anode is negative with respect to the cathode, no conduction occurs, and no signal voltage is produced across R. The resulting voltage seen across the resistor is called a half wave rectified voltage and the circuit is a half wave rectifier.

Figure 8-8B shows a full wave rectifier. Both the positive and negative swing of the input signal are seen across R as positive-going voltages, since each diode conducts for one alteration—one for the positive half cycle, the other for the negative half cycle.

A semiconductor diode consists of two crystals of germanium

Figure 8-8A. A diode functioning as a half wave rectifier (broken line indicates current path). From Terence Karselis, *Descriptive Electronics and Instrumentation,* 1973. Courtesy of Charles B. Slack, Inc., Thorofare, New Jersey.

Figure 8-8B. A full wave rectifier (broken lines indicate current paths). From Terence Karselis, *Descriptive Medical Electronics and Instrumentation,* 1973. Courtesy of Charles B. Slack, Inc., Thorofare, New Jersey.

or silicon chemically treated (doped) in such a way as to give one an excess of electrons (N-type semiconductor is a negative charge carrier) and the other a deficiency of electrons (P-type semiconductor is a positive charge carrier). The crystals are chemically bonded, and the bonding point is called the junction. When a voltage is placed across a semiconductor diode such that the P- and N-type material are connected to positive and negative potentials respectively (+ to P, — to N), the diode conducts. This is referred to as forward biasing the junction. When the polarity is reversed (+ to N, — to P), the junction is reverse biased and virtually no conduction occurs. Figure 8-9 shows a semiconductor full wave rectifier.

Figure 8-9. A semiconductor full wave rectifier.

Two additional types of specialized semiconductor diodes are the *Zener diode,* which is used as a voltage regulator or voltage reference source, and the *silicon controlled rectifier* (SCR), a rectifier with three elements (anode, cathode, and gate) that must be triggered by an external excitation voltage at the gate electrode before it will conduct, even though it may be forward biased.

TUBES, TRIODES, AND TRANSISTORS. When a third element is placed between the anode and cathode of a diode tube, the result is a triode. The third element is called the control grid, and it is used to control the amount of current flowing from cathode to anode. When the grid potential is made more positive or more negative, the current through the tube will increase or decrease respectively. In this way, a normally high current through the tube can be controlled by a small voltage applied to the grid. It is the application of this process that allows amplification to take place.

The biopolar transistor is the three-element analog of the vacuum tube triode. Transistors are of two types, NPN or PNP. In either case, the device is simply a sandwich of two P- or N-type semiconductor crystals between which a very thin slice of oppositely doped crystal is bonded. As noted previously, P- and N-type semiconductor material refers to where the crystal is an electron charge carrier (N-type for negative) or a proton charge carrier (P-type for positive). The center element of the sandwich is called the *base,* and the other two elements are the *emitter* and *collector.* Comparing the transistor to the vacuum tube, the emitter is analogous to the cathode, the base to the grid, and the collector to the anode. In much the same way that the grid-to-cathode potential controls current through a triode, the base-emitter potential controls transistor current flow. When emitter-base forward bias is increased, transistor current increases. When it is decreased, transistor current decreases. As with triodes, this effect can be utilized in using small signals to control large currents, thereby amplifying the signal.

Figure 8-10 shows the schematic symbols for NPN and PNP transistors. Note that the emitter arrow always points toward the N-type material. When used as amplifiers, the fact that a transistor is PNP or NPN has little effect upon the simplification process. One amplifier is just like the other; the only circuit characteristic altered is the direction of the circuit current.

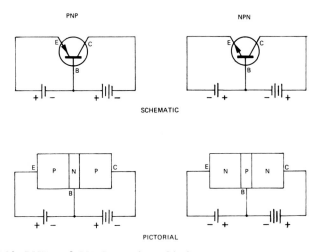

Figure 8-10. PNP and NPN transistor biasing. From Terence Karselis, *Descriptive Medical Electronics and Instrumentation,* 1973. Courtesy of Charles B. Slack, Inc., Thorofare, New Jersey.

A second-generation transistor called a Field Effect Transistor (FET) provides the same amplification capability as a bipolar transistor with the added advantage of exhibiting an extremely high input impedance. This makes it extremely useful in the input stages of amplifying instruments, since it prevents loading of the signal source. These devices find application in pH meters, EKG and EMG devices, and virtually all instruments that are required to amplify very small signals.

Adding a second grid to a triode tube yields a *tetrode*. The second grid is called the screen grid, and its principle action is to reduce interelectrode capacitance between the other tube elements at high frequencies. Tetrodes are the evolutionary dinosaurs of the vacuum tube family; they were just the bridge from triodes to pentodes. *Pentodes* are tubes with three grids: (1) a control grid, (2) a screen grid, and (3) a suppressor grid. Pentodes overcome the frequency and power handling limitations of the triode, yielding greater amplification, a capability to operate at higher frequencies, and the ability to yield greater power outputs.

In the last few years, as industry has attempted to provide smaller and smaller instruments with more reliability, the move has been away from vacuum tube devices to predominantly solid-state instruments. Semiconductor technology has provided the capability with more advanced components such that today virtually any electronic function previously performed by vacuum tubes can be accomplished in a smaller, less power-consuming way with semiconductors. For instance, solid-state rectifiers capable of handling 740 amps are now available; transistors capable of amplifying signals at frequencies as high as 2 gigahertz (2×10^{12} Hertz) are everyday items; a tubeless, flat television screen capable of being hung on a wall like a picture frame is within economically feasible range.

Integrated Circuits. A conventional glass envelope amplifier tube is about the size of a big man's thumb. A transistor capable of the same amplification would be about the size of a small pencil eraser. In both cases, each device consists of a single amplifier stage. On a square crystal chip about the size of the tip of a jeweler's screwdriver, an integrated circuit may contain as many as

200 stages of amplification, including all necessary transistors, resistors, and even capacitors! Figure 8-11 shows the equivalent circuit of a linear integrated circuit amplifier containing fifty-two transistors and diodes.

Figure 8-11. A typical integrated circuit—contains fifty-two transistors and diodes.

OTHER DISCRETE DEVICES. With vacuum tubes on the way out in electronics, bipolar transistors, FETs and I.C.s make up the bulk of active devices found in instrument circuits. There are, however, other devices that find use in special applications.

It was mentioned in a previous section that an SCR (silicon controlled rectifier) is a three-element device that will conduct in one direction but only after it has been "gated" or triggered. A *triac* is much like an SCR except it will conduct in *either* direction after it has been triggered. The big problem inherent in both SCRs and triacs is that once triggered, they will not shut off until the anode-cathode voltage across them is virtually zero. This led to the development of the silicon controlled switch (SCS), which is basically an SCR with a second gate terminal added. This device can be turned off by shorting the anode gate to the anode momentarily. It is turned on by conventional gate triggering. SCRs, SCSs and triacs all find application in areas involving turning on and controlling high current loads, such as motors, power supplies, etc.

Power Supplies and Amplifiers

The material previous to this point dealt with individual components and simple circuits and how they operate. This section will "put it all together" and look at how multiple-stage circuits function in examples of practical application.

The functional stages of a power supply were noted previously to consist essentially of three components: a transformer, a rectifier, and a filter network. Figure 8-12 shows a schematic diagram of a typical instrument power supply. Note that there are more components than previously indicated in the simplified discussion.

The AC input to a power supply is derived from commercial "wall" power, consisting of 115 VAC, 60 Hz. When an instru-

Figure 8-12. A typical power supply schematic.

ment is plugged into a wall receptacle and turned on, the 115 VAC
is fed by way of the line cord into the instrument, through the
on-off switch (S_1) and line fuse (F) appearing at the primary of
the transformer (T_p). The transformer has multiple secondary
windings supplying three different circuits: (1) high voltage—
regulated, (2) high and low voltage—unregulated, and (3) filaments. Each winding supplies a specified group of circuits.

The high voltage regulated supply is obtained by way of a
full wave rectifier employing two gas-filled diodes. The AC
voltage appearing at the transformer secondary is rectified by the
diodes and appears across R_B, a bleeder resistor. Gas diodes are
used in circuits requiring good regulation and high current loads.

The capacitors $(C_1$ and $C_2)$ and inductive chokes $(L_1$ and $L_2)$
filter the pulsating DC into a pure DC voltage. The capacitors
function as follows: As the supply voltage pulse rapidly reaches
its peak value, the capacitors charge up to that value. As the
voltage rapidly drops off, the capacitors are unable to discharge
rapidly due to R_B, hence the voltage tends to remain high; the
capacitors are "opposing a change in voltage." In a like manner,
the inductive chokes "oppose current changes" that tend to appear
due to the supply pulsations. The result is a relatively pure DC
output voltage appearing across the voltage regulator tube (V_R)
and its dropping resistor (R_D).

The voltage regulator, a gas-filled cold cathode diode, operates
with the gas in the ionized state. In this way, a constant voltage
is felt across the tube, even though current through the tube may
vary because of the demands of the load. This is accomplished
due to the fact that ionization requires that a specific potential be
maintained (the V_R potential). Current changes, on the other
hand, are absorbed by the degree of ionization. An increase in
load current means a decrease in regulator current; hence, a lesser
degree of gas atoms are ionized.

The high voltage unregulated section of the power supply
utilizes indirectly heated high vacuum diodes and employs only
RC filtering with no voltage regulation; however, an additional
circuit is made up by resistors R_1, R_2, R_3, and R_4. This is a voltage
divider used to provide more than one voltage from a single HVDC

source. Since they are hooked in series, the full DC output is "divided up" by the resistances into voltage drops proportional to their resistance. Hooking a circuit from ground to any of the points marked will yield the indicated voltage. In this manner, multiple circuits having individual voltage requirements can be driven off a single rectifier.

Figures 13A and 13B show two other types of power supplies common to instrumentation. Figure 13A shows a metallic bridge rectifier with RC filtering and electronic voltage regulation as opposed to a V_R tube. The advantage of this type of supply is threefold: (1) no filaments are required; (2) higher DC output voltages are possible without correspondingly higher transformer voltages since the full secondary voltage is used rather than one half, as with centertapped rectifiers; and (3) voltage regulation is obtained over a wider range of load currents. The electronic voltage regulator is a type of feedback sensing network; the voltage divider (R_1, R_2, R_3) senses the output voltage of the circuit. Should load current demands change, V_0, the sensed voltage, would also tend to change. This voltage in turn controls conduction of Q_2, which controls conduction of Q_1, through which all circuit current (load and sensing) flows. For example, if load current decreases, divider current tends to increase, increasing sensed voltage (V_0) at Q_2 base. This in turn increases Q_2 conduction, thereby decreasing the potential at Q_1 base. Consequently, Q_1 conducts less and V_0 remains stable. The Zener diode in Q_2 emitter circuit provides a constant reference potential for Q_2.

Figure 8-13B is a power supply finding increasing use in instrumentation today. It is a dual polarity ($\pm$ 15 VDC) supply used to drive operational amplifier circuitry. The circuit is a bridge rectifier with a center tapped transformer, and RC filtering and Zener regulation at each of the outputs.

A unique power supply often encountered in instrumentation is the full wave voltage doubler. It is unique in that it requires *no* transformer (although it can be used with one). The circuit as shown in Figure 8-13C operates as follows: On the negative alternation of the input, D_1 conducts and C_1 charges to the peak voltage (V_p). On the positive swing of the input, D_2 "sees" not

Figure 8-13A. A full wave bridge rectifier with electronic voltage regulation.

Figure 8-13B. A double-ended power supply with Zener regulation.

Figure 8-13C. A voltage doubler.

only the peak input voltage but also the voltage of C_1 since C_1 is, in effect, in series with the input. As a result, C_2 charges to $2\,V_p$, or *double* the peak input voltage.

The application of diodes as rectifiers relies principally upon conduction or nonconduction of the device. On the other hand, the process of amplification depends upon (1) a variation in conduction that is proportional to the input signal and (2) the process of voltage division.

An amplifier, in the simplest sense, is a signal-sensitive voltage divider. In order to understand amplification, a simple analogy is often used: a voltage divider with one fixed resistance and one variable resistance in series (Fig. 8-14A). The law for voltages in a series circuit states that the applied voltage will be dropped proportionally across the resistances R_1 and R_2. If R_1 and R_2 are initially equal, the potential at point A will be 5 volts. However, if R_2 increases in value, the potential at A increases. If R_2 decreases, the voltage at A decreases. In an amplifier circuit, R_2 is represented by a triode or bipolar transistor, which in turn changes conduction in response to an input signal at grid or base, respectively. The change in conduction represents a relative change in the resistance of the device. For example, in Figure 8-14B, as the signal at the base of the transistor goes positive ($+100$ mv), the conduction of the device increases (increase forward bias means an increase in conduction) such that the voltage drop across the transistor decreases to 3 volts. As the input signal goes negative (-100 mv) the conduction of the transistor decreases (decreasing forward bias means a decrease in conduction) and the voltage across the transistor increases to 7 volts. Thus, a signal voltage variation of 200 mv has produced an output voltage variation of 4 volts, a gain or amplification of $4/.2 = 20$. It should be noted also that in addition to amplification, a phase reversal has occurred. As V_{in} goes positive, V_o goes negative, etc. This circuit is called a common emitter amplifier. If the input signal were injected at the emitter, no phase reversal would occur and the circuit would be a common base amplifier

A vacuum tube amplifier functions in much the same way as the previously discussed transistor common emitter amplifier. The

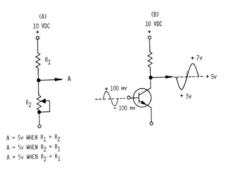

Figure 8-14A&B. Amplification.

signal is injected at the grid and taken off the anode or plate, and a 180-degree phase reversal takes place. The major difference is in the high voltages used in tube circuits; as a result, more power dissipation occurs.

Having seen how an individual transistor (or tube) amplifies, it is now possible to examine a typical transistor amplifier circuit (Fig. 8-14C). Each component shown has a specific function, and each will be discussed in turn.

Figure 8-14C. A correctly biased transistor amplifier.

Q_1 and R_1 constitute the basic amplifier (voltage-sensitive divider) circuit. A signal appearing at the base of Q_1 will be amplified and appear at the collector lead. R_2 and R_3 are a biasing network; they constitute another voltage divider (in this case not voltage sensitive), in parallel with R_1 and Q_1 and used to provide the correct bias at the Q_1 base lead. R_4 and C_2 are used to provide a steady potential at Q_1 emitter (if C_2 were absent, current variations through R_4 caused by Q_1 responding to the input signal would result in Q_1 emitter voltage changes and a loss of amplification). C_1 and C_3 are coupling capacitors that block any DC voltages from appearing at the input and output, respectively, but allow the AC signal voltages to pass. Why does one want the DC voltage blocked? Consider the case of passing the signal from the collector of the amplifier shown to another amplifier's base. The collector of a transistor amplifier is at a DC potential of anywhere from 5 to 10 volts. If this were applied to the base of a transistor (normally at a DC voltage of 0.1 to 1.0 volt), the device would be constantly in a state of high conduction (saturation) and would be unable to respond to small signal voltage changes. By using coupling capacitors, this effect is negated, and many stages of amplifications can be coupled (the technical term used is cascaded) to provide an overall amplification far in excess of a single stage. Such is the case with integrated circuit amplifiers as shown in Figure 8-11.

Wave Generators and Logic Circuits

Although a majority of circuits in most instruments are concerned with amplifying a signal, the instrumentation found in physical therapy utilizes a wide variety of wave-generating circuits from sine wave ultrasonic circuits to square wave and trapezoidal wave circuits.

All wave-generating circuits employ as a control device, in one way or another, the charge-discharge activity of a capacitor. The rate at which the capacitor charges and discharges is in turn a primary factor in determining the frequency at which the waveform is generated. The simplest form of oscillator is a "tank" circuit consisting of a capacitor, an inductor, a power source, and a switch. In Figure 8-15, with the switch in position 1 the capacitor charges (A) as shown. When the switch is in position 2, the capacitor discharges (B) through L, generating a magnetic field. As the capacitor completes its discharge, the inductor's magnetic field collapses (C) and in doing so induces a current that charges the capacitor with a polarity opposite to the original condition (D). When the magnetic field is fully collapsed, the capacitor begins to discharge in the opposite direction (E), and the sequence is repeated in reverse (F and G) until the capacitor is charged as it was originally (H). It appears (to the uninitiated) that this represents an apparent perpetual motion device; obviously such is not the case. The effects of reversing the capacitor's electrical field and the inductor's magnetic field both lead to energy loss; consequently, the oscillations would appear as shown in Figure 8-16. In order to obtain undamped oscillations, some form of *regenerative feedback* is required. If the switch were rapidly thrown back to position 1, at step H the capacitor could re-

Figure 8-15. LC tank circuit oscillation. From Terence Karselis, *Descriptive Medical Electronics and Instrumentation*, 1973. Courtesy of Charles B. Slack, Inc., Thorofare, New Jersey.

charge, replacing its lost energy, resulting in constant amplitude oscillations.

A practical oscillator circuit requires the three items referred to in the above description. These are as follows:

    1. A frequency-determining network
    2. Regenerative (in phase) feedback
    3. A tuned switching device

Figure 8-16. Ideal versus practical oscillations. From Terence Karselis, *Descriptive Medical Electronics and Instrumentation*, 1973. Courtesy of Charles B. Slack, Inc., Thorofare, New Jersey.

Tuned LC tank circuits, quartz crystals, and RC circuits provide item 1 in practical oscillators. Transformers (one winding of which is part of a tank circuit) provide the necessary phase shift (as can groups of RC networks) to bring about regenerative feedback when used in conjunction with transistors or tubes. For example, as an input signal to an amplifier from a tank circuit goes positive, the amplifier output goes negative (180° phase shift). When coupled back to the input by way of a transformer (180° phase shift), the feedback is positive going, in phase with the original signal. The process is *switched* by way of the amplifier reaching saturation or cutoff, resulting in a reversal of the voltage changes. Figure 8-17 shows three transistor oscillators—a Hartley LC oscillator, an RC phase shift oscillator, and a quartz crystal oscillator.

Relaxation oscillators are characterized by output waveforms that change suddenly from one condition to another, the most common type being *multivibrators*. Free-running multivibrators are basically square wave generators consisting of two complementary coupled amplifiers, meaning each output is coupled by way of an RC circuit to the other amplifier's input (Fig. 8-18). Since in a given amplifier, input-output waveforms are 180 degrees out of phase, this complementary coupling requires that when one

Figure 8-17. Hartley (upper left), phase shift (upper right), and crystal controlled (lower) oscillators. From Terence Karselis, *Descriptive Medical Electronics and Instrumentation,* 1973. Courtesy of Charles B. Slack, Inc., Thorofare, New Jersey.

amplifier is "on," the other must be "off." The action of the RC networks is such that they determine the on-off time and also effect the change that reverses the amplifier's conditions. The result is an output as shown in Figure 8-19. By changing the values of the RC network, waveforms such as those shown in Figure 8-20 can be provided.

Two other multivibrator types are (1) the monostable or one-

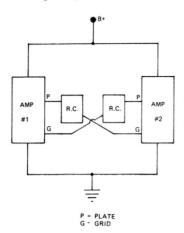

Figure 8-18. An astable (free-running) multivibrator. From Terence Karselis, *Descriptive Medical Electronics and Instrumentation,* 1973. Courtesy of Charles B. Slack, Inc., Thorofare, New Jersey.

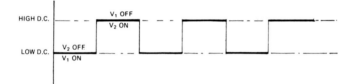

Figure 8-19. Output waveform of an astable multivibrator. From Terence Karselis, *Descriptive Medical Electronics and Instrumentation,* 1973. Courtesy of Charles B. Slack, Inc., Thorofare, New Jersey.

Figure 8-20. Results of varying conduction times of a free-running multivibrator by changing the coupling circuit R and C values. From Terence Karselis, *Descriptive Medical Electronics and Instrumentation,* 1973. Courtesy of Charles B. Slack, Inc., Thorofare, New Jersey.

shot multivibrator, which generates a single pretimed pulse when externally triggered, and (2) the bistable or flip-flop multivibrator, a circuit that will remain in one condition until triggered, when it will "flip" to the other condition. It will remain in that state until another trigger "flops" it back to its original condition. This circuit is used extensively in computers since it can be used to store information (on = 1, off = 0) as well as count and divide when coupled with other flip-flops. Free-running multivibrators find use as "time clocks" in computer circuitry.

Another group of relaxation oscillators are the blocking and ringing oscillators. Blocking oscillators and ringing oscillators are both characterized by two common factors: (1) both types contain, in some form or another, an LC resonant circuit to provide oscillation, and (2) resonant oscillations occur only when the tube or transistor is in the off (cutoff) condition. Blocking oscillators are characterized by the fact that they produce a single, sharp sinusoidal pulse at preset intervals. They may be free running, producing a single pulse constantly at a predetermined interval, controlled by a charging or discharging capacitor, or they may be triggered, producing a pulse only when an input trigger is present.

Ringing oscillators generate a series of dampened sinusoidal pulses when "shocked" into oscillation by an external signal; hence, they are more generally termed shock-excited oscillators. Figure 8-21 shows a typical circuit. When no input signal is present, Q_1 is conducting and the tank circuit ($L_1 C_2$) coil constitutes a low DC resistance. All transistor current flows through it; therefore, no voltage is felt across C_2 (the output). When a negative

Figure 8-21. A shock-excited ringing oscillator.

input pulse cuts off Q_1, the magnetic field generated around L_1 due to the high transistor current flow now collapses, charging C_2, and oscillations are set up in the tank circuit, generating a series of output pulses. As soon as the negative input pulse is removed, Q_1 begins conducting and oscillations cease. If the input signal kept Q_1 cut off long enough, the tank circuit oscillations would eventually dampen, since no regeneration is provided.

Another group of interesting wave generators are the trapezoidal, sawtooth, or ramp generators. These circuits are characterized by an output waveform resembling the teeth of a saw—a slowly rising voltage followed by a rapid drop back to zero. All of these circuits use the charging and discharging of a capacitor to yield the required waveform. The simplest sawtooth generator is the neon glow tube generator. Figure 8-22A shows the neon tube (V_1) in parallel with a capacitor (C_1), both being in series with resistor (R_1). Since conduction through the neon tube only occurs when the gas is ionized, the tube acts as a switch, allowing the capacitor to discharge. When circuit power is applied, C_1 begins to charge through R_1. The output voltage is the charging voltage across the capacitor. When the capacitor voltage reaches the firing potential of the neon gas, the tube conducts and the capacitor rapidly discharges (the tube acts as a short circuit between the capacitor's plates). When the capacitor's voltage drops below the extinction voltage of the neon gas, the tube de-ionizes, acts like an open circuit, and C_1 begins to charge again. Note that the circuit is free running; it requires no input trigger. Figure 8-22B is a triggered (synchronized) sawtooth generator. It differs from the previous circuit in operation in one aspect only—the input trigger turns on the transistor, thereby yielding a discharge path for the capacitor. In all other aspects, circuit operation is identical.

Microwave Oscillators

It was mentioned in a previous section that the "Q" or selectivity of a tuned circuit dropped off drastically above 20 MHz. This occurs because the "lumped" reactance of individual capacitors and inductors is overcome by the *distributed* reactance of

Figure 8-22A. A neon tube sawtooth generator.

Figure 8-22B. A ramp function (sawtooth) generator. From Terence Karselis, *Descriptive Medical Electronics and Instrumentation,* 1973. Courtesy of Charles B. Slack, Inc., Thorofare, New Jersey.

component interelectrode capacitance and circuit wiring, such that at approximately 100 MHz, circuit efficiency can be as low as 50 percent. As a consequence, high frequency (microwave) oscillators and amplifiers of special design are required.

The unique feature of microwave oscillators is the incorporation of the resonant circuit directly into the design of the tube itself. This is accomplished by reducing a resonant circuit down to its simplest form. The simplest form of an inductor would be a short straight segment of wire. When other parallel segments are added, the inductance is further decreased, and the result is somewhat like a squirrel cage. The simplest capacitor is two plates separated by air. If these two simplified components are put together, the result is a round, flat, cagelike structure; if an infinite number of inductor segments are then added, the result is a flat drum or cavity. This is the resonant circuit of a microwave tube.

The walls of the drum constitute as small inductance, with the top and bottom as the resonant circuit capacitance. The overall device is termed a "cavity resonator."

The Klystron (Fig. 8-23) is a vacuum tube with a cathode, control grid, two buncher grids, two catcher grids, and a collector. Resonant cavities are connected to the buncher (1) and catcher (2) grids. When the tube conducts, electrons approach the buncher grid and start the first resonant circuit oscillating. Due to this, electrons tend to leave the buncher grid in cluster groups or "bunches," hence the name. Upon approaching the catcher grid, the first "bunch" of electrons starts the second resonant circuit oscillating; the subsequent groups of electrons that arrive maintain the oscillations. An inductive feedback loop from the second to the first cavity maintains the oscillations required for the buncher electrodes' action. The high efficiency and improved power output of the Klystron over conventional tubes makes them useful at frequencies above 1,000 MHz.

Figure 8-23. Simplified diagram of a Klystrom ultra high frequency amplifier-oscillator.

A second, somewhat different resonant cavity RF tube is the *magnatron*. A magnatron is essentially a diode with a superimposed magnetic field and a series of resonant cavities. Figure 8-24 shows the construction of a typical magnatron. The centrally located cathode emits electrons which are acted upon by both the cathode-anode electric field and the superimposed magnetic field such that they travel along a spirallike path towards the anode. As the electrons pass the cavity slots, they transfer energy into the cavity energy field, causing the cavity to generate oscillations (the

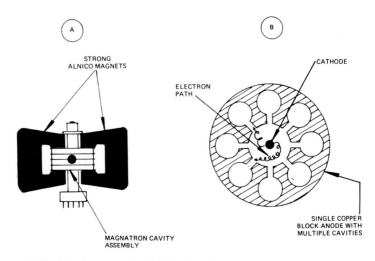

Figure 8-24. (A) shows a simplified drawing of a magnatron. (B) is a cutaway top view of the cavity assembly with spirallike electron paths. From Terence Karselis, *Descriptive Medical Electronics and Instrumentation*, 1973. Courtesy of Charles B. Slack, Inc., Thorofare, New Jersey.

basic principle is similar to that employed to generate sound in tin whistles). The microwave oscillations can be picked up by an inductive probe and fed to a transmitting device (actually an antenna) by way of coaxial cable or a formed wave guide. Magnatrons are considered as self-excited RF oscillators, as they convert pulsed HVDC into pulsed RF energy, and they are used extensively as the power output stage of microwave diathermy units.

THE ELEMENTS OF THERAPEUTIC INSTRUMENTATION
Instrument Systems

How to Get the Best of Them

The average instrument user in a typical medical facility tends to view biomedical instruments as mysterious and unfathomable devices put together by some wild-eyed mad scientists kept locked away in the basement of a large instrument company. The user is quite happy to turn switch (A) and push button (B) and see the instrument "percolate" as it is supposed to, without having to worry himself or herself about *how* it performs its esoteric duty. Herein lies the single most difficult problem for those working with medical instrumentation! "If you don't know *how* it works, how do you know it is working properly?" The solution to this problem can be found in a number of different ways, from obtaining an engineering degree to ignoring the problem completely. An easier, practical, and more useful technique involves not so much learning about instrumentation in a specific sense but rather adapting existing knowledge and common sense into the right approach. To find the right approach, the following question must be asked: Just what is the primary function behind *all* instrumentation? Answer: To extend man's capabilities! Whether it is meant to measure a specific parameter or apply a therapeutic process, instrumentation only enhances the man's ability to perform the function. Since instrumentation extends man's senses and capabilities, it must function in a somewhat similar way. In assaying a particular situation or problem, man must (1) observe, (2) evaluate, and (3) act; when he does so, signal transmission takes place in a definite direction. For example, while driving an automobile, an approaching obstacle would send a visual stimulus, generating electrical excitation, which is transmitted to the brain. The signal is then evaluated, and evasive action (turning the steering wheel) occurs as a result of muscular motor activity caused by the electrical excitation. It is important to note that two signals were involved—the stimulus (received signal) and the response (transmitted signal). All instruments function exclusively to handle one or both of these signal forms, i.e. an EKG handles a received signal, a diathermy unit transmits a signal. With this point of view in mind, one can visualize a simplified medical instrument in one of two ways as shown in Figure 8-25 (A and B). In (A), the signal is sensed, processed, and displayed, while in (B), the signal is generated, processed, and transmitted. Consequently, whichever is the case, most instrument systems can be simplified into a block diagram consisting of (1) a sensing or transmitting unit (the transducer), (2) a processing unit (most often an amplifier), and (3) a generating unit (signal generator) or display unit (meter or oscilloscope, etc.). In addition, all in-

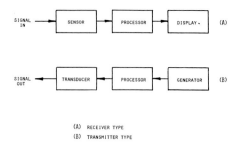

(A) RECEIVER TYPE
(B) TRANSMITTER TYPE

Figure 8-25. Typical instrument systems.

strument systems require power to function, so a fourth unit, a power supply, can be considered as requisite. If one approaches instrumentation in this way, it will tend to be used more efficiently with consequently less "downtime" due to operator error. Whenever malfunctions or breakdowns do occur, the better informed, more knowledgeable operator can troubleshoot or give sound symptomatic fault information to the biomedical electronics technician, once again reducing down-time.

In applying the above technique, the most crucial items required are (1) a thorough understanding of *what* the device should do, (2) a modicum of knowledge of *how* it does it, (3) familiarity with the instrument controls, and (4) a strong mental picture of the instrument in functional but simplified block diagram form. To obtain two of these four tools, it becomes necessary to rely upon the instrument manufacturer. His operating manual will most often yield items 1 and 2. Item 4 may or may not be present; however, a clue to the "functional" blocks within an instrument can be drawn from the controls on its front panel. For example, an on-off switch indicates a power supply. Each operation performed by the device requiring an individual control or adjustment indicates a functional unit. A multiple-position switch allowing various outputs indicates a common output system. With careful observation and a little imagination, a simplified block diagram of even the most sophisticated instrument can be obtained.

Some Additional Points on Signal Processing

Once a signal has been generated within an instrument, it must be fed from the signal source to the output. In addition, some form of modification of the signal may be required. The most common forms of signal processing are rectification and amplification. However, other forms of signal manipulation can occur, such as *modulation, gating,* and *clipping.*

Modulation can be accomplished in two ways: amplitude modulation and frequency modulation. The latter process involves varying the frequency of a signal in proportion to the amplitude of a second signal and is most often used in communications-type circuitry. *Amplitude modulation* is used extensively in therapeutic instrumentation. The term amplitude modulation is self-explanatory; the amplitude of the primary signal is modulated, i.e. varied in proportion to the magnitude of the secondary or modulating signal. In all cases involving AC signals, the primary signal *must* be of a higher frequency than the modulating signal. Four general methods of modulation are used in therapeutic instruments. These are as follows:

1. Opening and closing the filament circuit of a vacuum tube so that its condition occurs in smoothly rising and falling surges.
2. Varying the amplitude of a pulse generator's output signal by way of a motor- or cam-driven rheostat.
3. Varying the plate supply to an oscillator, accomplishing the same result.
4. Varying the conductance of a tetrode or pentode by applying the modulating signal to the screen grid.

Each of these techniques can be found in various instruments commercially manufactured for physical therapy. An examination of the first technique indicated above will provide a general understanding of how modulation takes place.

Figure 8-26 is a Switch Modulated Vacuum Tube Armstrong Tickler Coil Oscillator. The plate coil shown provides regenerative feedback to the LC tank circuit, thereby maintaining oscillations. If the filament voltage and V+ were kept constant, the output signal would be a constant voltage, constant frequency sine wave. As switch S_1 (this could be a set of relay contacts) is periodically opened then closed again, the conduction of the tube varies due to the filament alternately being heated and cooled. The result is periodic surges of oscillation at the output as shown in Figure 8-26. The reader should note that the maximum rate at which surges can be generated is limited by the maximum rate at which the filament can cycle from hot to cold and back. If variable rate capability is necessary, the modulating signal can be obtained electronically from an (RC) oscillator, the frequency of which can be altered by changing the time constant of the circuit. This is accomplished by switching in various resistances (since $t = RC$), which in turn controls the rate at which the capacitor can charge or discharge, thereby changing the oscillator's frequency. The output of this oscillator is then used to *modulate* the output of the primary oscillator circuit by one of the previously mentioned methods.

Figure 8-26. A switch modulated oscillator.

Probably the most common modulating technique used in electronics is the mixing tube technique. A pentode or tetrode oscillator is used to provide the primary signal, which originates in the tube's control grid circuit. The modulating signal is applied to the second (screen) grid, altering the tube's conduction. If the second grid is relatively positive, the control grid's oscillations are allowed to pass to the plate. If the screen grid is relatively negative, the oscillations are suppressed and no output occurs.

Gating can be considered as a type of all-or-none modulation in which the output from the primary oscillator or pulse generator is turned on and off. The action is analogous to switching the circuit on and off, and in fact, this is exactly how such circuits function. A typical example is as follows: The primary oscillator is placed in series with a gating amplifier. In order for oscillations to occur, *both* circuits must be conducting. However, the gating amplifier is normally kept cut off. Positive gating pulses when applied to the gating amplifier input cause it to conduct, thereby allowing the primary oscillator to operate. In contrast to a modulating signal, gating pulses must be square waves and are most often obtained from multivibrator circuits, particularly when variable gate periods are desired. A 60 Hertz gating signal can be obtained directly from line frequency voltage by use of *clipping circuits.*

A clipping circuit does exactly as its name implies; it "clips" the peaks off waveforms. Figure 8-27 shows a simple power frequency neon tube clipping circuit, which operates as follows: The neon gas tube will not conduct until its firing voltage (approximately 50 volts) is reached. During that time the voltage from the secondary of the transformer is felt at the output. When the neon tube fires, the output voltage is the ionization voltage of the tube. The same process occurs on both the positive and negative alternations of the transformer voltage; hence, the output is a somewhat less than perfect square wave.

Figure 8-27. A simple neon tube clipper.

Other types of clipping circuits involve the use of biased diodes or triodes. The overall effect, however, is the same; predetermined peaks of the input waveform are clipped.

Basic Principles of Transducers

In most types of electronic instrumentation, it is the *transducer* that acts as the transmitting or receiving element of the instrument system. However, in some instances of therapeutic medicine, the transmitting device is not really a transducer in the strict sense of the word; it may act as nothing more than an electrode (a terminal point of an electrical circuit). Nevertheless, an understanding of some of the principles involved in the application of transducers is required of anyone involved in therapeutic medicine.

Any device capable of converting one form of energy into another can be classified as a transducer. Case in point: a typical household light bulb. This electrical transducer converts electrical energy into electromagnetic radiation, i.e. light and heat energy. A somewhat more sophisticated form of transducer is the common chemical pH electrode—a device that converts chemical activity into electrical energy. Most transducers are classified based on the type of energy required to "excite" them. Hence, the common light bulb is an *electro-optical* transducer, while a pH electrode is considered a *chemoelectric* transducer.

The three energy forms primarily employed in physical medicine are (1) low and medium high frequency electrical currents, (2) radio frequency electrical and electromagnetic radiation, and (3) ultrasonic mechanical energy. The application of low and medium high frequency electrical currents requires little more than metallic electrodes as transducers, while RF energy employs the use of basic electrical and electromagnetic principles in its application. The only "true" transducer used in physical medicine is the ultrasonic or *piezoelectric* transducer.

The piezoelectric effect is a bidirectional phenomenon first discovered in certain crystalline materials. If a crystal of Rochelle salt (quartz SO_2) is mechanically distorted, stresses within its lattice structure result in surface charge polarization such that one side of the crystal becomes positive and the other negative. However, it is the reverse action that finds its application in physical medicine—the fact that when a crystal is excited by an AC electrical signal it will distort or vibrate, producing sound waves of the same frequency as the stimulating signal. Since quartz and Rochelle salts are dependent upon careful and correct cutting of the crystal to yield satisfactory results, ultrasonic elements of barium titanate (molded ceramics) are becoming more common. These commercial substances have the dual advantages of less cost and wider temperature stability. Figure 8-28 shows an example of the piezoelectric effect; the reader should note that the process is a reversible one; an alternating current voltage applied to the crystal produces mechanical vibrations.

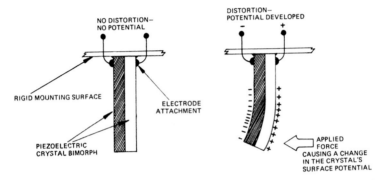

Figure 8-28. A simplified diagram showing the piezoelectric effect. From Terrence Karselis, *Descriptive Medical Electronics and Instrumentation,* 1973. Courtesy of Charles B. Slack, Inc., Thorofare, New Jersey.

Piezoelectric crystals also find application in oscillator circuits, since their resonant vibrations are inherently stable, providing exceeding stable output frequencies from the oscillator.

In either of the above applications, the piezoelectric crystal is mounted between two metallic plates, enabling the application or withdrawal of mechanical energy.

Medical diathermy utilizes both electrical and electromagnetic fields to provide deep tissue heating. The "transducers" used to apply the energy to the patient in these applications are not energy-transforming devices but rather more like oversized electrical components. In the application of *electrical fields,* the patient becomes the dielectric in large capacitor made up of the application plates with the patient sandwiched between them. When *electromagnetic* energy is employed, an applicator coil is wound around the patient (on the leg, for example), thereby making the patient the "core" of an oversized inductor. In both instances, it is the fundamental electrical activity of these oversized components that provides the therapeutic energy to the patient. The patient is in effect immersed in the appropriate energy field.

The use of muscle stimulating currents requires the least sophisticated transducer of all; in fact, the applicators used in this mode of therapy are little more than simple contact electrodes or terminals. The patient, when placed between the electrodes, simply becomes a resistive element in a series circuit network. When a voltage is generated across the electrodes, current flows out from one electrode through the patient and into the other electrode. This form of physical medicine is the only one in which "electrical current" flows from instrument to patient. In the previous methodologies noted, the patient is immersed in or becomes the target of some form of *energy field*.

Electromagnetic Radiation

Generation and Transmission of Electromagnetic Radiation

The previous section discussed the use of "energy fields" as the therapeutic agent in physical medicine, indicating that both electrical and electromagnetic fields are used. More specifically, electromagnetic energy was related to high frequency (short wave and microwave) diathermy. The use of electromagnetic radiation, however, is not restrictive to diathermy wavelengths. Radiations falling into and around the visible spectrum are also employed in physical medicine.

The dualistic nature of electromagnetic energy came to light in the early nineteenth century when the Danish physicist, Oersted, accidentally observed its effect on a magnetic compass during a lecture demonstration. Today, it is known that magnetic effects are a result of charges in motion. Since the electrons in an atom are in motion, both orbital and spin in nature, they act as minute coils carrying current and hence generate minute magnetic fields. If the substance is such that the effects of the various fields are cancelled, the net result is that the material is nonmagnetic. If the minute magnetic fields are such that they are additive, the substance will have a net magnetic field.

In an earlier section, with the discussion of electromagnetism, through a conductor, a magnetic field was generated around that conductor. One can take this example and expand upon it in order to see how it relates to the generation of electromagnetic energy fields in space.

Radio frequency oscillations are produced by electronic oscillator circuits. When such alternating currents are applied to an appropriate length of conductor ($\frac{1}{2}$ or $\frac{1}{4}$ wavelength of the oscillating frequency), an antenna is produced. The antenna segment has two ends, (1) the transmitter end, attached to the oscillator output, and (2) the open end. During one *half* cycle of oscillation current will flow from the transmitter end to the open end. During the next half cycle it will flow from the open end back to the transmitter end. As the current tends to be maximum at the center, it is at this point around the conductor that a doughnut-shaped magnetic field is generated, the lines of force of which are perpendicular to the antenna. This constitutes the *magnetic* portion of the radiated electromagnetic field. The *electrical* field is produced by the capacitance that exists between the two ends of the conductor. As charges alternately pile up at the open and transmitter ends of the antenna, electrical lines of force are produced parallel to the antenna. This constitutes the electrical field. Note that the two fields are 90 degrees of phase *in time* and *in space* (Fig. 8-29A). When the electrical field is at maximum intensity, electrons are piled up at one antenna end and current is zero; therefore, magnetic field is nil. Magnetic lines of force are perpendicular to the antenna, electrical lines of force are parallel to it. The wave field radiated into space constitutes a series of alternating magnetic and electrical waves moving outward from the antenna as shown in Figure 8-29B.

As the LC values of an oscillating tank circuit become smaller, the frequency of oscillation becomes higher, and the wavelength of the radiated energy becomes shorter. At wavelengths above 0.1 mm (3,000 MHz), it is not possible to construct circuitry to accomplish oscillation. Radiation at these wavelengths comes from molecular and electronic vibrations in molecules and atoms which

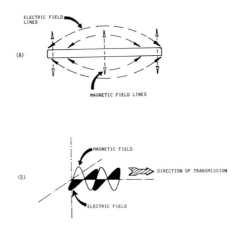

Figure 8-29. Antenna energy fields.

can be made to "oscillate" by appropriate stimulation, such as heating and electrical discharge. The waves that are generated in this manner constitute the so-called visible spectrum of *infrared, visible,* and *ultraviolet* light.

Wavelengths in the x-ray and gamma regions require still smaller "oscillators," and these are found within the atomic nucleus as a result of high energy particle collisions.

In evaluating the transmission of electromagnetic radiation and its effect upon other materials, two general items must be considered: (1) the intensity and frequency of the transmitted energy and (2) the properties of the receiving material.

The intensity of the radiated energy, with antenna characteristics constant, is a function of the current in the antenna. The antenna current is in turn dependent upon the antenna *reactance* for a given frequency and applied power. From this, it is possible to conclude that since reactance is frequency dependent (as previously discussed), at some frequency, reactance will be zero and the antenna will be at resonance. It is at this frequency at which maximum energy is radiated.

The reaction of a given receiving substance to radiated energy is determined primarily by the frequency (or wavelength) of the transmitted signal. At longer (radio) wavelengths, it is the bulk electrical and magnetic properties that will determine the result. For example, an insulator has few movable charges; therefore, no counteracting fields can be produced. Hence, electromagnetic waves travel easily through electrical insulators, while they are absorbed by the human body which has an abundance of movable charges with which to react.

At shorter wavelengths, atomic properties begin to take an effect and in fact play a significant role, while at very short wavelengths, the receiver interaction is a result of elementary particle, i.e. electrons, neutrons, and protons, interaction.

As a general rule, it can be said that the longer the wavelength, the more predominant will be the "wave properties" of electromagnetic radiation, while the shorter the wavelength, the more predominant will be its "quantum properties."

It is the wave properties of visible light that help the student to understand its behavior when passing from one medium into another. One should keep in mind, however, that the laws governing this action remain just as valid when applied to other regions of the electromagnetic spectrum. If it is remembered that the shorter the wavelength of a photon or wave of energy, the greater its energy and hence its potential penetrating ability, the basic laws of *reflection, refraction,* and *absorption* can be used to predict the behavior of any electromagnetic wave whether visible or invisible.

One may predict, for example, the behavior of two separate wavelengths of radiation passing from one medium (air) into a second medium (a polished glass plate). If wavelength (A) is visible light and (B) is x-ray energy, since (B) is shorter in wavelength it is therefore higher in energy. Thus, the majority of (A) will be *reflected,* while the majority of (B) will pass into the glass medium. Any photons entering the glass will alter their direction in accordance with the law of *refraction.* In general the higher the energy of the photon, the less the refractive effect. Finally, all radiant energy entering the glass will be decreased in magnitude *exponentially* according to the law of absorption. The higher the photon energy, the greater its penetrating ability and the less its chance of being absorbed.

The Electromagnetic Spectrum

In the previous section, the generation and radiation of electromagnetic energy fields were discussed with little mention of the method of classifying them. In most instances, regions of the spectrum are in fact distinguished on the basis of how a particular wavelength is produced or detected. Radio waves are produced and detected by radio circuits, while infrared waves are generated or detected by heat.

An overall view of the electromagnetic spectrum can be based on classification as to wavelength as shown in Table 8-I. It should be noted, however, that the boundaries between regions overlap and the figures given are approximate.

The speed of radiation in free space is 300 million meters per second, and this figure can be used to find the wavelength or frequency of the radiation if one or the other is known, in the following manner:

$$\text{(meters)} = \frac{300{,}000{,}000 \ \text{(meters/sec.)}}{\text{Frequency (Hertz)}}$$

For example, a 30,000 MHz radio wave has a wavelength of 0.01 meter or 1.0 cm, while a 27 MHz diathermy wave has a wavelength of approximately 11 mm and a 10 KC radio wave has a wavelength of 30,000 meters. Although the above measurement of wavelength is given in meters, the standard classical method used gives wavelength in Angstroms (Å): $1\text{Å} = 1 \times 10^{-10}$ meters. Another wavelength unit used extensively in clinical analysis is the nanometer (nm): $1 \text{ nm} = 1 \times 10^{-9}$ meters.

ULTRAVIOLET RADIATION DEVICES
Ultraviolet Radiation

Sources

The most commonly known natural source of ultraviolet radiation (1,800 to 4,000 Angstroms) is sunlight, but its therapeutic capability is limited by not only quantity (ultraviolet constitutes a small fraction of the total solar radiated energy) but in some cases also by quality, since certain regions of the ultraviolet region are absorbed by the oxygen molecules of the air. Hence, it is no

TABLE 8-I

	Cosmic Rays	Gamma Rays	X-Rays	Ultra-violet	Visible	Infra-red	Radio Short Wave	Radio Long Wave
WAVELENGTH (cm)	10^{-12}	10^{-10}	10^{-8}	10^{-6}	10^{-4}	10^{-3}	10	10^5
FREQUENCY (hertz)	10^{17}	10^{15}	10^{13}	10^{10}	10^9	10^8	10^5	10

accident that high mountain "air" is thought to be more therapeutic than that in the low-lying damp valleys. The ultimate
source of the sun's ultraviolet radiation is in the heated gaseous
envelope surrounding the sun, which has an average temperature
of approximately 5,000°C. These heated gases are continuously
being ionized, with the resulting emission of discrete "particles" of
energy when displaced orbital electrons regain their normal position. The energy content of these *photons* is related to frequency
and wavelength as follows:

$$E = \frac{hv}{\lambda}$$

Where $E =$ energy in ergs
$\lambda =$ wavelength in Angstroms
$v =$ frequency in Hertz
$h =$ Planck's constant

In general, it can be said that the shorter the wavelength, the
higher the energy.

To insure adequate intensities of ultraviolet radiation for
therapeutic application, artificial ultraviolet sources must be used.
Like the ultraviolet radiation generated by the sun, artificial ultraviolet generation is due to ionization of the substance employed
as the "emitter." The two most common methods of producing
ionization are (1) the application of heat and (2) arcing due to
an electric current. The latter technique is the method of choice
in most cases; however, an example of the former technique is
found in the common incandescent tungsten bulb. An electric
current passed through a tungsten filament generates heat, which
increases the kinetic energy of its atoms. Increased collisions of
the atoms generates infrared, visible, and ultraviolet radiations.
To provide this wide range of radiation, the filament temperature
must be operated at approximately 3,100° C; below 500° C, only
infrared radiation is produced. Of the total energy emission
of a tungsten bulb, approximately 0.5 percent is in the ultraviolet
region. Needless to say, incandescent sources are rarely used in
therapeutic applications involving UV energy.

As noted previously, the spectrum of energy produced by an

incandescent source is a *continuous* one. When elementary substances such as xenon gas are ionized, they produce radiations that are *not continuous* but in specific narrow lines (Fig. 8-30). These *line spectra* are characteristic of the substance in question since each element has its own unique set of orbital electrons and, therefore, emission quanta. While ionization can be brought about by heating, it is impractical at the temperatures necessary to ionize those substances that will emit ultraviolet radiation; hence, an alternative technique is used. When a gas is enclosed in a suitable container with an electrode at each end, and sufficient voltage is impressed across the electrodes, at some point the gas will ionize and an electric current will arc between the electrodes. By sustaining the current and adding in vapor form a substance capable of ultraviolet emission, i.e. mercury, a practical ultraviolet generator can be made. The arcing current provides high velocity particles which by way of collision cause atoms of the emitting substance to radiate ultraviolet energy. This gas discharge or electric arc process is the most common technique used in commercial ultraviolet-generating devices.

Figure 8-30. Typical line spectra.

Physical Behavior of Ultraviolet Radiation

The clinical aspects of ultraviolet energy behavior are covered elsewhere in this volume; consequently, this section will deal lightly with some of the physical aspects that are directly related to the application of ultraviolet therapy.

The transmission of radiant energy is governed by various physical laws, and two of the most important in the application of therapeutic radiation are the inverse square law and the cosine law. Briefly, the inverse square law states that the intensity of radiation from a *point source* decreases inversely with the square of the distance from the source. Hence, doubling the distance between source and target will decrease the intensity of the radiation to one quarter of its former value. The cosine law shows that minimum reflection from a surface occurs when the angle between *incident ray* and reflecting surface is 90 degrees; hence, at this angle, maximum absorption will occur. Radiation intensity is then proportional to the cosine of the angle of radiation and a perpendicular to the target surface.

The interaction of electromagnetic radiation and matter was mentioned previously indicating that the reactions that took place were at the (1) bulk, electrical, and electromagnetic, (2) molecular and atomic, or (3) subatomic or elementary particle level. Such reactions take place, however, only *after* the radiation has crossed the interface between the transmitting medium (air) and receiving or absorbing medium (the patient). Like visible light, ultraviolet radiation is subject to the laws of optics governing reflection, refraction, and absorption. At the interface between two mediums, reflection and absorption take place, and the ratio of reflection to absorption for a given amount of transmitter radiation is directly dependent upon (1) the wavelength of the radiation, (2) the angle at which it strikes the medium (angle of incidence), and (3) the physical nature of the medium. This data is important in the design of ultraviolet therapeutic devices, particularly in the design of reflectors, as well as affecting the quality of ultraviolet application as a therapeutic agent.

Once absorbed by the target medium, penetrating ultraviolet radiation undergoes one or more of the interactions mentioned previously. Since the absorbed energy represents an increase in the net energy of the system, in order for the system to return to its normal or "ground" state, the excess energy must be dissipated. This can take place via ionization, chemical reactions, or heat or light emission (fluorescence). Whatever the case, the absorbed energy is absorbed in an exponential manner until all the energy has been transferred to the medium or the residual radiation exist into another medium.

A Typical Ultraviolet Generating Device

Just like any other device or instrument, an ultraviolet radiation generator can be subdivided into specific functional parts. A typical device consists of the component parts as listed below:

1. An ultraviolet radiation source (lamp)
2. A reflecting device with shutters
3. An applicator column or arm
4. A support base with enclosed transformer or ballast circuitry

Specific ultraviolet sources will be discussed in the next section; this section will briefly consider the remaining three areas.

As noted previously, ultraviolet radiation is subject to all the physical laws of visible light, i.e. reflection, etc. Considering that an ultraviolet source of radiation emits its energy omnidirectionally (in all directions), the use of such a source without some type of reflecting device would be highly inefficient, since most of the energy would be dissipated into the air. Use of an appropriate reflector concentrates and redirects most of the diffusing radiation onto the patient. Parabolic and terrace-type reflectors of smooth, polished metallic surfaces are used to accomplish concentration of radiation. Figure 8-31 shows typical parabolic and terrace-type reflectors.

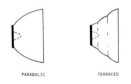

PARABOLIC   TERRACED

Figure 8-31. Typical reflectors.

In order to facilitate application of ultraviolet radiation to patients in various positions and to various surfaces of the body, the source and reflector (the head of the device) must be mobile and capable of great flexibility and adjustment with minimal effort. To accomplish this, counterbalanced telescoping columns with adjustable joints are used, such as those shown in Figure 8-32.

Figure 8-32. Burdick U.V. 800 ultraviolet lamp. Courtesy of The Burdick Corporation, Milton, Wisconsin.

To provide maximum stability in ultraviolet lamps, the transformer or ballast circuitry required to control the line voltage to "fire" the ultraviolet source is usually housed in the base of the lamp. Wheels or casters are fixed to the base to provide maximum mobility.

Mercury Lamps

Low Pressure Mercury Arc Lamps

The most efficient method of producing ultraviolet radiation is by way of a sustained electric arc. Open carbon arcs were used previous to the invention of the mercury lamp; however, mercury arc lamps are the most common type of therapeutic ultraviolet generators used today.

The basic mercury arc lamp consists of (1) an envelope transparent to ultraviolet radiation (2) electrodes which furnish the voltage to create the arc, (3) a support gas to maintain the electric arc and provide ionizing temperatures, and (4) liquid mercury, which acts as the ultraviolet emitter when ionized. Two types of low pressure mercury lamps are obtainable, cold cathode and hot cathode lamps. The cold or hot designation refers to the method by which electrons are emitted from the cathode in order to initiate ionization of the support gas. In hot cathode lamps, the electrodes are preheated and a low voltage is impressed across the electrodes. The increased kinetic energy of electrons in the electrode material plus the energy of the low voltage is sufficient to cause emission of electrons ionizing the support gas and establishing current flow between the electrodes. Once initiated, the current through the support gas generates heat which vaporizes the mercury. The mercury atoms then collide with high velocity electrons, are ionized, and thereby emit ultraviolet radiation. The greatest concentration of ultraviolet energy is generated in the 2537 and 1849 Angstrom lines as shown in Figure 8-33.

Figure 8-33. Mercury (low pressure) spectrum.

Ordinary borasilicate glass is not suitable for ultraviolet source envelopes since it absorbs in the ultraviolet region; therefore, ultraviolet transmitters such as quartz, fused quartz, and silicon dioxide as well as some high phosphate glasses are used. Fused quartz is commonly used, as it has other physical advantages besides being transparent to ultraviolet. It is physically strong, has low thermal conductivity (and hence has a low sensitivity to thermal shock), and is also an electrical insulator. A low pressure mercury arc lamp with a fused quartz envelope is often referred to as a cold quartz lamp.

The cold cathode variety of lamp (which may *also* be called a cold quartz lamp) required no heating of the electrodes. However, in order to initiate electron emission and generate an arc, a high voltage (1,500 v) must be placed across the electrodes. Once ionization occurs and the arc is generated, the operation of the lamp is the same as its hot cathode brother. Figure 8-34 shows the schematic diagram of a typical cold quartz lamp. Note that the secondary of the transformer is in series with the lamp providing ballast (current limiting) capability.

Figure 8-34. Simplified schematic of a Birtcher Spot Quartz Lamp. Courtesy of The Birtcher Corporation, Los Angeles, California.

High Pressure Mercury Arc Lamps

The basic operating principles of the low pressure mercury arc lamp, including arcing, heating, and ionization, extend to the high pressure lamp. The major difference is in the *behavior* of the high pressure lamp. When the vapor pressure of the atomized mercury in a lamp exceeds one atmosphere, the lamp is a high pressure device. The mercury spectrum is generated by the initiation process previously discussed; however, it differs from the low pressure mercury spectrum in that the typical spectral lines broaden and "shoulder" or "wing" lines appear on both sides of the characteristic lines. In addition, a weak continuous spectrum is generated. The majority of emitted energy is in the lines from 2967 to 3660 Angstroms. Due to the increased mercury vapor in the tube, the 2537 Angstrom line is almost totally self absorbed by the vapor and not emitted by the lamp.

Fused quartz envelopes are most often used due to the advantageous characteristics previously noted. The high pressure lamp envelope is normally at a high temperature; however, it can be air or water cooled since both air and water transmit ultraviolet radiation. The use of fused quartz envelopes along with the high operating temperature produced has led to the use of the term *hot quartz lamps* in referring to these devices.

In comparing high and low pressure mercury lamps, the following items are the most important. High pressure mercury lamps require several minutes to reach full intensity, while low pressure lamps reach full intensity almost immediately. After turnoff, low pressure lamps can be immediately restarted, while high pressure lamps must be "rested" for a few minutes prior to restarting.

Two important factors that determine the operating efficiency of a mercury lamp are cleanliness and lamp deterioration. Keeping a lamp and the surrounding reflector clean prevents deterioration of the envelope and loss of ultraviolet radiation. Deterioration of the lamp itself can be caused by aging of the envelope, internal blackening of the envelope, and operation of the lamp at excessive voltages and/or unnecessary use.

Other Artificial Sources

Carbon Arc Lamps

In the latter part of the nineteenth century, carbon arc lights were introduced as an alternative method of street illumination to gas. Shortly after that, Niels Finsen originated artificial therapeutic radiation using carbon arc lamps.

The basic principle of the carbon arc is the production of radiation by vaporizing and ionizing inorganic salts in an electrical arc. Two carbon electrodes are opposed to each other, in series with a ballast resistance or choke coil. The electrodes are initially touching when a voltage is applied, then separated slightly. An arc is maintained between the electrodes, and three forms of radiation are generated. The heated electrode tips become incandescent and as such emit a continuous visible and infrared spectrum. The arc heats the inorganic salts and metals of the electrodes, causing characteristic line spectra to be emitted. To provide radiation at specified wavelengths, iron, strontium, aluminum, nickel, and rare earth metals such as cesium are placed in the electrode core. Carbon arcs, however, are low efficiency ultraviolet emitters, and the major radiation peak in all types of carbon arc lamps falls between 3500 and 4000 Angstroms. Other disadvantages include noise (sputtering), fumes, and ashes produced, as well as the high power consumption (15 to 20 amps) of these devices.

Fluorescent Ultraviolet Lamps

The so-called 'black light" lamp is an example of a fluorescent ultraviolet lamp. These lamps are generally low pressure mercury devices in which the ultraviolet transmitting envelope is coated on its inner surface with a fluorescing substance called a phosphor. The specific type of phosphor used determines the wavelength of energy radiated. When "fired," the photons of the high energy mercury lines generated by the arc strike the phosphor and are absorbed. The process of fluorescence then takes place, and *longer* wavelength radiation is emitted by the phosphor.

Some "sun" lamps and the typical office fluorescent lamp belong to the same family of devices as the black light, all of which are low powered lamps and therefore must be used in groups to provide any degree of intensity.

Other Ultraviolet Lamps

The xenon arc lamp was previously mentioned as being a usable ultraviolet source; however, the potentially dangerous high pressure (20 atmospheres) and high power (1000 watts) necessary for its use make it less than desirable for routine use.

Molecular hydrogen and zirconium arc lamps are also used as ultraviolet generators but are not routinely found in typical institutions.

INFRARED GENERATORS

Therapeutic Heat

Luminous and Nonluminous Radiation Sources

The use of heat as an agent to relieve sore and aching muscles originated, in all probability, sometime during the stone age when the first caveman noticed that lying in the sun on a warm rock did wonders for a body fatigued by chasing (or being chased by) dinosaurs. In more recent times, Roman baths and hot springs have found similar acceptance. Today, the popularity of health club sauna and steam baths is no less common.

Unbeknownst to him, the caveman mentioned above was enjoying the two most common forms of therapeutic heat application, luminous heat (the sun) and nonluminous heat (the warm rock).

Heat is defined as a measure of the kinetic energy of the molecules in a particular substance or system. Cold, in contrast, is not a separate entity but rather the loss of or absence of heat.

An object heated to a higher temperature than its surroundings will give off heat in one or more of three ways: (1) by electromagnetic radiation, (2) by conduction, and (3) by convection. All of these modes are used in physical therapy in the form of lamps (radiation), hot packs (conduction), and water and paraffin baths (convection and conduction).

Luminous and nonluminous heat therapy uses electromagnetic radiation in the infrared and near-infrared region of the spectrum, from 7,000 to 120,000 (approximately) Angstroms. Natural sunlight consists of nearly 60 percent infrared energy, the remainder being visible and ultraviolet, and hence represents the most abundant natural source of radiant infrared energy.

Infrared radiation can be generated by two types of sources, the so-called luminous and nonluminous heat energy. The nonluminous sources do generate some visible radiation but mostly in the near-infrared region.

Nonluminous generators employ some form of resistive element through which an electric current is passed. Remembering some basic electricity, when a current is passed through a resistance, energy is dissipated in the form of heat (P_{watts} $I^2_{current}$ $\times$ $R_{resistance}$). The temperature of the element is approximately 500° to 600°C. The energy dissipated is in the form of infrared radiation. A typical nonluminous generator consists of a resistance wire coil wound around a porcelain support rod. The rod is mounted in a reflective head and held on a support arm. Nonluminous generators operate from 50 to 1500 watts of power and come in various sizes.

Luminous infrared generators utilize the same resistance heating principle. However, due to the higher temperatures attained by the heating element, two problems arise: (1) the filament must be placed in an evacuated or inert gas atmosphere to prevent oxidation, and (2) a large part of the radiation generated is visible energy and therefore produces little heating.

Luminous infrared sources consist of tungsten or carbon filaments in glass or conical quartz bulbs with reflective metal back surfaces. Quartz is superior to other materials due to its insensitivity to thermal shock; contact with cold surfaces during operation will not cause it to crack or crystallize. In addition, quartz bulbs heat up and cool very rapidly.

Incandescent tungsten filament gas-filled bulbs (so called heat lamps) are also used as infrared generators of the low wattage variety, as are ordinary household bulbs of the 25 to 50 watt type. The latter are often employed in bakers, where two or more bulbs are mounted in a reflective housing which can be placed over a patient's leg, arm, or body.

Conductive Heating Devices

Hot water bottles, which replaced the older heated stones or bricks as conductive heating devices, are still in use today in many places. The most recent form of conductive heating device, however, is the electric blanket. Once again, the basic principle employed is resistive heating, and the temperatures attained are low (maximum 110°). A typical heating blanket consists of a flexible heating element within an electrically insulated covering which is sewn between two layers of cloth. Temperature control is by way of a multiple-position switch and transformer or a variac. Temperature regulation is obtained by way of a bimetallic strip or other type of thermometer. High temperatures cause the switch to open, breaking the circuit and preventing current flow through the heating element. Once the temperature drops, the switch closes and heating resumes.

NERVE AND MUSCLE STIMULATING GENERATORS

Introduction

Low voltage electrotherapy constitutes the *only* form of therapy in which current flows *directly* from the therapeutic device into the patient. All other therapeutic modalities involve the transfer of *energy* from devices to patient without *direct* connection. Because of this direct connection between patient and current source, the therapist should be acutely aware of all the possible implications that arise by making the patient an integral circuit element. A firm understanding of the instrumentation involved is a necessary prerequisite in producing such an awareness.

Types of Current and Terminology

The low voltage currents employed in electrotherapy are no different than the currents found in any typical electrical instrument. They can be direct (DC) or alternating (AC) in nature, or a combination of both. The specificity of electrotherapeutic currents is due primarily to the type of waveform employed, more so than to the basic form of current. The terminology used in describing low voltage currents is far from standardized; however, all the terms used describe modifications of one or both of the two basic current forms.

Direct current is also termed galvanic current or continuous current, since it is characterized by the steady flow of charges in *one direction* through an electrical circuit (which, in this application, includes the patient).

Alternating current, as its name implies, periodically reverses its direction. The charges constituting the current flow migrate in one direction for a specified amount of time and then reverse their direction of migration.

The three basic *waveforms* used with alternating currents are as follows:

1. Sinusoidal
2. Rectangular (including pulsed square waves)
3. Trapezoidal (sawtooth)

The terms faradic, sinusoidal, and pulsed are used in describing specific types of AC waveforms based on the way in which the wave changes with time.

When a current is suddenly turned on and off at periodic intervals, it is termed an *interrupted* current. If, on the other hand, its magnitude is *gradually* increased and decreased, it is called a *surging* current. As noted previously, any alteration of the magnitude of a waveform is called *modulation;* hence both interruption and surging are forms of modulation. Both AC and DC currents can be interrupted and surged.

Figure 8-35 shows some of the more common waveforms used in electrotherapy. From the physiological point of view, the overall effects of steady DC currents tend to be *chemical* in nature, producing ionic migration between the positive and negative terminals of a circuit. Alternating currents or interrupted DC result in *muscular contraction,* while pure AC (the positive and negative alterations supply equal energy) produces no net ion movement.

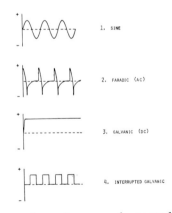

Figure 8-35. Common low voltage waveforms used in electrotherapy.

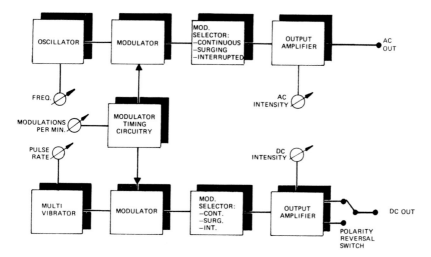

Figure 8-36. Block diagram of an electrotherapeutic generator. From Terence Karselis, *Descriptive Medical Electronics and Instrumentation,* 1973. Courtesy of Charles B. Slack, Inc., Thorofare, New Jersey.

The *frequency* of an alternating current is defined as the number of cycles or complete alternations (positive to negative and back again) generated in one second. Hence, a 60 Hz current yields sixty cycles per second. The frequency of an AC current is an important criteria of classification, due primarily to the physiological effects it elicits. An AC current below 20 Hz applied to a healthy skeletal muscle will yield clonic contractions which are in proportion to the applied frequency. If, however, the frequency is greater than 20 Hz, tetanus occurs. As a result, frequencies bleow 20 Hz are called *pulse* frequencies and frequencies above 20 Hz are called *tetanizing* frequencies.

A Simplified Instrument

A block diagram of a simplified low voltage generator capable of delivering AC and DC currents of various forms is shown in Figure 8-36. Although individual manufacturers provide their own unique design features and specialized controls, a number of common characteristics can be found in virtually all instruments. They are as follows:

1. A power input cord consisting of three wires: a "hot" current carrying conductor which is at a potential of 115 VAC when plugged in, a "cold" current carrying conductor which is at ground potential and serves as a "return" for the "hot" side, a safety *ground* wire which under *normal* conditions *does not* carry current but serves as a path to ground for unwanted charges appearing on the instrument cabinet.

2. A fuse located electrically on the input side of the power supply circuit. The fuse is placed in this position to ensure that if any excess current is drawn it will be felt immediately at the power supply and power will be interrupted. The physical placement of the fuse socket is generally at the rear of the instrument cabinet.

3. A main power switch and indicator or pilot light. The power switch, like the fuse, is also on the primary or input side of the power supply circuit. A neon indicator bulb is hooked across the instrument side of the power supply to show that power is applied when the switch is closed.

4. Some form of output energy monitoring device, to allow continual observation of the current being passed through the patient. In most instances, this is accomplished by placing a milliampmeter in series with the patient electrodes and positioning the meter on the face of the instrument.

5. A timer which is used to automatically cut off power to the electrodes after therapy has been applied for a preset time period. The timer is generally mechanically or electrically activated and provides capability for the operator to select periods of therapy from a few minutes to an hour.

6. Female electrode jacks, into which the insulated male electrode conductors are plugged. The jacks are marked as to polarity (+ and −) and may also be color coded, positive being *red*, negative being *black*.

7. A frequency control knob, which in most instances is

actually the shaft of a variable resistance or, in some cases, a multiple position switch connected to a series of capacitors. The resistance or capacitance changes result in changes in the pulse generator frequency.

8. An intensity control for varying the current intensity being applied to the patient. This component is generally a wire-wound variable resistance acting as a rheostat, increasing the resistance in series with the patient leads and thereby decreasing the circuit current.

9. A switch which, when activated, can reverse the polarity of the electrode jacks.

Every muscle stimulating device may not incorporate all of the above design features, but most will be found in the better, well-designed commercial instruments.

A Closer Look at an Actual Instrument

Figure 8-37 shows a block diagram of a commercial muscle stimulating device, the Burdick MS/600 (The Burdick Corporation, Milton, Wisconsin). The device is capable of delivering faradic (AC) current in either continuous, interrupted, surging, or pulsed form, as well as various levels and polarities of galvanic (DC) currents. The essential circuits are shown in the block diagram and are analyzed below. Figure 8-38 is the schematic diagram.

Figure 8-37. Burdick MS/600 muscle stimulator (faradic current). From information supplied by The Burdick Corporation, Milton, Wisconsin.

Power Supply

The power supply is a conventional, solid-state, full wave rectifier (CR1 and CR2) with RC filtering (C7, R18, C8), delivering two output voltages: 400 VDC for the output amplifier and 250 VDC for the pulse generator and surge blocking oscillator. The power supply also generates the galvanic current voltages.

Pulse Generator

The pulse generator (V1) is essentially a plate-coupled, free-running multivibrator. The pulse rate control (R20) is a variable resistance which controls the bias to one side of the multivibrator, and this, in conjunction with the time constant of the multivibrator coupling circuits, controls the pulse frequency.

Surge Blocking Oscillator

The blocking oscillator (V3) surge rate is controlled by way of a single fixed capacitance (C5) and a series of timing resistances connected by way of the surge rate switch. The discharge of the

Figure 8-38. Burdick MS/600 schematic. Courtesy of The Burdick Corporation, Milton, Wisconsin.

capacitor can be rapid (low resistances switched in), yielding eighty-five pulses per second, or it can be slow (high resistance switched in), yielding one pulse per second. In the nonsurge mode, the function switch removes power from the blocking oscillator.

Cathode Follower—Modulator

The cathode follower (V2-A) circuit is used to impedance match the pulse generator and blocking oscillator circuits to the output amplifier (V2-B). In the nonsurge mode, the pulse generator signal is simply fed through the cathode follower by way of C4 and R8 to the output amplifier. In the surge mode, the blocking oscillator's surge signal modulates the pulse generator output at the grid of the cathode follower by providing a varying bias.

Output Amplifier

The high voltage output amplifier (V2-B) couples the faradic output signal at its plate circuit through a pulse transformer (T2) across the secondary of which a variable resistance (R9A) is hooked. This is the faradic output level control. The signal is then fed to the output jacks by way of the function selector switch (S3).

Galvanic Circuitry

In the galvanic mode, the 250 VDC output of the power supply is fed through a variable resistance (R31), which functions as the galvanic (fine) output control, then on the high-low function switch, through the output current meter and out the electrode jacks. In the (+) galvanic mode, the red jack is internally grounded. In the (−) galvanic mode, the black jack is grounded. In either case, the electrodes must be connected to a load (the patient or a load resistance) before the meter will indicate, since the patient, electrodes, and meter constitute a series circuit. Figure 8-39 shows a simplified diagram of the galvanic circuitry.

Figure 8-39. Block diagram of the Burdick MS/600 galvanic circuit. From information supplied by The Burdick Corporation, Milton, Wisconsin.

Transducers—Electrodes

When energy is transmitted from an instrument system into a biological system or vice versa, some form of transducer (a device that changes energy from one form to another) is generally required. For example, body temperature is transduced into an electrical signal by way of a thermistor in an electronic thermometer; electrical energy is transduced into sound waves by a piezoelectric crystal in ultrasound therapy. In electrotherpy, the transducer provides electrochemical contact between the patient and the instrument system, and since the energy on both sides of the interface is electrical, the transducer is termed an *electrode*.

Electrodes constitute the interconnecting element between the therapeutic device and the patient. The form or shape of the electrode is dictated by its use or application. Since it must transfer the current or voltage across the instrument-patient interface, its characteristics must provide optimal conditions for that transmission. Whether they are used to detect signals and transmit them to an instrument or, as in the case of therapeutic applications, transmit current into the patient, all contain one common denominator: they are biphasic electrochemical elements consisting of a metal-electrolyte system. In the case of electrodes used in physical therapy, the electrolyte can be as simple as a normal saline solution or special electrode paste formulations. The actual charge transfer across the instrument-patient interface involves complex electrochemical gradients and physiochemical processes. Although these processes are of primary importance in "sensing" and recording bioelectric potentials, the single most important factor in therapeutic electrode application is the concept of "current density." If one remembers that current measurement is based on the number of charges that pass a given point in a circuit (remembering that the point has some cross-sectional area) in a given amount of time, the current density will vary as the cross-sectional area of that point changes. Hence, if the current flow passing a point having a 1 mm area is 15 milliamps, cutting the area in half will result in a current of 30 milliamps; the current density has increased. It is this principle which is *one* of the governing factors in the use of the so-called dispersive electrode in therapeutic applications. By use of a large area electrode placed distal from the application point of the active electrode, the current is dispersed throughout a large tissue volume and the exit current density is also lowered. Accidental conditions in which the dispersive electrode is making contact at a few points of small cross-sectional area, or if the patient is touching a grounded metallic object (a metal bed or table), can cause severe necrotizing burns due to excessively high current density.

The electrodes used in electrotherapy run the gamut from bare metallic sheets to specially designed metal-impregnated rubber or plastic. The active electrode is of smaller area than the dispersing electrode and usually is mounted on the end of a handle into which a switch has been incorporated to allow the therapist to interrupt the current. An absorbent material such as felt, gauze, or cotton, soaked with the appropriate solution, provides the electrolyte phase.

The Burdick Corporation of Milton, Wisconsin, has developed molded, metal-impregnated electrodes called Conductrodes™ which have no sharp edges or exposed metal. A well-moistened gauze pad provides the electrolyte phase between the patient and the Conductrode surface. These electrodes have the advantage of being noncorrosive and easily cleanable as well as being flexible. They can easily be cleaned with alcohol or even autoclaved. They are available in 5", 3", and 1" diameter sizes.

SHORT WAVE DIATHERMY GENERATORS
Introduction

As noted in the previous section, the use of heat as a therapeutic agent is as old as man himself. However, it was not until the late nineteenth century that high frequency radiation was discovered to cause heating of the tissues through which it was passed.

Although both ultraviolet and infrared heating involve the absorption of electromagnetic radiation to produce heating, their effects are characteristically different from diathermy in that diathermy produces a dispersive deep tissue heating while the former two are restricted to superficial tissue effects.

The total energy of any system is the sum of its potential energy plus kinetic energy. In turn, the amount of kinetic energy within a system is indicated by its temperature (in short, the amount of heat in the system). From this, one can conclude that any alteration of the kinetic energy of the system will result in a heating or cooling effect. Energy absorbed by a molecular system must be utilized in one of a number of ways: (1) by chemical reaction, (2) by reemitting the energy (fluorescence, phosphorescence), (3) by transfer due to molecular collision, or (4) by conversion to vibrational, rotational, or translational kinetic energy. This latter method is the basis for deep tissue heating via diathermy.

Types of Diathermy

Historically, the two early forms of diathermy were "long wave" and "short wave" diathermy, designations based on the relative wavelength of the radiation employed. Long wave diathermy utilized a wavelength of approximately 300 meters (1 megahertz) and short wave diathermy from 3 to 30 meters (10 to 100 megahertz). Today, the predominant form of diathermy is microwave diathermy (a form of therapeutic radar). However, short wave diathermy is still in use. Short wave diathermy has operating frequencies between 10 and 100 MHz, while microwave diathermy has an operating frequency in the 2,000 megahertz region and wavelengths of approximately 12 cm.

It was noted in a previous section that the higher the frequency of radiation, the greater its penetrating capability. Hence, the ability to provide deep tissue heating and the resulting efficiency is directly proportional to the frequency of the radiation employed. The major practical difference between short wave and microwave diathermy is in the transmission of the energy to the patient. Short wave transmission requires the patient to become an integral part of the output circuit, even though he is not *directly* in a conduction path. In contrast, microwaves, due to their higher energy and shorter wavelength, assume qualities resembling visible light and as such can be projected, reflected, and focused. Hence, in applying this mode of therapy to a patient, direct contact is *not* required between patient and instrument.

A Simplified Short Wave Diathermy Unit

A simplified block diagram of a short wave diathermy unit is shown in Figure 8-40. The unit has essentially four subcircuits.

Figure 8-40. Block diagram of a simple short wave diathermy unit.

1. A *Radio Frequency Oscillator* provides stable, drift-free oscillations at the required frequency. Since oscillators are prone to drift as load conditions upon it change, it must be isolated from the patient circuit. Isolation is provided by way of the following circuit.

2. The *Output Power Amplifier* serves not only as a buffer between the oscillator and the patient circuit but also as an amplifier capable of generating the power required to drive the electrodes.

3. The *Output Resonant Tank* circuit is an LC circuit made up of the *secondary* winding of the output transformer (the primary serves as the load for the output power amplifier), in parallel with a tuning capacitor, both of which are in parallel with the patient. With the patient between the electrodes, the output tuning capacitor is adjusted until the circuit is at resonance, at which time maximum power can be transferred to the patient.

4. The *Power Supply* provides the voltages required to drive the RF oscillator and power amplifier. In addition, a timer is incorporated which must be activated to turn on the unit. After the prescribed treatment time has elapsed, the timer automatically removes AC power.

Patient cables and electrodes used with short wave diathermy must be of the shielded cable type. This ensures maximum energy transfer to the applicator electrode with minimal loss of energy.

The controls and indicators found on the type of device listed above would be as follows:

1. A main *Power Switch* for applying AC line power to the unit.

2. A *Timer* for controlling the duration of the therapeutic dose. Most timers are designed so that the timer shuts off power when the time runs out.

3. An *Output Intensity* control allowing variation of the power applied to the patient.

4. A *Tuning Control* which tunes the output circuit, including the patient (the load), for maximum energy transfer from RF oscillator circuit to the output.

5. An *Output Power Meter* enabling the operator to monitor the relative energy being applied to the patient.

It should be noted that in this type of instrument, the output meter monitors only the current drawn by the output amplifier and *not* the output power in the patient circuit; hence, it is only an *indirect* measurement of energy reaching the patient and not a true measurement.

Figure 8-41A. Block diagram of the Burdick MF/490 short wave diathermy unit—27.12 MHz. From information supplied by The Burdick Corporation, Milton, Wisconsin.

Some Actual Instruments

Two commercially available short wave diathermy units that are basically the same as the simplified instrument outlined above are the Burdick Model MF/490 and the Birtcher Model 800 Crystal Bandmaster. These devices, although they operate at different frequencies, are sufficiently alike from a general viewpoint to warrant that a comparative analysis be undertaken. Each of the circuits outlined in the simplified discussion above will be discussed in more detail for each unit (Figs. 8-41 and 8-42).

Power Supplies

BURDICK MF/490. The power supply consists of a power transformer (T_1) which is energized only when a timer, an overload circuit breaker, a cabinet door interlock, and a power on switch are all activated. All these interlocks are on the primary side of the transformer. The high voltage secondary windings of the transformer supply high AC voltage to the RF oscillator (812A) and the power amplifier (810). The 10 and 6.3 low voltage secondaries supply filament voltage to the same two tubes. AC voltage is used as plate supply to these tubes, since no modulation is required and therefore DC is unnecessary.

BIRTCHER 800. The Birtcher power supply contains (1) a function switch (Sw2), (2) a filament transformer (TR1), (3) a power transformer (TR2), and (4) rectifier tubes (T1 and T2). The function switch serves to provide either diathermy or surgical

BURDICK MODEL MF-490
27,120 MC DIATHERMY
SER #8001—

Figure 8-41B. Burdick Model MF/490 diathermy schematic diagram. Courtesy of The Burdick Corporation, Milton, Wisconsin.

Figure 8-42. Birtcher 800 Crystal Bandmaster short wave diathermy schematic. Courtesy of The Birtcher Corporation, Los Angeles, California.

modes of operation by energizing either both TR1 and TR2 or TR1 alone. The filament transformer provides outputs of 5 volts, 6.3 volts, and 10 volts for rectifier filaments, oscillator filaments, and amplifier filaments, respectively. The power transformer yields a 600 volt output for a full wave rectifier (T1-T2) and a 1500 volt output for a half wave rectifier (T3). The full wave rectifier DC output supplies the operating voltages for the RF oscillator (T4), while the half wave rectifier serves the output amplifier (T5) through an RF choke (RFC3).

Oscillator Circuits

BURDICK. The tuned, plate-tuned grid RF oscillator (812A) is a conventional RF oscillator utilizing interelectrode capacitance between plate and grid to provide regenerative feedback. The oscillating frequency is 27.120 MHz $\pm$ 21.5 KHz and is factory set by adjusting C13.

BIRTCHER. A crystal-controlled, tuned, plate-tuned grid tetrode oscillator (T4) provides the RF energy with feedback from the plate tank circuit (C7-L1) by way of interelectrode capacitance. The crystal (Y-1) provides stable oscillations at 6.78 MHz, and the oscillator output is tuned to 13.56 MHz (1st even harmonic).

Amplifier Circuits

BURDICK. The oscillator signal is loop coupled from the oscillator output tank circuit (C12-L2) to the RF amplifier grid tank circuit (L3-C14). The signal is amplified and fed by way of the plate tank circuit (C15-L4) and coupling loop to the resonant output circuit. A neutralizing capacitor is factory tuned to prevent plate-to-grid feedback from producing self-oscillation of the amplifier. The output meter monitors the grid current in the amplifier which is maximum at resonance.

BIRTCHER. The oscillator signal is capacitive coupled by way of C-3 to the grid of the amplifier tube (T5), where it is amplified and passed through the output resonant tank circuit (L2-C8) to the secondary coil (L3). C-12 is a neutralizing capacity to prevent self-oscillation of the amplifier.

Output Circuits

BURDICK. A parallel tuned circuit (C16-L5), two series inductors (L6-L7), and the applicator electrodes constitute the resonant output circuit. C16 is the tuning element, which is adjusted to peak the plate current at reasonance. L5 is then adjusted to select the appropriate output power by varying the coupling ability of the tank.

BIRTCHER. The output circuit is a series resonant circuit consisting of inductor L3, capacitors C9 and C10, and the applicators.

Adjusting C10 resonates the patient circuit with the amplifier tank circuit. Output energy is adjusted by altering the coupling ability of output coil L3. It should be noted that both output circuits are tuned by matching the output circuit impedance to the amplifier tank circuit impedance with tuning controls, i.e. peaking the output meter to maximum. At that time, maximum energy is transferred from amplifier to output. This adjustment must therefore be made with the output control at a minimal or low *after* the output circuit is tuned to resonance. The amount of energy coupled to the output circuit is varied by the output control.

Another Birtcher short-wave diathermy unit is the Birtcher Model 860 Crusade II, having an output frequency of 27.120 MHz. Figure 8-43 shows a block diagram of this instrument. The power supply contains essentially a fuse, a combined timer/on-off switch, and a transformer. The transformer supplies AC filament and plate voltage to the oscillator stage. The oscillator is a tuned plate, push-pull RF generator utilizing interelectrode capacitance regenerative feedback to sustain oscillations. The grid current drawn by the oscillator tubes is used as an indicator of output power by the output meter. The *oscillator* plate circuit resonant tank couples energy to the output circuit parallel tunable tank, which controls the power applied to the applicators. A single control (output) is used to provide both tuning of the tank and output energy intensity. This is accomplished by tuning the circuit for increased output and *detuning* for less output.

Figure 8-43. Block diagram of the Birtcher 860 diathermy unit. From information supplied by The Birtcher Corporation, Los Angeles, California.

Many new commercial diathermy units are now providing the capability of automatic or self-tuning. This is advantageous in instances where patient movement causes the output circuit to go out of resonance. In such instances, some units employ a type of feedback control system (servomechanism) to retune the output. The unit shown below constantly monitors the output, which contains not just the 27.120 MHz primary frequency but two side band frequencies, an upper 27.22 MHz and a lower 27.02 MHz. When the output is tuned, the side band frequencies are equal in magnitude, causing no response in the servodetector (a form of differential detector). Should the system *not* be in resonance, the difference between the side band signals activates a servomotor, which returns the circuit until the side band signals are again equal and the output is once again resonance.

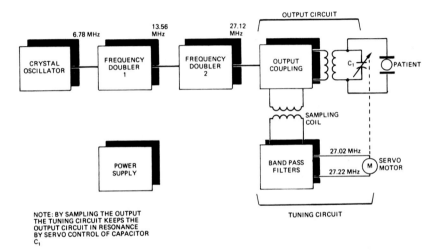

Figure 8-44. Block diagram of a short wave diathermy unit with automatic tuning. From Terence Karselis, *Descriptive Medical Electronics and Instrumentation,* 1973. Courtesy of Charles B. Slack, Inc., Thorofare, New Jersey.

A Unique New Device

Figure 8-45 shows a photograph of a relatively new commercial short wave diathermy unit, the Mettler Electronics "Auto-Therm." Some of the more unique features of this device are (1) it is self tuning, (2) the output meter indicates the relative energy dose absorbed by the patient, and (3) it is compact and light in weight.

Figure 8-46 shows a block diagram of the functional circuits of this device. As shown in Figure 8-45, the unit consists essentially

Figure 8-45. Mettler Autotherm™short wave diathermy unit. Courtesy of Mettler Electronics Corporation, Anaheim, California.

Figure 8-46. Block diagram of the Mettler Autotherm™ short wave diathermy unit. From information supplied by Mettler Electronics Corporation, Anaheim, California.

of two parts: a mobile stand with controls and meter plus a RF unit/applicator drum head. A solid-state high voltage power supply plus a unique absorbed dose meter circuit constitute the major portion of the circuitry contained in the stand, along with a filament transformer for the RF oscillator and a timer. In the power supply, AC line voltage is rectified into 600 volts DC by way of a *full wave quadrupler.* This voltage is fed through the meter circuit to the *RF oscillator* in the drum head enclosure. The *meter circuit* monitors the voltage at the RF oscillator plate and screen grid circuits and by computing the difference indicates the true relative power absorbed by the patient. With no patient in the ouptut circuit field, the meter will indicate zero, regardless of the intensity control setting.

The drum head enclosure houses the RF oscillator, which is a dual pentode class C tuned plate-tuned grid, push-pull oscillator circuit. Oscillations are sustained by interelectrode capacitance feedback. Adjustment of the output intensity is controlled by varying the screen grid voltages. The circuit's design is such that it creates little RF interference noise and consequently requires minimal shielding. This permits its use directly on the patient, whereas in *all other short wave diathermy units, the primary generator is enclosed in a strongly shielded cabinet* and is coupled to a secondary patient circuit. In addition, the patient circuit is a self-tuning multiple capacitor tank and is always in resonance with itself.

Transducers—Applicators

The interfacing element between an instrument system and a human system is the transducer. However, in therapeutic applications involving the application of energy, they are more generally termed *applicators.* Short wave diathermy applicators are either of the capacitive or inductive type, based on the type of energy used to apply the therapy. When an *electrostatic* field is used, the patient becomes an integral part of the output circuit. He is placed between two applicator surfaces and consequently becomes the dielectric material between the plates of a capacitor. Therapeutic energy then passes from plate to plate via the patient.

When the transmitted energy is electromagnetic in nature, the patient is positioned within the RF magnetic field generated around copper-braided insulated wires. These wires may be coiled around a limb or "pancaked" onto the body surface. Figure 8-47 shows three types of short wave diathermy applicators.

Figure 8-47. Short wave diathermy applicators. From Terence Karselis, *Descriptive Medical Electronics and Instrumentation,* 1973. Courtesy of Charles B. Slack, Inc., Thorofare, New Jersey.

MICROWAVE DIATHERMY GENERATORS

Introduction

One of the most important inventions to emerge during the World War II era was radar. Initially, it was developed and used as a ground-based defense system to detect enemy aircraft; later, it was further sophisticated and placed in aircraft. The requirements for airborne radar necessitated smaller systems and higher frequencies; this in turn led to the final development of *microwave* radar. From this military development came the therapeutic agent *microwave diathermy*. The single most important advantage of microwave diathermy is its capability to produce rapid, localized deep heating. This is in contrast to the somewhat dispersive type of heating produced by short wave diathermy.

The ability to generate microwave frequencies necessary in airborne radar systems originated with the development of the multicavity magnatron, a complete RF oscillator-amplifier in one package.

The Multicavity Magnatron

The higher the frequency an oscillator is required to generate, the greater the associated circuit effects of interelectrode capacitance and inductance. Consequently, conventional tubes are incapable of efficient operation above 20 MHz. The search for high frequency power circuits led to the development of special devices called cavity resonators. Two of these are the *reflex-klystron* and the *magnatron*. The latter is the heart of all microwave diathermy units.

A magnatron is essentially a diode tube with a cylindrical hollow block acting as the anode around a centrally located cathode. Circular cavities (hence the name cavity resonator) are cut out of the anode, resulting in multiple anode segments separated by cavities. Each cavity functions electronically as an individual resonant circuit of a single inductor coil segment (the diameter) and a single capacitor (the top and bottom walls). In a conventional tube, an applied electric field existing between cathode and anode causes electrons to flow in a straight path from cathode to anode. In a magnatron, an electric field is present, but in addition, a magnetic field is also applied. The electric field is produced by keeping the anode at zero potential and the cathode at a high negative. The magnetic field is applied perpendicular to the electric field by way of heavy alnico magnets. Electrons flowing from cathode to anode therefore follow a helical spirallike path due to the combined effects of the two fields. As they pass the cavity slots, energy is transferred to the energy field of the cavity, causing the cavity to oscillate. Figure 8-48 shows a cavity magnatron and the path of an electron. The resonant oscillations occur-

Figure 8-48. (A) shows a simplified drawing of a magnatron. (B) is a cutaway top view of the cavity assembly with spirallike electron paths. From Terence Karselis, *Descriptive Medical Electronics and Instrumentation,* 1973. Courtesy of Charles B. Slack, Inc., Thorofare, New Jersey.

ring within the cavity result in magnetic variations which are picked up by an inductive probe and coupled by way of a coaxial cable to the transmitting antenna and reflector. The magnatron provides high frequency oscillations with high output power; it is analogous to a combination oscillator-amplifier system. Magnatrons used in radar systems are capable of generating RF energy in megawatt amounts; however, the maximum output of any medical microwave magnatron is limited to approximately 150 watts.

A Simplified Microwave Generator

Figure 8-49 shows the block diagram of a typical microwave diathermy unit.

The *power supply* furnishes power for energizing the magnatron oscillator and the timing circuitry. Since the cathode voltage of a magnatron is a large negative potential (3000V), some form of rectification is necessary.

The *magnatron control circuit* controls the output power of the system by way of varying the magnatron operating voltage.

Figure 8-49. Simplified block diagram of a microwave diathermy unit. From Terence Karselis, *Descriptive Medical Electronics and Instrumentation,* 1973. Courtesy of Charles B. Slack, Inc., Thorofare, New Jersey.

Safety circuitry is necessary to prevent excessive output. This can be accomplished by an overload circuit monitoring the magnatron current.

The *magnatron oscillator* provides high power RF energy which must be coaxially coupled to the applicator head. The current drawn by the magnatron when monitored by an output meter is a direct measure of the energy *transmitted* to the patient. This is not, however, a measure of *absorbed* energy.

An Actual Instrument

An example of a typical commercial microwave diathermy unit is the Burdick Model MW/225 (Fig. 8-50). This device has essentially the same substages as the previous simplified instrument, with various additions.

The front panel controls and indicators are as follows:

1. An on-off power switch controlling AC line power to the instrument.
2. A timing control allowing the operator to adjust the time of applied therapy. This timer automatically cuts power to the unit after the preselected time has elapsed.
3. An *output* level control which controls the amount of energy being transmitted to the patient. This control is not calibrated since the output is monitored by the operator using the output meter.
4. An *output* meter which indicates the relative output energy in watts. As noted previously, this is the transmitted energy, *not* the absorbed energy.
5. Two colored indicator lamps: an *amber* "standby" in-

Figure 8-50. Burdick Model MW/225 microwave diathermy unit. Courtesy of The Burdick Corporation, Milton, Wisconsin.

dicator, showing that power is applied to the unit, and a *red* "output" lamp, showing that microwave output is available.

In addition to the obvious visible controls, a built-in safety feature is the reset function of the *output* level control. After therapy has been applied for a given amount of time and the timer has cut power, in order to reactivate the system, the output control must be turned back to zero in order to reset the safety lock-out relay. It can then be adjusted to give an output. The same reactivation procedure must also be followed to restore power if the overload relay has deenergized the system.

A closer look at the instrument can be obtained by looking at the block diagram in Figure 8-51.

The input *power control circuit* contains the timer, power

Figure 8-51. Block diagram of the Burdick MW/225 microwave diathermy unit. From information supplied by The Burdick Corporation, Milton, Wisconsin.

switch, and output control, along with a cooling fan. The output control is a variac located in the power supply which permits adjustment of the voltage fed to the magnatron cathode high voltage transformer primary. Adjusting this control effectively changes the voltage at the magnatron cathode. The timer, overload relay, and power switch interrupt voltage applied to the variac and hence to the high voltage transformer.

The magnatron filament transformer is energized at all times after the power-on switch is closed, thereby maintaining the magnatron in a standby condition.

The solid-state half wave rectifier provides a negative DC voltage to the magnatron cathode of approximately 3500 volts. This is sufficient to cause oscillations. An output current limiting (overload) relay senses the magnatron cathode current and shuts off power if it exceeds 74 mA (equivalent to 130 watts output). The output energy is inductively coupled from the magnatron to the reflector head by way of coaxial tubing.

Transducers—Antennas/Reflectors

The application of microwave energy requires specialized devices known generally as reflectors. These elements are in reality directional antennas since microwave energy, as noted previously, due to its short wavelength has optical properties in that it can be reflected, refracted, and focused. Put simply, microwaves follow a line-of-sight propagation path, while short wave RF energy is omnidirectional in nature.

The energy fed into a microwave applicator is first coaxially coupled to a radiating element and then focused and directed by a reflecting element. The electrical energy transmitted along the coaxial cable terminates at the radiating device, where it is transformed into electromagnetic waves. The radiating device is actually a small antenna, which, when matched by correct manufacture to the wavelength of the energy to be propagated, acts like a resonant circuit, exhibiting no reactance, just pure resistance. The radiated energy emitted from the antenna propagates according to a definite pattern; therefore, a reflecting element is used to focus the energy in the desired direction. The reflectors used in microwave diathermy may be parabolic hemispheres or rectangular "corner" types, as shown in Figure 8-52. Dose information and spacing data is generally printed on the outside of the reflectors.

Figure 8-52. Microwave diathermy applicators. From Terence Karselis, *Descriptive Medical Electronics and Instrumentation,* 1973. Courtesy of Charles B. Slack, Inc., Thorofare, New Jersey.

In comparing the instrument systems used for applying short wave and microwave diathermy, a major advantage that the latter system appears to have is its simplicity of application and control. Since the factors influencing the energy dosage received by the patient are output power, time of application, and distance between applicator and patient, once the reflector is aligned and set, application requires little more than adjusting the output power (generally calibrated in percentages of maximum output) and setting the timer (between 20 and 30 minutes). No output circuit tuning is required, and the need for continual monitoring to determine if the output circuit remains tuned (or, alternatively, automatic tuning circuitry) is removed. A second advantage is patient comfort and ease. With microwave therapy, no component of the instrument system touches the patient. This small fact is in itself greatly comforting to patients who tend to be nervous and hypersensitive.

The disadvantages of this type of diathermy are the limited effect of one-sided application of the energy stream, and the skin reflection that occurs due to the optical nature of microwave energy.

ELECTRODIAGNOSTIC DEVICES
Introduction

The now-famous "twitch" of Galvani's frog in the eighteenth century heralded the birth of the field of electrophysiology, one subdivision of which is the modern specialty of electrodiagnosis. Electrodiagnosis can be defined as the diagnosis of disease states associated with the neuromuscular system by (1) studying the mechanical response to externally applied stimulation, termed *myography*, (2) analysis of the electrical signals generated by way of externally applied stimulation or spontaneous activity, termed *electromyography (EMG)*, or (3) studying the speed at which action potentials are passed along a particular segment of the nervous system, termed *conduction velocity analysis*. Under (1) fall the so-called classical techniques of faradic (AC) and galvanic (DC) stimulation to observe the *reaction of degeneration* (RD) of a damaged neuromuscular unit, as well as the more modern techniques of *strength-duration* analysis and chronaximetry. A brief description of the instrumentation used with each of the above modalities will be given in the following section.

Classical Electrodiagnosis Instrumentation

Classical Myography (RD Studies) Devices

As noted above, the primary function of classical faradic/galvanic myography is the determination of *reaction to degeneration*. The instrumentation required for this technique can vary from extremely simple combinations of components to complex pulse generators. Whatever its shape, size, or level of sophistication, the essential requirements for such a device are as follows: (1) the ability to deliver a continuous DC current at variable magnitudes and (2) the ability to supply alternating current pulses of approximately 1 millisecond duration at repetition rates of 50 to 200 per second. These functions can be accomplished by two crude but utterly simple circuits. The variable DC current can be generated by a 45 VDC battery or series of batteries together with a variable resistance. The AC current can be obtained by using a DC voltage source together with a faradic coil. The faradic coil is actually a combination relay/transformer in which the DC, energizing current as it flows in the *primary* winding, activates a set of its own contacts. The relay contacts open, thereby removing power from the primary circuit and causing the coil to deenergize. The constantly energizing-deenergizing sequence induces pulses of energy into the secondary winding, which serves as the output circuit to the patient. Both of these circuits are shown in Figure 8-53. E and E_2 refer to the electrodes. The pulse repetition rate can be adjusted by adjusting the gap of the relay contacts.

Figure 8-53. Galvanic and faradic generators.

The currents generated by the above circuits, or suitable substitutes, can also be obtained from most commercial therapeutic instruments, as well as from some chronaximeters, as will be discussed.

Strength-Duration/Chronaxie Analysis Devices

While classical myography can assess *qualitatively* the response of a neuromuscular unit to stimulation, the two factors of importance in attempting to assess such response *quantitatively* are the *strength* of the stimulating current and the *duration* of its application. These two factors are of primary importance due to the fact that effective stimulation of a biological cell requires that a specified *charge mass* cross its membrane in order to generate an action potential. The practical consequence of this fact is that a short duration pulse of high current intensity can produce the same result as a lower intensity pulse of longer duration. A lower limit of intensity, however, is produced by charge diffusion across the cell membrane which opposes the low level stimulating current. The minimal stimulus intensity below which no response is produced in neuromuscular tissue, even if the stimulus is applied continually, is called the *rheobase*. By applying pulses of varying amplitude and duration, strength-duration curves can be constructed for a particular muscle or nerve, as shown in Figure 8-54. When the amplitude of the rheobase is doubled, the pulse width capable of eliciting the same response as the initial amplitude is termed *chronaxie*. This arbitrary index of excitation is actually the reciprocal of neuromuscular excitability since as the excitability of a nerve or muscle is impaired due to disease or injury, its chronaxie would increase. The two parameters of chronaxie and rheobase are studied collectively, since the former cannot be determined without first measuring rheobase.

Figure 8-54. Strength-duration curves with chronaxie points.

The instrumentation required to perform the above measurements can be specifically designed for such application (for example, the TECA CH3 Chronaxie Meter and Variable Pulse Generator, manufactured by TECA Corp., White Plains, New York), or the same results can be obtained by using any pulse generator or stimulator having the capability of providing precise pulse amplitude, duration, and repetition rate selection. Earlier chronaximetry devices utilized capacitive discharge RC circuits to generate pulses of the required duration. As discussed in an earlier section, the charge-discharge time for a capacitor for a given amount of charge is determined by the size of the capacitor and the resistance through which it must charge or discharge. The period in which 63.2 percent of the applied charge accumulates or is discharged is called the *time constant,* and it can be calculated from the following formula. Since t only represents 63.2% charge or discharge, in calculating pulse duration, 5t should be used.

$$t = RC$$

Where t = time in seconds
       R = resistance in ohms
       C = capacitance in farads

It can be seen that by manipulating either R or C, the rate at which the capacitor charges or discharges can be precisely controlled. In earlier chronaximeters of capacitive discharge design, a series of capacitors of ranging approximately in value from 10 microfarads to 100 picofarads (0.001 MFD) were discharged through a fixed resistance of 10 kilohms (1×10^4 ohms), yielding pulses ranging in duration from 500 milliseconds to 5 microseconds. The *amount* of charge in the capacitors could be accurately regulated, thereby providing capability to determine chronaxie. The technique involved determining the minimum voltage at which excitation occurred using DC (galvanic) current of 500 to 1000 millisecond pulses. This value was then doubled and the capacitors charged. The capacitors were then individually discharged in sequence, smallest to largest, until the same excitation occurred.

Electronic stimulators used for strength/duration analysis and chronaxie determination consist essentially of two major circuits. The first is a pulse generator capable of generating rectangular pulses of selectable amplitude and duration. In most instances, this circuit will be a triggered monostable multivibrator. The second circuit is a pulse repetition rate oscillator, which is used to provide the selection of precise time intervals between the output pulses. In addition to the automatic pulse repetition provided by this circuit, generally a manual trigger is included to allow generation of a single pulse. The pulse repetition rate oscillator can be any type of oscillator generating short duration trigger pulses. One type of circuit used is a free-running multivibrator.

The two circuits work in conjunction as follows: each time the pulse repetition rate oscillator triggers the pulse generator, the monostable circuit goes through one full cycle of operation, generating an output pulse. When its cycle is completed, the circuit remains "off" until the next pulse repetition rate oscillator trigger sends it into operation. A power amplifier may be used as an output circuit, or the signal may be taken directly from the pulse generator. Figure 8-55 shows a block diagram of a typical pulse generator/chronaximeter.

Figure 8-55. Block diagram of a chronaxie pulse generator.

The controls and indicators associated with a typical chronaximeter/pulse generator are as follows:

1. An AC power switch, which furnishes AC power to the instrument.
2. A power-on indicator—a neon bulb indicator most often placed across the input transformer primary winding indicating AC power is available.

3. A function selector switch, allowing the operator to select the appropriate circuitry for DC (galvanic) and/ or rheobase/chronaxie testing. In addition, some devices provide an internal calibration circuit which can be hooked into this switch.

4. A pulse duration selector, allowing the operator to select pulse durations from 0.1 millisecond to 500 milliseconds. Some instruments provide additional adjustments for vernier adjustment between the fixed switch positions.

5. A pulse interval selector, providing variation of the time interval between pulses.

6. An output intensity control for adjusting the output current intensity.

7. An output indicator bulb which is driven by the current flowing to the patient. The indicator will pulse in intensity along with the output pulses.

8. Electrode jacks for attaching the electrode cables to the instrument.

An important difference between pulse generators used in strength-duration/chronaxie testing is the type of output current control a particular device generates. Two types of instruments are in present use, constant voltage/variable current and constant current/variable voltage. With a constant voltage source, the units output impedance should be less than 50 ohms; with a constant current generator, the output impedance should exceed 10 kilohms. It should be noted that use of either type, generally dictated by personal preference of the operator, provides no *accurate* predication or measurement of the charge actually passing through the various areas of treated tissue. This is due primarily to the effects of contact resistance at the electrodes and the electrical characteristics (resistance and capacitance) of the tissue under treatment, which varies with individuals. Arguments for the use of both types of devices are strong, but no definitive evidence proving one better than the other presently exists, and satisfactory data can be obtained from both.

Electromyography Instrumentation

The EMG System

Electromyography is basically a physiological monitoring process in which the muscle potentials of skeletal muscle activity, whether voluntary or by way of external stimulation, are monitored and/or recorded. Although other methods are used, the method predominantly in use today for monitoring EMG signals is by way of oscilloscope tracings. Because of this, the typical EMG instrument is essentially a special-purpose oscilloscope with various attachments dictated by specific application. The design features incorporated into electromyography systems are dictated by the various characteristics of the biopotentials it is required to detect. An understanding of these parameters will facilitate the analysis of the instrument system used to detect them. Voltage, frequency, and signal source impedance are the three most important factors that must be considered in selecting the correct instrument system.

Muscle potentials in electromyography range from 100 microvolts (mv) to approximately 1 millivolt. These potentials are monophasic or biphasic pulses with an approximate frequency range between 15 Hz and 10 KHz. The variability of source impedances found in bioelectric potential recording requires that the input circuitry of the recording or monitoring device be high in order to prevent circuit loading.

An EMG recording system can be produced using individual components such as preamplifiers, amplifiers, recorders, and stimulators, but generally, a combined system functioning within a single cabinet and utilizing interrelated controls exemplifies a typical commercial system.

Figure 8-56 shows a block diagram of a complete EMG system. Each section will be discussed individually.

Figure 8-56. A typical EMG system.

Electrodes

EMG electrodes can be of two basic types, *surface* type or *needle* type. In routine clinical electromyography, the needle electrode is predominant. Needle electrodes can be unipolar and coaxial in construction. Unipolar electrodes are simple, fine needles, insulated except for a small segment at the tip. Coaxial needle electrodes are essentially hypodermic needles through which a single insulated wire, with a bare tip, is passed; in the case of some systems, two wires are used. The needle itself may be one active element of the electrode system, or it may just be the grounded shield as in the case of the two-wire or differential electrode noted above. Surface electrodes are silver or silver chloride discs in specially designed attachment cups or adhesive pads. These electrodes are applied to the skin, over the area of interest, after the skin has been prepared by cleansing and applying electrode paste. Such electrodes are not capable of detecting some of the low amplitude, high frequency signals important in EMG analysis and hence are not used extensively.

Concerning electrode materials, since most metals generate polarization and offset voltages due to metal-electrolyte reactions, chemically non reactive or inert metals such as platinum and silver are used extensively in physiological monitoring techniques. Other factors, such as drift, recovery time, etc., are included in the evaluation and choice of electrodes by researchers and designers. A detailed analysis of such factors is beyond the scope of this section; however, one should be aware that the use of the wrong type of electrode generates problems and signal distortion that even the most sophisticated amplifier system cannot rectify.

Signal Amplifiers

The type of amplifier necessary in monitoring biopotentials must have the following characteristics: (1) an overall gain of approximately 100,000, (2) a frequency response of DC to 10 KHz, (3) an input impedance of at least 1 megohm and, preferably, greater than 100 megohms, and (4) a differential input with a high (250,000) common mode rejection ratio (CMRR). Items (3) and (4) are obtained by use of a *differential amplifier*. Such an amplifier has three input leads, two signal leads, and a ground lead. Electrical noise or interference will appear in equal magnitude and phase on both signal leads; hence, it is "common" to both inputs. The amplifier is constructed to cancel common signals; therefore, the noise will not appear at its output. A biopotential will appear at the two signal leads, but it will be *out of phase,* due to the fact that the ground electrode is located between the two signal electrodes on the patient; consequently, it *will* be amplified. Figure 8-57 shows this principle diagramatically. The high gain of the amplifier is obtained by the use of multiple stages of amplification.

Figure 8-57. An example of common mode rejection.

Preamplifiers are designed as high sensitivity, high gain devices used to couple electrode systems to instrument systems providing gain and impedance matching. In EMG systems, the preamplifiers are generally located close to the electrodes in chielded containers. The signal is then coupled via coaxial cable to the main EMG cabinet. Remote preamplifiers are also of the differential type.

Cathode Ray Tube Display

The EMG signal, once amplified, is fed into the display system, terminating at the cathode ray tube deflection plates. The cathode ray tube consists of an electron gun which projects a beam of high velocity electrons at the phosphor-coated inner face of the tube. To reach the screen, the beam passes between two sets of deflection plates (horizontal plates causing horizontal deflection, etc.). Horizontal deflection is time calibrated, and the vertical deflection system is voltage calibrated; hence, the result is a time/amplitude graph of the vertical input signal (Fig. 8-58). The horizontal amplifier of the cathode ray tube system is calibrated in sweep times to allow precise measurement of the input pulse durations. A typical unit may have selectable sweep times from 1 millisecond to 200 milliseconds. The horizontal sweep signals are generated by varying the frequency of a ramp function generator. To provide the sweep at just the right time to monitor an action potential, the sweep is triggered at the same time and by the same stimulating signal that causes the action potential.

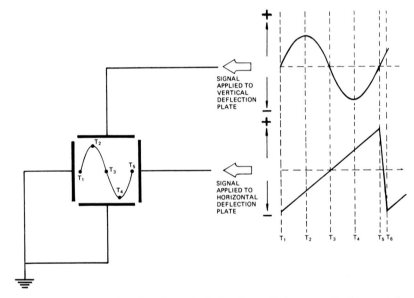

Figure 8-58. Sweep signal and vertical signal applied to a cathode ray tube. From Terence Karselis, *Descriptive Medical Electronics and Instrumentation*, 1973. Courtesy of Charles B. Slack, Inc., Thorofare, New Jersey.

Special cathode ray tubes are now available that allow an image to be maintained on the face of the scope. Such devices are called "storage scopes," and they allow the operator to hold a particular action potential for prolonged study or photography. The image can be removed by the operator simply by depressing an "erase" button.

Stimulator

The stimulator section found in a typical EMG system is generally physically incorporated into the horizontal amplifier section of the oscilloscope. In this way, the horizontal trace is triggered just prior to the muscle being stimulated. This ensures that the evoked response will appear during the trace and not prior to it. The stimulator should have the capability of supplying repetitive or single pulses of variable magnitude, time, and repetition frequency. Pulse duration should be variable from 50 microseconds to 2 or 3 milliseconds, with pulse repetition rates between 0.5 and 50 per second. Some systems incorporate integral timing markers into the trace and elapsed time indicators to provide nerve conduction velocity testing capability.

The above requirements constitute the basic items necessary for a physiological stimulator. Additional modifications may include a stimulus isolation unit and the capability to generate double, triple, and biphasic pulses. *Stimulus isolation* is generally used to eliminate differential (noise currents, due to the stimulating signal, occurring in the tissues around sensing electrodes as a result of tissue impedance). This can be accomplished by isolating the stimulator from ground and providing a high input impedance into the amplifier. The ideal system provides both of these. *Biphasic stimulation* is necessary when rapid cell recovery is required. When a cell is stimulated by a short duration, high energy pulse, a following pulse of long duration, low intensity, *and* opposite polarity will make the next charge through the cell zero. This form of stimulation also tends to eliminate electrode polarization.

Nerve Conduction Velocities

The velocity at which a nerve can propagate an impulse can be indicative of the physical condition of the nerve, and any complete electrodiagnostic procedure should include some motor and sensory nerve conduction velocity studies. In general, healthy nerves exhibit conduction velocities in the range of 40 to 60 meters per second, while abnormal values below that indicate injury or disease. Specific values are determined by the particular nerve under consideration.

The instrumentation required for conduction velocity studies is the basic EMG system, with the added requirement of a stimulus isolation unit. This unit is necessary because of the relatively high stimulating voltages (50 to 150 volts) employed close to the sensing electrodes which are measuring millivolts. An elapsed time indicator (as noted in the previous section) and/or visible timing markers on the trace are also required. Some systems provide two or four sweep capability (called a step-sweep), allowing the operator to observe four times the usual amount of information. For instance, a single stimulus at the little finger can be observed at four points along the ulnar nerve and all the potentials observed on the screen at once.

ULTRASONIC INSTRUMENTATION

Introduction

Just as the origin of microwave diathermy can be traced to the development of military airborne radar during World War II, therapeutic ultrasound shares a similar mode of origin. Sonar (*sound navigation and ranging*) was developed during the same time period as radar, and during the postwar years the field of medical ultrasonics was born. Whereas microwave finds application primarily as a therapeutic agent, ultrasound is finding wide application in the area of diagnosis as well as therapy, principally because of its relatively safe noninvasive nature. Whatever its application, diagnostic or therapeutic, ultrasonic energy and the instrumentation required for its generation requires the following basic elements.

Basic Concepts and Instrumentation

Sound energy, whether audible or ultrasonic, is essentially nothing more than mechanical vibration of a physical body within some type of continuous system or phase. A drum head vibrates, causing mechanical vibration of the air in contact with it, and the vibrations are passed through the air as waves—sound. A ship's sonar transducer vibrates, producing sound waves in the sea water surrounding it. From these examples, two requirements for the transmission of sound become obvious: a *source* or *transmitting* element and a *medium* through which the sound travels. Sound is divided into subgroups based on its frequency. Subsonic sounds are those frequencies below approximately 15 Hz. *Audio* sound frequencies range from 15 Hz to 20 KHz. Frequencies above 20 KHz are classed as *utrasonic*. The two characteristics of ultrasound that make it a useful medical tool are (1) its ability to penetrate tissue without producing injury and (2) its ability to reflect "echoes" when passing between mediums having different densities. The former characteristic is employed in therapeutic ultrasound, the latter in diagnostic ultrasound. Frequencies in the range of 0.8 MHz to 1 MHz have proven experimentally to be preferable for therapeutic use, with effective energy outputs in the range of 0.5 to 3 watts per square centimeter. The effective energy output is determined by dividing the total instrument output power by the area of the transducer in contact with the patient. For example, an instrument with a 10 cm^2 transducer head generating 6 watts of output power has an effective output of 0.6 watts per cm.^{2}

Figure 8-59. Block diagram of a simple ultrasonic generator. From Terence Karselis, *Descriptive Medical Electronics and Instrumentation,* 1973. Courtesy of Charles B. Slack, Inc., Thorofare, New Jersey.

The basic instrumentation required to provide therapeutic ultrasound is shown in Figure 8-59. Ultrasound is basically RF electrical energy converted to mechanical vibrations. The key element in the instrument system generating ultrasound is the transducer, an electromechanical converter. The element at the heart of an ultrasonic transducer is a *piezoelectric crystal.* Certain natural and man-made crystals when placed in an electrical field will be mechanically distorted. By applying an alternating electrical field at the resonant frequency of the crystal, it can be made to vibrate, thereby generating alternate compression and refraction of the medium around it. The phenomenon is a reversible one in that if one mechanically distorts such a crystal, a potential will develop across its structure. The former effect of electromechanical conversion is used in therapeutic devices, while both methods of conversion are used in diagnostic transducers.

The type of crystal originally used as piezoelectric devices was natural quartz. However, these crystals have a high inherent impedance and, consequently, require extremely high driving voltages, on the order of 4000 volts at maximum output. Lithium sulfate salt crystals require less driving voltage; however, the materials of choice in present-day transducers are barium titanate ($BaTiO_3$) and lead zirconate titanate (PZT). These man-made polycrystalline ceramic devices have low impedance and, consequently, require lower driving voltages. For example, a PZT crystal requires approximately 30 volts driving energy.

In the transducer head used to apply therapeutic ultrasound, the crystal is cemented into a mounting and driven by RF pulses at its natural resonant frequency and the appropriate amplitude. The face portion of the applicator head and crystal mounting is designed such that it will also resonate at the natural frequency of the crystal.

The therapeutic effects of ultrasound are threefold: (1) thermal effects due to the vibrational energy being converted into heat, (2) mechanical effects within the tissue (termed micromassage), and (3) chemical effects due to changing cell permeability and ionic diffusion. Some tissues tend to absorb increased amounts of ultrasonic energy selectively, such as bone cartilage and tendon. In the case of tendon, the gross effects are an increase in its tensile strength.

A Typical Ultrasonic Generator

The basic elements of an ultrasonic generator were shown in Figure 8-59. In the case of typical therapeutic devices used today, a slightly more complex instrument is required. Its construction should allow selection of pulsed or continuous ultrasound. Such a simplified device is shown in Figure 8-60. In this instrument, a gate circuit has ben added which allows either pulsed or continuous operation of the RF oscillator.

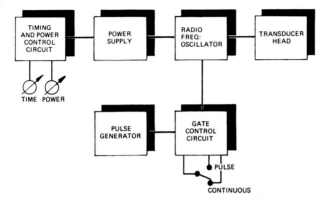

Figure 8-60. Block diagram of an ultrasonic generator with continuous or pulsed operation capability. From Terence Karselis, *Descriptive Medical Electronics and Instrumentation*, 1973. Courtesy of Charles B. Slack, Inc., Thorofare, New Jersey.

The controls and indicators usually found on a typical ultrasonic generator are as follows:

1. A timer, to allow selection and control of the time of therapy. Such devices generally cut off power to the oscillator circuits or interrupt output power when the duration of therapy has elapsed.
2. Output intensity or power control, providing the capability to select zero to maximum power output.
3. Transducer cable jack, to pass energy to the transducer. Some units provide automatic power interruption when the output cable is disconnected.
4. An operation mode selector switch, allowing the operator to select pulsed or continuous operation.
5. An output power indicator, usually a milliampmeter, so the operator can monitor the relative transmitted power.

6. Some form of "power on" indicator, either a neon bulb or LED, to indicate wall power is applied to the device.

Operation of the device would be as follows: When power is applied, the RF oscillator is activated, generating continuous ultrasonic oscillations. This signal is directly coupled to the transducer. The pulse generator, generally having a 60 Hz output frequency, is used to control a gating amplifier, which in turn controls the oscillator. The gating action is such that the oscillator is allowed to generate an output *only* when the gate pulse is present. In the continuous mode, the gating signal is isolated from the oscillator circuit, allowing it to free run. Output power is controlled at the oscillator, and duration of therapy is controlled by a timing unit that shuts off the AC input to the instrument after time has elapsed.

Two Actual Instruments Compared

Two commercial ultrasound therapy units are the Burdick UT/420, operating at 870 KHz, and the Birtcher Megason XV, operating at 1MHz. These two devices are representative of the instruments employed in ultrasound therapy, and the various circuits of each will be discussed in more detail. A block diagram of each unit is shown in Figure 8-61 and schematic diagrams in Figure 8-62.

Power Supplies

Burdick UT/420. AC power is applied to the primary of the transformer (T4) by way of the timer cutout switch (S1), a fuse, and an RF filter. The two high voltage secondary windings provide, by way of half and full wave rectifiers (CR8 through CR17), the various DC bias and plate voltages for the tubes (V5, V8, V9). Filament voltages are supplied by a low voltage secondary. A power indicator lamp (DS1) is in parallel with the transformer primary.

Birtcher Megason XV. The primary circuit of the power supply is virtually the same as in the Burdic device, employing an RF filter, a combined power/timer switch (S1), and a power indicator lamp (DS1). A half wave voltage doubler (CR101 through

Figure 8-61A. Burdick UT/420 ultrasonic unit. From information supplied by The Burdick Corporation, Milton, Wisconsin.

Figure 8-61B. The Birtcher Megason XV ultrasonic unit. From information supplied by The Birtcher Corporation, Los Angeles, California.

CR104) supplies the high voltage for the oscillator tube (V1). A half-wave rectifier (CR105) generates a negative bias voltage for the output control tube (V101).

Oscillator Circuits

BURDICK. The Burdick RF oscillator (V5) is a tuned plate oscillator, feedback being taken from the plate tank circuit (T5 and C16) by way of inductive coupling (T5 pins 6 and 7). The output frequency is adjusted by tuning the coil segment in parallel with C16. V9 is the gate control tube providing current for the oscillator cathode. Its conduction is in turn controlled by the gate amplifier (V8). Output power is varied by adjusting R30 which adjusts the screen grid voltage thereby effectively controlling the oscillator's conduction.

BIRTCHER. An electron coupled oscillator (V1), utilizing screen grid feedback and having good stability, provides the 1 MHz RF oscillations. The grid tank circuit (C7, C8, L2) is temperature compensated and tuned by adjusting L2. Output power

Figure 8-62A. Burdick UT/420 ultrasound unit schematic. Courtesy of The Burdick Corporation, Milton, Wisconsin.

Figure 8-62B. Birtcher Megason XV ultrasound schematic. Courtesy of The Birtcher Corporation, Los Angeles, California.

is controlled indirectly by the tuning control (R2), which effectively controls V1 screen voltage and therefore the oscillator's conduction. The two sections of V101, the power control tube, act as a variable resistor whose conductor is in turn controlled by R2.

Pulse Generator and Gate Circuit

BURDICK. The Burdick gate circuitry is controlled by a 60 Hz pulse generator (V6, V7), which supplies negative going 50 volt pulses of 3.3 millisecond duration to the gate amplifier (V8) grid. The pulses are amplified and inverted, and passed to the gate control tube (V9). When continuous operation is selected by switch S4, the negative bias present at V9 grid is removed and the tube conducts continually, i.e. the gate is "open". In the pulse mode, switch S4 places a negative bias of 50 volts on V9 grid. The positive 3.3 millisecond pulses from the gate amplifier overcome the bias and turn on V9 sixty times per second, which in turn allows the oscillator to fire during that time. The result is a series of RF oscillations of 3.3 milliseconds duration every 16 milliseconds.

BIRTCHER. The Birtcher unit provides only continuous operation; therefore, no pulse generator or gate circuitry are required.

Output/Transducer Circuit

BURDICK. The output of the RF oscillator (V5) is inductively coupled and impedance matched by T5, C14 to the coaxial connector (T4). The energy is then passed via coaxial cable to the applicator head and hence to a ceramic crystal. Output power is monitored by monitoring the current through the gate control tube and RF oscillator. During continuous operation the meter indicates average power; in the pulsed mode, it indicates peak power. R38 provides a dummy load for the oscillator when the applicator is disconnected.

BIRTCHER. An impedance matching network of L1, C5 connects the RF oscillator circuit to the coaxial applicator jack (J1). This is necessary due to the normally high output impedance of the oscillator and the low impedance of the coaxial cable and barium titanate ceramic crystal. The output meter (M1) monitors the plate current of the oscillator.

The applicators employed with the above devices are heavy metal chambers, with the piezoelectric crystal cemented to the resonance-matched applicator face. Two electrodes are cross mounted on the crystal to which the RF signal is applied. An impedance-matched coil may also be included. An energy absorbed baffle plate absorbs stray energy, and the whole assembly is sealed to ensure it is watertight. A coupling medium is necessary to transmit energy to the patient, since the ultrasonic waves will tend to be reflected by air. A typical unit is diagrammed in Figure 8-63.

Figure 8-63. Simplified diagram of an ultrasound therapy applicator. From Terence Karselis, *Descriptive Medical Electronics and Instrumentation,* 1973. Courtesy of Charles B. Slack, Inc., Thorofare, New Jersey.

ELECTROANESTHESIA AND ELECTROPROSTHETICS

The use of electricity and electronics in the medical sciences has mushroomed in recent years. Conventional applications such as electrotherapy, electrodiagnosis, electroencephalography, and electrocardiography constitute the major areas of medical electronics. Recently, however, the uses of electrical and electronic devices in the areas of electrically induced anesthesia (electroanesthesia or electrosleep) and electrically controlled and operated prosthetic devices (electroprosthetics) has increased.

Electroanesthesia

The inducement of surgical level anesthesia by electrical means is termed electroanesthesia. This definition is by no means a universal one, since many individuals exhibit a resistance to the effects of the sleep-inducing currents. To produce anesthesia via electrical means, a current is passed between bitemporal electrodes through the skull and hence the brain of the patient. The first sensation felt by the patient is a slight tingling in the area of the electrodes, which leads into a state of relaxation, then sleep or anesthesia. This technique is still primarily experimental and is used mostly in research applications due to the side effects its use produces. The major objections against the use of this technique at present are the production of hypertension, tachycardia hyperexia, cutaneous burns, and excessive secretions of mucus and saliva. Recently, scientists have attempted to produce a preinduction drowsiness by the use of pulsed electrostatic fields prior to the application of actual transcerebral low currents.

The technique and instrumentation for inducing electronarcosis is as follows: A pulse generator capable of generating frequencies from DC to approximately 20 KHz with pulse durations around 1 millisecond is adequate for most applications, since the most useful frequency appears to be around 100 Hz. Initially, a low DC current is applied to electrodes placed bitemporally (although anterior-posterior location is also used) on the patient's skull, after which a selected pulse pattern is superimposed. A typical sequence involves a 10 to 15 milliamp reference upon which 5 to 10 milliamp pulses are added. Overall current range used to date has been from 5 to 110 milliamps in both continuous and pulsed patterns. A major problem in the technique is obtaining adequate current density in the selected area of the brain without causing electrode site burns. The problem is due to the intervening bone and tissue resistance preventing most of the current from reaching the brain. If the voltage is increased to overcome this, the magnitude of the side effects is increased.

A typical instrument is shown in Figure 8-64. The electrodes used are comparable to any typical surface electrode employed in physiological monitoring. In most cases, noble metals (silver,

Figure 8-64. Block diagram of an electroanesthesia unit. From Terence Karselis, *Descriptive Medical Electronics and Instrumentation,* 1973. Courtesy of Charles B. Slack, Inc., Thorofare, New Jersey.

etc.) are used to eliminate polarization. In addition to the automatic voltage and current controls incorporated into its design capability, adjustment of the pulse duration and repetition rate are also included.

The physiological mechanism by which electroanesthesia is induced is presently unclear; however, various theories have been postulated including one which suggests that the currents may effect enzyme systems. Another theory indicates the possibility that the currents may cause the release of some type of generalized inhibitory substance into the bloodstream. Whatever the specific mechanism of action, electroanesthesia is today still a research tool for the most part.

A less dramatic but nevertheless medically useful application of electrotherapy is in the area of healing ischemic ulcers. Researchers at the University of Missouri Medical Center found that application of low intensity direct currents ranging in magnitude from 200 to 400 microamperes increased the amount of healing and rate at which ischemic ulcers healed by 24 percent. The instrumentation consisted of a low voltage, low current source with an output range of 200 microamperes to 1 milliamp. The output jacks allowed cable connections to copper mesh electrodes. The negative electrode was placed on the wound for the first few days, and its effect was to reduce or inhibit pathogenic bacterial growth. The positive electrode was then used over the wound to accelerate the healing process, which appears to work by way of stimulating proliferation of fibroblastic cells and microcirculation into the traumatized area.

Another therapeutic application of low intensity currents is in assisting fractures to heal. Inactive metal screws driven into bone on both sides of a healing fracture are used as electrodes between which a low intensity current is passed. Microampere currents appear to accelerate the healing process significantly.

Both of these applications of electrotherapy are examples of the possibilities that abound in the field of electromedical currents.

Electroprosthetics

Any device or component used to replace a missing *part* or *function* of the human body is a *prosthesis*. Prostheses may be temporary or permanent, internal or external, and as such can be powered or operated by way of residual neuromuscular activity, or they may function by way of an electrical or electronic power pack. Pacemakers, artificial limbs, and braces fall into this category.

In the area of prosthetic limbs, the critical area of design in producing an effective device is the patient-device-patient feedback network. This network is a servocontrol mechanism of the type found in many null balance systems such as chart recorders. Electroprosthetic devices are electromechanical systems that mimic the body's system of neuromuscular activity and hence require the same type of closed-loop sensory-motor system. Figure 8-65 is an example of a basic system. The activity necessary for limb or body motion requires a three stage process: (1) *sensory* activity and transmission of *stimulus,* (2) evaluation and decision for command, (3) *motor* activity following *command.* In electroprosthetic devices, a *transducer* of some type takes the place of missing or injured sensory nerves. A complex system of electronic circuits, often analog and digital computer subcircuits, performs the evaluation, decision, and command activity, while carefully designed electromechanical, pneumatic, and hydraulic systems provide the rotation, extension, and flexion capability to the mechanical limb. External power packs supply the energy to

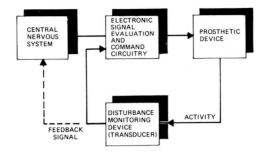

Figure 8-65. Block diagram of an electroprosthetic system. From Terence Karselis, *Descriptive Medical Electronics and Instrumentation,* 1973. Courtesy of Charles B. Slack, Inc., Thorofare, New Jersey.

drive the hydraulic and electrical systems of the prostheses, while the *triggering* energy is usually a signal derived from some residual voluntary muscular activity remaining in a partially amputated limb or joint. Other activating signal sources are the eyelids, ears, neck, and even the tongue. Transducers used are mercury strain gauges and microswitches.

The following devices are typical examples of some recently developed electroprosthetic systems. An alarm system designed to prevent self-inflicted injury and provide improved motor control to its user was constructed, employing (1) a mercury strain gauge to detect pressure at the fingertips. The resulting electrical resistance change causes (2) a variable frequency oscillator to increase its output frequency, which in turn alters the (3) audible tone heard by the individual wearing the device. The electronics are of the integrated circuit (I.C.) type that require little power and are extremely rugged. The small size of the circuitry allows it to be worn on the wrist like a wristwatch.

A feedback control system providing a patient with increased sensitivity in grasp control has been developed using a noise transducer. Figure 8-66 shows the system. When an object is grasped or lifted and inadequate force is applied, the noise transducer generates a signal which is processed and integrated into a motor-drive command, thereby increasing the grasping power. When no further slippage occurs, the noise signal is absent and the motor remains at the point where it previously stopped. In order to activate the system into releasing the object, a voluntary trigger signal can override the system and drive the servomotor in the opposite (release) direction.

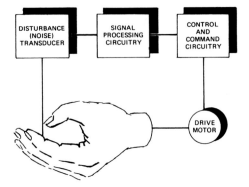

Figure 8-66. Block diagram of the adaptive control mechanism of an electroprosthetic hand. From Terence Karselis, *Descriptive Medical Electronics and Instrumentation,* 1973. Courtesy of Charles B. Slack, Inc., Thorofare, New Jersey.

The field of electroprosthetics is in its infancy, but, with the increasingly sophisticated developments in electronic materials and circuits design, there is no question that the physical therapist will see increasingly more wondrous and surprising man-made miracles.

REFERENCES

1. *Basic Electricity.* Navpers 10026-A, Washington, Bureau of Naval Personnel, U.S. Government Printing Office, 1960.
2. *Basic Theory and Application of Transistors.* Training Manual 11-690, Department of the Army, Washington, U. S. Government Printing Office, 1959.
3. Bellville, J.W. and Weaver, C.S. (eds.): *Techniques in Clinical Physiology.* Toronto, Collier-Macmillan Ltd., 1969.
4. *Biophysical Measurements.* Tektronix Measurement Concepts. Beaverton, Oregon, 1971.
5. Brown, J.H.N.; Jacobs, J.E.; and Stark, L.: *Biomedical Engineering.* Philadelphia, F.A. Davis, 1971.
6. *Burdick Syllabus — A Compendium on Electromedical Therapy.* Milton, The Burdick Corporation, 1969.

7. Buchsbaum, Walter H.: *Buchsbaum's Complete Handbook of Practical Electronic Reference Data.* Englewood Cliffs, Prentice-Hall, Inc., 1975.
8. Camishion, R.C.: *Basic Medical Electronics.* Boston, Little, Brown, 1964.
9. Clement, P.R. and Johnson, W.C.: *Electrical Engineering Science.* New York, McGraw Hill, 1960.
10. Cromwell, Leslie: *Biomedical Instrumentation and Measurements.* Englewood cliffs, Prentice-Hall, Inc., 1973.
11. Dart, Francis E.: *Electricity and Electromagnetic Fields.* Columbus, Charles E. Merrill Books, Inc., 1966.
12. Diefenderfer, James A.: *Principles of Electronic Instrumentation.* Philadelphia, W.B. Saunders Co., 1972.
13. *Digest of the 7th International Conference on Medical & Biological Engineering.* Almquist and Wiksell, Stockholm, 1967.
14. Dummer, G.W.A. and Robertson, J.M. (eds.): *Medical Electronic Equipment.* Vol. I-IV, Oxford, Pergamon Press, 1970.
15. *Electronic and Electrical Fundamentals.* Vol. I-IV, Fort Washington, Philco Ford Corporation, Tech. Rep. Division, 1960.
16. *Fundamentals of Transistor Electronics.* Fort Washington, Philco Ford Corporation, Education and Tech. Services Division, 1967.
17. Geddes, L.A. and Baker, L.E.: *Principles of Applied Biomedical Instrumentation.* New York, John Wiley and Sons, 1968.
18. Grossman, C.C.: *The Use of Diagnostic Ultrasound in Brain Disorders.* Springfield, Charles C. Thomas, 1966.
19. Grob, B. and Kiver, M.S.: *Applications of Electronics.* New York, McGraw Hill, 1960.
20. Karselis, Terence: *Descriptive Medical Electronics and Instrumentation.* Thorofare, Charles B. Slack, Inc., 1973.
21. Malmstart, H.V.; Enke, C.G.; and Benjamin, W.A.: *Electronics for Scientists.* 1962.
22. Markus, John: *Source Book of Electronic Circuits.* New York, McGraw Hill, 1968.
23. Offner, F.F.: *Electronics for Biologists.* New York, McGraw Hill, 1962.
24. Light, S. (ed.): *Electrodiagnosis and Electro-Myography.* Baltimore, Waverly Press, 1961.
25. Light, S. (ed.): *Therapeutic Electricity and Ultraviolet Radiation.* Baltimore, Waverly Press, 1967.
26. Simpson, Robert E.: *Introductory Electronics for Scientists and Engineers.* Boston, Allyn and Bacon, Inc., 1974.
27. Segal, B.L. and Kilpatrick D.G. (eds.): *Engineering in the Practice of Medicine.* Baltimore, Williams and Wilkins, 1967.
28. Smith, D.A.: *Medical Electronics Equipment Handbook.* Indianapolis, Howard W. Sams, 1962.
29. Watkins, A.L.: *Manual of Electrotherapy.* Philadelphia, Lea and Febiger, 1958.
30. Yanof, H.M.: *Biomedical Electronics.* Philadelphia, F.A. Davis, 1965.

Chapter 9

INSTRUMENTATION AND POWER DISTRIBUTION WIRING SYSTEMS

INSTRUMENTS, GROUND, AND TERMINOLOGY

NOTWITHSTANDING that they are considered to be places of healing, it has been proposed more than once that hospitals and medical care facilities in general are unhealthy places in which to reside. When one considers the potential hazards concentrated into the shell of a typical hospital, the statement takes on more than slight credibility. Considering that a typical hospital contains concentrated pockets of hazardous organisms, chemicals, nuclear energy, and electrical energy, the thesis becomes alarmingly real to the average layman. However, the problem is of even more importance to the individual required to spend his total working experience within that environment. Such a situation calls for extreme and continual care, vigilance, *and* awareness on the part of the medical worker. From the point of view of physical therapy, the electrical energy area is of prime consideration. Not only should the therapist be aware of the theory and operation of the devices he uses, but he also should have some knowledge of the way in which they function as integral parts of the power distribution system of the hospital and as potential hazards. Since the generally accepted value of current capable of causing ventricular fibrillation and possible death in patients whose normal skin resistance has been circumvented by way of an external pacemaker or catheter is in the micro-ampere region, therapists should be cognizant of sources and conditions capable of eliciting such currents. The two major divisions of electrical hazards are classified by the source of the poten-

358

tially dangerous currents. These are (1) line voltage and (2) leakage currents. To properly understand the ways in which these hazardous conditions can arise first requires an understanding of the concepts of electrical ground and power distribution.

Ground, or Earth, or What?

A correct understanding of electrical ground requires a knowledge of the items and connections that constitute an electrical circuit. The essential components and current paths in a typical electrical circuit are shown in Figure 9-1. They are (1) a power source (the battery), (2) a load (R_2), (3) a source conductor, and (4) a return conductor. It is as a "return" conductor that electrical ground can find application, but more important is its function as a safety valve. This concept can be clarified by referring to Figure 9-2. If one regards ground or earth (which is what the term *ground* originally referred to) as an infinite electrical charge accumulator or source, it then has the ability to either give up or accept charges without itself becoming charged. Consequently, any object that is electrically charged and in turn touches or is connected to ground will give up or take on the appropriate charges until it is the same potential as ground, i.e. until it has become neutral. It is this fact that makes earth ground the reference point for electrical zero potential. Any object connected by a very low resistance path to ground is said, for all practical purposes, to be at zero volts; in addition, any

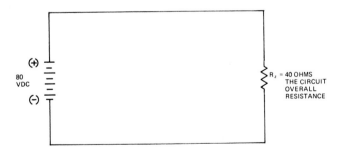

80 VDC (+) (−)

R_2 = 40 OHMS
THE CIRCUIT
OVERALL
RESISTANCE

Figure 9-1. Essential components of an electrical circuit. From Terence Karselis, *Descriptive Medical Electronics and Instrumentation*, 1973. Courtesy of Charles B. Slack, Inc., Thorofare, New Jersey.

Figure 9-2. The action of grounding a charged object. From Terence Karselis, *Descriptive Medical Electronics and Instrumentation,* 1973. Courtesy of Charles B. Slack, Inc., Thorofare, New Jersey.

hazardous charge that may appear on the object is immediately shunted to ground. If the object were not grounded and an individual touched both it and ground simultaneously, he would become the path to ground and hence receive an electrical shock (which may or may not be perceptible, depending upon the magnitude of the current flow).

From the above discussion, it can be seen that electrical ground serves two purposes: (a) it acts as a reference point for electrical zero potential and (b) it functions as source or sink for hazardous electrical charges. Both of these functions are utilized in the circuits which supply power to homes and businesses as well as medical facilities. In addition, these functions take on specialized application in instrumentation. It is in this application that the confusion between "true" earth ground and "instrument" ground can arise.

"True" Ground Verses "Instrument" Ground

As noted above, an electrical circuit requires the essentials of a power source, a load, and a source and drain conduction path. A majority of instruments are built on chassis or frames of conductive metal. In addition, each circuit within these devices must be provided with a source and drain path, connecting it to the device's power supply. In many instruments, it has become common practice to use the chassis or frame of the instrument as a ground "return" path from each circuit back to the power supply circuit. In instruments supplied by a two-conductor power cord and using a chassis return, the instrument circuit ground is *not* a true "earth" ground. This is shown in Figure 9-3. This type of device constitutes a potential hazard, for (a) if some fault within the instrument power supply primary side causes the instrument ground to be raised to a potential above true ground and (b) its human operator touches it while simultaneously touching another device whose chassis *is* at true ground, current will flow through the operator with uncomfortable consequences. If, however, the device is served by a three-conductor power cord *and* the building power distribution system is adequately ground-ed (Note: taking either one of these requirements for granted can be hazardous to one's health), the instrument ground *will* be at true earth ground and hence will provide the safety valve action noted previously (Fig. 9-4). Both of these examples are based on the assumption that the power distribution system is a grounded system. As will be discussed later, *all* distribution systems in medical facilities are *not* grounded.

Figure 9-3. Diagram of a two-wire device with chassis ground (*not* true ground).

Figure 9-4. Diagram of a three-wire device with the chassis connected to true ground.

Terminology and Coding in Wiring Systems

Power distribution into commercial and residential buildings follows a similar pattern. A transformer steps down the utility voltage from 2200 volts to 240 or 120 volts at the main service or distribution panel. In modern wiring systems, three conductors originate from there and supply the sub– or branch circuits within the building. These conductors are color coded and named in accordance with the National Electrical Code (NEC), which is published by the National Fire Protection Association, Boston, Mass. The *hot* current carrying conductor is insulated with *black* covering and is at a potential of 120/240 volts with respect to ground. The *cold* (or neutral) current carrying conductor is insulated with *white* covering and is at the same potential as ground. It is generally attached to a ground wire at the service box. The *safety ground* conductor is also attached to ground at the service box and color coded by way of *green* insulation (or is a bare wire). The grounding conductor *does not*, under normal circumstances, carry current. It is there only to provide a path to ground for fault currents.

From the service distribution box, the three-conductor system is connected to each individual branch wall outlet. The way in which the connections are made at the outlet is, once again, outlined in the N.E.C. Using the round grounding pin as the key, the N.E.C. requires the following method of connection: If the grounding pin is located *below* the two parallel blade receptacles, the left-hand slot houses the cold or neutral lead, while the right-hand slot houses the hot lead (if the ground pin is above the blade slots, they are reversed). Within the outlet box, the black (hot) conductor should terminate at the brass-colored terminal, the white (cold) conductor at the silver (nickel plated) terminal, and the green (ground) wire at a lug screw coded green which is located at one end of the plastic outlet assembly.

Although these requirements are law where the N.E.C. is used as the local electrical code, sloppy workmanship and cost-cutting shortcuts can lead to hazardous construction methods, such as not using a third conductor for grounding so that the ground terminal of the outlet is connected to the cold power lead or just simply *not* connecting the ground terminal within the outlet box. (The author has *seen* examples of both such techniques). The key to safety is suspicion; one should be skeptical and suspect any system until proven safe! That way both the therapist and the patient will live longer.

Types of Distribution Systems

Since 1962, the National Electrical Code has required the use of three-wire electrical systems. However, many buildings and facilities contain outdated and unmodified wiring systems, or systems that have been modified in a here-and-there method, leaving half of a system adequate and half of it inadequate. Some knowledge of the types of wiring systems that can be found in medical facilities can be useful to those who work in them.

Figure 9-5 is a simplified diagram of a typical two-wire distribution system. The cold or neutral conductor is grounded on the secondary side of the utility distribution transformer, and the distribution system is therefore referred to as a "grounded" system. Hazardous situations can and do occur with this type of system; for example, in an instance of accidentally reversing the two-bladed plugs commonly found on many electrical devices. In

Figure 9-5. A power distribution system (two-wire). From Terence Karselis, *Descriptive Medical Electronics and Instrumentation,* 1973. Courtesy of Charles B. Slack, Inc., Thorofare, New Jersey.

such a case, a fault within a device can allow hazardous voltage to appear on its chassis or case, even though its power on-off switch is in the open position. This occurs because power switches are by convention placed in the hot conductor side of the input power leads, and when the plug is reversed at the receptacle, the hot power line is connected to the device's cold lead.

Hazards such as those above led to the adoption of the three-wire distribution system, which is identical to the two wire system but for the addition of the third safety "grounding" conductor. Not only does the three-wire system automatically prevent accidental plug reversal, it also ensures that any fault currents occurring on an instrument's chassis will immediately be shunted to ground. Close observation of a typical three-prong plug will show that the ground blade is longer than the two power blades. This ensures initial contact by the ground conductor, reducing the possibility to arcing in the case of fault within the instrument.

Figure 9-6 illustrates the hazards that can occur with the two-wire power distribution system and the safety features inherent in the three-wire system. In the diagram, an individual working with instrument A, which is correctly grounded (it may be individually grounded or served by way of a three-wire system), and also touching instrument B, an ungrounded device in which faulty insulation has placed line voltage on its case, receives a possibly fatal electrical shock. By touching both devices, he becomes a low resistance pathway to ground. If instrument B had been connected by way of a three-wire power cord to a three-wire distribution system, the hazard voltage would have been shunted to ground by way of the safety ground lead, since it offers less resistance than the human body. Current is lazy — it always takes the path of least resistance. An additional point to be emphasized here is that a cheater plug, the infamous three-wire-to-two-wire-plus-pigtail converter, can easily circumvent the safety ground lead of a three-wire device if not used correctly. Needless to say, they rarely *are* used properly. The pigtail on the cheater is designed to be attached to the screw on the outlet box but rarely is attached simply because people are too hurried or lazy to take the time, or a screwdriver is not readily at hand. In such instances, the hazard shown in Figure 9-6 is once again present. A golden rule to use with cheater plugs in medical facilities is *DON'T* — just do not use them.

Figure 9-6. (1) shows a grounded two-wire distribution system. (2) shows how a fault in an ungrounded instrument can shock an individual touching both the faulty device and a grounded device simultaneously. From Terence Karselis, *Descriptive Medical Electronics and Instrumentation*, 1973. Courtesy of Charles B. Slack, Inc., Thorofare, New Jersey.

EQUIPMENT HAZARDS AND THEIR CAUSES

The Hazards—Macro- and Microshock

The previous three sections dealt with power distribution and ground, emphasizing its safety function. How do equipment hazards arise, and just how many types of electrical shock are there? This section will briefly discuss these items.

Electrical shock can be of two types, perceptible or imperceptible. In scientific terms, they are referred to as macroshock and microshock, respectively, and are characterized by the magnitude of current involved. Authorities in the field of electrical safety are continually at loggerheads concerning whether it is voltage or current that is the dangerous culprit in electrocution. The case is simplified if one always considers Ohm's Law: $I = V/R$. The *magnitude of current* in a circuit depends upon both the applied *voltage* and the circuit *resistance*. Since the resistance involved in electrocution varies according to the particular circumstances, then so will the current produced by a given voltage. The need then arises to establish the definitions of macro– and microshock. The normal human dry skin resistance can vary from tens of thousands of ohms (10 KΩ) to hundreds of thousands of ohms (100 KΩ), depending upon the contact area. As a general rule of thumb, current across the intact dry skin of less than 1 milliampere will cause no perceptible response and is therefore referred to as *microshock* current. Above 1 milliampere, up to approximately 15 milliamperes, the response varies from minimal perception of a tingle to muscle spasm at the higher currents. Values in the 100 to 200 milliampere range can cause death due to respiratory paralysis and cardiac fibrillation. Any current above the threshold of perception (1 ma) is termed *macroshock* current. Whatever its characterization, under the appropriate circumstances, both micro– and macroshock can kill. For example, a patient who is catheterized for an external pacemaker becomes an extremely susceptible individual, since conductors circumvent the normal body resistance to the point that direct contact with the myocardium is present. A microshock fault current, inperceptible to an attending nurse or doctor adjusting the patient electrodes (say 100 microamperes from a faulty electric bed), can pass through the attendant and cause the patient to go into fibrillation — and the attendant is totally unaware of having caused the accident! It is obvious that any medical worker required to use electrical apparatus near or on patients should be acutely aware of the possible hazards that may be involved and how they arise.

The Hazards—Their Causes

The most obvious way in which a person can receive an electrical shock is by coming into contact with both the hot and cold conductor of a power line (obviously a case of hair-straightening macroshock). Although obvious, it is not the most common cause of electrocution. The most common accident involves an individual who touches a hot conductor, or the case of a faulty device which is at line (120 volts) potential and also a good electrical ground simultaneously. The ground may be a damp basement floor (concrete is notorious for drawing and holding moisture), a cold water faucet, or a second, properly grounded, device. Whichever the case, the result is the same.

An all-too-common occurrence in electrical instruments is insulation breakdown of the input power cord such that the instrument chassis becomes charged. Although in many cases the safety ground will provide the protection necessary, use of improper extension cords and three-to-two cheater plugs can provide the breakdown in the safety system. It is important to note that *two* criteria must be met in order to set up a macroshock hazard, (a) the instrument fault and (b) the operator error (whether conscious or unconscious). Such is the case with most electrical hazards occurring with the use of electronic instruments.

Hazards in which voltage is directly applied to an instrument chassis (as above) are referred to as *leakage* voltage due to *voltage division*. Depending upon where in the instrument circuit the fault occurs, the point of contact can be anything from one volt to hundreds of volts. As noted above, insulation breakdown is the cause most often encountered, followed by loose terminal connections, moisture bridges between terminals, and component failure. Leakage by voltage division is most often encountered in cases of macroshock. In the case of microshock, the cause can arise from two other sources, capacitive coupling leakage and inductive coupling leakage. *Capacitive coupling* can cause leakage between any two metallic conductors (due to interelectrode capacitance), which increases with the frequency of the voltage involved. Because of the frequency dependence of capacitive leakage, some authorities question its potential as a hazard. However, in the case of medically susceptible individuals, no possible dangers should be neglected, especially in the case of ultrasonic and higher frequency devices.

Inductive coupling is responsible for leakage in most motor-driven devices (beds, cast saws, etc.) as well as in instruments using transformers. Inductive coupling is like capacitive coupling, a frequency-dependent phenomenon, but unlike the latter, it does not require especially high frequencies to be effective. Sixty cycle power line frequencies are adequate to produce significant amounts of inductive leakage.

Whatever its source, leakage current cannot endanger anyone if the device it arises in is *adequately* grounded. If not, the hazard is there whether perceptible or not to the operator.

RECOMMENDED SAFETY PRACTICES
The Individual and the Institutional Environment

The effects of electrocution are curable — by prevention. Although it is possible to resuscitate a patient sent into fibrillation or respiratory collapse by electrocution, it is not always successful. Hence, prevention is the key word in eliminating electrical accidents. Prevention within the hospital environment, although generally considered to be the responsibility of the maintenance branch of hospital engineering, is in reality the responsibility of each and every medical worker. It has been stated by safety experts in the field (D. Roveti and M. H. Aronson, Medical Electronics and Data, #25, Jan.-Feb. 1974) that a larger proportion of technical workers are killed due to accidental electrocution than lay persons because of the following facts: (a) technical and scientific workers are by the nature of their work exposed to more electrical and electronic equipment than the lay person and (b) these individuals tend to have no more knowledge of the hazards associated with electrical apparatus than the layman. If such is the case (and the authors tend to agree with the experts), then there must be a reason for professional medical workers to ignore the warnings so often expounded concerning electrical safety. It appears that the average human psyche contains some small segment bent on self-destruction. It is made obvious when a person sees others taking unnecessary chances but, as is most often the case, fails to see the same tendency in himself. A case in point is the heavy drinker who chides his friend for being overweight, telling him that excessive food is slowly occluding his vascular system with sclerotic deposits, while all the time excessive alcohol is reducing the drinker's own liver to a fibrotic ball. The point is that one sees other people's mistakes, but not his own. This is acceptable for the average individual, but the mark of a professional, whether medical or not, is the characteristic of keeping up to date in his own discipline *and* those fields which are closely related to it. This includes being aware of not only the new treatment or diagnostic techniques in his field but also of the many characteristics of the *tools* he uses. The responsibilities of an individual required to work with electronic instruments can be summarized as follows:

1. Be professional. Study and stay up to date with the problem of safety and electrical hazards.
2. Be professional. Know your instrument! A device cannot be used either effectively or safely if the operator is not thoroughly familiar with its operation and idiosyncrasies.
3. Be skeptical. Ground everything to true ground but the patient, and remember, instrument ground return is *not* necessarily true ground.
4. Be skeptical. Insist that engineering initially check and then periodically recheck all wiring systems for correct wiring and adequate ground as outlined in the N.E.C. Article 517, Health Care Facilities.
5. Be sensible. Avoid absolutely the use of extension cords and cheater adapters.
6. Be suspicious. Consider everything as a potential hazard until proven otherwise.

These few guidelines are by no means the end-all to electrical hazards, but following them will help to develop an awareness for possible problems, and they may promote the growth of safe habits in using electrical equipment.

The Institution and Its Responsibilities

Beyond the professional responsibilities expected of medical workers operating electronic instrumentation is the necessity to request and expect of the hospital administration and staff a safe environment, not only for the medical workers but also for the patient. It is a safe bet that updating and modifications of various plumbing and wiring systems in a relatively old institution (circa 1920?) have over the years contributed to at least some poor ground connections and miswired receptacles. A majority of electrical accidents occur when instrument faults occur simultaneously with wiring system faults, due either to loss of ground integrity or to the development of voltage differentials between ground systems. The hospital's responsibility in the reducing of such hazards begins with employing *qualified* clinical engineers (or biomedical engineers, whichever title is applicable, since no nationally accepted definition is presently predominant and backing them up by giving them *full authority* to enforce safety regulations. Today's typical general hospital civil engineer is not sufficiently qualified in areas such as leakage current and microshock to accomplish this.

With an appropriate engineer on its staff, the next responsibility of the hospital is the development of an inhouse bioengineering department to provide (a) initial testing and verification of all new equipment, (b) maintenance and calibration of all inhouse equipment, and (c) repair and inspection of all equipment as well as house wiring. Such a department could also provide inhouse education for the medical, nursing, and other professional hospital staff in the area of medical safety as well as consultation and expertise in the choice and purchase of medical equipment.

The Home or Private Office

The use of medical electronic equipment in a home or office is a hazardous practice unless the user is absolutely sure of the safe and correct wiring of his wiring system. How many of those who plan to utilize private offices are? How many of them have also planned to have their wiring systems verified for (a) correctness of wiring to the receptacles and (b) integrity and quality of the ground or the instruments for grounding integrity and/or leakage current values? These items are the minimal requirements necessary for ensuring a safe electrical environment for the therapist and the patient.

Some guidelines to follow in nonhospital areas to ensure a degree of electrical safety are given below. These are in addition to the items noted above and in the previous section.

1. Be sure there are sufficient outlets in any given room to service all necessary equipment.
2. Be sure all outlets in a given room are on the same branch circuit and served by the same transformer.
3. Avoid placing items that are good conductors and that *might* be accidently grounded, i.e. a metal cart touching a cold water pipe, within reach of the patient.
4. Do not use extension cords or cheater plugs.
5. Keep fluids and chemicals away from the patient and equipment.
6. Do not use equipment supplied with molded three-way plugs. It is not unusual to find that the ground pin is *not* connected to the grounding conductor within the plug itself.
7. Use instruments with cabinets that are insulated (plastic rather than metal) or ensure grounding.
8. Continually check power cords for fraying and broken insulation.
9. Know where the main circuit breaker for a given room is to ensure that power can be interrupted in case of an emergency.

The home or office can be a safe or hazardous electrical environment in which to treat a patient and work; it depends upon the therapist.

Medical Device Legislation

The increasing cost of health care to the individual and the expanding activity of third-party agencies to paying these costs have long ago reached the obvious stage at which governmental interest and action was stimulated. Many individuals foresee a National Health Insurance Plan, i.e. The Kennedy Plan, being instituted within the next few years, while others see prepayment plans similar to the Kaiser Foundation plan in California. Whatever the fate of health insurance or its mode of payment, one needs no law degree to foresee the eventual control and regulation of state and national agencies over allied health workers' licensure, certification, and continuing education. In addition, device legislation will also become a fact of life. Device legislation as proposed by the United States Senate (Bill S 2368, Medical Devices Amendment)* could become law in the very near future. At that time, any medical device, including all electronic and other devices used in physical therapy, will be classified into special categories by the Federal Drug Administration's Bureau of Medical Devices and Diagnostic Products. From that point in time onward, each and every instrument that is manufactured for medical use will be screened to determine if it is (a) new or not, (b) custom-made, (c) life-sustaining or (d) life-supporting, or even (e) a prescription device. The law will require premarketing scientific review to assure effectiveness and will reduce or eliminate possible risk of injury with exposure or use of the device. The FDA's Bureau of Medical Devices and Diagnostic Products will have the authority to enforce product recall as well as premarketing clearance and mandatory reporting of failures or defects.

The problems associated with device legislation that appear to be causing the most concern among practitioners and industry representatives are the legal vagueness and ambiguities of S 2368. Areas of uncertainty include such things as the definitions of classes of devices and failure to include provisions within the bill to prevent marketing of unclassified devices. A more practical problem to consider might be the lag time that intervenes between development of a device and its entrance into the competitive marketplace. Today's drugs undergo lag times of from ten to fifteen years, depending upon the FDA tests required. Some industry leaders predict that the lower the risk requirement dictated by the FDA, the longer will be the lag time; therefore, the volume of new devices will drop.

Whatever and whenever device legislation appears as law, its impact will be felt by any individual using medical instrumentation. The only question that remains is, how big an impact? The physical therapist can, however, be sure of one thing, his/her instrumentation *will* be safer!

---

*Now Public Law 9-1-295 (1976).

REFERENCES

1. Buchsbaum, Walter H.: *Buschsbaum's Complete Handbook of Practical Electronic Reference Data.* Englewood Cliffs, Prentice-Hall, Inc., 1975.
2. Cromwell, Leslie: *Biomedical Instrumentation and Measurements.* Englewood Cliffs, Prentice-Hall, Inc. 1973.
3. Karselis, Terence: *Descriptive Medical Electronics and Instrumentation.* Thorofare, Charles B. Slack, Inc., 1973.
4. Simpson, Robert E.: *Introductory Electronics for Scientists and Engineers.* Boston, Allyn and Bacon, Inc., 1974.
5. Medical Electronics and Data. Vols. VI and XIII, Measurement Data Corp., Pittsburgh, 1974.
6. Newsletter. Association for the Advancement of Medical Instrumentation, Vol. XII, #4, 5, 6. Arlington, 1976.

INDEX

375